COMPREHENSIVE
RADIOGRAPHIC
PATHOLOGY

COMPREHENSIVE
RADIOGRAPHIC
PATHOLOGY

RONALD L. EISENBERG, M.D.

Chairman, Department of Radiology
Louisiana State University School of Medicine
Shreveport, Louisiana

CYNTHIA A. DENNIS, R.T.

Director, School of Radiologic Technology
Louisiana State University School of Medicine
Shreveport, Louisiana

with 684 illustrations

The C. V. Mosby Company

ST. LOUIS • BALTIMORE • PHILADELPHIA • TORONTO   1990

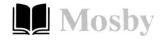

Editor: Anne Patterson
Developmental Editor: Maureen Slaten
Assistant Editor: Jo Salway
Book Design: Liz Fett

Printed in the United States of America
The C.V. Mosby Company
11830 Westline Industrial Drive, St. Louis, Missouri 63146

Library of Congress Cataloging-in-Publication Data
Eisenberg, Ronald L.
    Comprehensive radiographic pathology/Ronald L. Eisenberg,
  Cynthia A. Dennis.
      p. cm.
    Includes bibliographical references.
    ISBN 0-8016-6142-0
    1. Diagnosis. Radioscopic. 2. Pathology. 3. Medical
  technologists.   I. Dennis, Cynthia A.   II. Title.
    [DNLM: 1. Pathology. 2. Radiography. 3. Technology, Radiologic.
  QZ 4 E36c]
  RC78.E533   1990
  616.07′57—dc20
  DNLM/DLC
  for Library of Congress   89-14466
                                                     CIP

GW/MV/MV 9 8 7 6 5 4 3 2

*To all students and radiographers
wishing to better understand
the value of the profession
of radiologic technology*

Preface

An understanding of basic principles of pathology and an awareness of the radiographic appearances of specific diseases are essential parts of the training of a radiologic technologist. It enables the radiologic technologist to become a more competent professional and a knowledgeable member of the diagnostic team. An understanding of disease processes can aid the technologist in selecting proper modalities and in determining the need for retaking a radiograph that might be acceptable under different circumstances.

Unfortunately, most teaching programs currently use textbooks designed only for high school or college students or for medical students, or they use a set of teaching slides that require the active participation of a radiologist. Our solution has been to develop a well-illustrated, comprehensive textbook of pathology designed specifically for students of radiologic technology and as a reference guide for graduate radiographers.

An introductory chapter discusses basic pathology (including the immune reaction and AIDS) and introduces the pathologic terms that are used throughout the book. It also describes the advantages and limitations of three widely used new modalities: ultrasound, computed tomography, and magnetic resonance imaging. Each of the remaining chapters is a systematic approach to the diseases involving a specific organ system, organized in a manner that is conducive to progressive lesson planning. For each of the most common pathologic conditions there is a brief description of the disease itself and its clinical manifestations, followed by the imaging findings. Specific information relative to radiologic technology is included, such as the changes in technique needed for patients with specific conditions and any special handling of the patient that may be required. If multiple imaging modalities can be used, the most appropriate initial procedure is indicated, as well as the sequence in which various imaging studies should be performed.

Each chapter opens with a listing of goals and objectives designed to show the student what information should be thoroughly understood. This is followed by radiographer notes, which offer helpful suggestions for producing optimal radiographs of the specific organ system. Each chapter ends with a series of review questions to help readers assess their degree of comprehension of the material.

Several appendices include material that is valuable to the radiologic technologist but applies to multiple chapters. There is an extensive glossary and a list of major prefixes, roots, and suffixes that will enable the reader to decipher the meaning of unfamiliar words. In addition, there is a table detailing the diagnostic implications of abnormal values of important laboratory examinations.

RONALD L. EISENBERG
CYNTHIA A. DENNIS

Acknowledgments

Figures 4-1 to 4-24, 4-26 to 4-61, and 4-63 to 4-93 were borrowed with permission from Eisenberg RL: Gastrointestinal radiology: a pattern approach, ed 2, Philadelphia, 1990, JB Lippincott Co.

The unnumbered figures in chapters 2 through 10 were borrowed from Thibodeau GA: Anatomy and physiology, St Louis, 1987, The CV Mosby Co.

Contents

COMPREHENSIVE
RADIOGRAPHIC
PATHOLOGY

CHAPTER 1

Introduction to Pathology

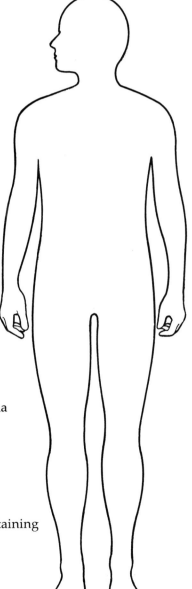

PREREQUISITE KNOWLEDGE

The student should have a basic knowledge of the normal anatomy and physiology of the human body. A good foundation in medical terminology, including word roots, prefixes, and suffixes (see Appendix A) will be most helpful in digesting the somewhat difficult information presented in this and future chapters. In addition, proper learning and understanding of the material will be facilitated if the student has some clinical experience in all areas of radiography of the human body and film evaluation, including a concept of the changes in technique required to compensate for density differences produced by underlying pathologic conditions.

GOALS

To acquaint the student radiographer with basic medical terminology used to describe various pathologic conditions occurring in the human body (including hereditary diseases, immune reactions, and AIDS) and to introduce the student to some specialized imaging techniques

OBJECTIVES

1. Describe edema, ischemia, infarction, hemorrhage, and neoplasia
2. Describe the various alterations of cell growth
3. Be able to describe the various hereditary diseases and their radiographic manifestations
4. Be able to describe the various immune reactions of the body
5. Be able to describe AIDS and the precautions necessary when radiographing patients who have AIDS
6. Be familiar with the changes in technical factors required for obtaining optimal quality radiographs in patients with various underlying pathologic conditions
7. Be able to describe briefly the theory of image production with ultrasound, CT, and MRI

RADIOGRAPHER NOTES

Radiography of patients with underlying pathologic conditions can present problems for even the most experienced radiographers. Adjustments in patient position may be necessary to prevent excessive pain due to the body's response to trauma or certain disease processes. A change in routine projections may be indicated to visualize subtle alterations in the normal radiographic appearance. Many disease processes also alter the density of the structures being radiographed and therefore require changes in technique. For example, extensive edema

---

Table 1-1. Penetrability to x-rays of pathology of body systems, for far-advanced disease states

SKELETAL SYSTEM

Additive (hard to penetrate)
  Acromegaly
  Acute kyphosis
  Callus
  Charcot joint
  Chronic osteomyelitis (healed)
  Exostosis
  Hydrocephalus
  Marble-bone
  Metastasis (osteosclerotic)
  Osteochondroma
  Osteoma
  Paget's disease
  Proliferative arthritis
  Sclerosis
Destructive (easy to penetrate)
  Active osteomyelitis
  Active tuberculosis
  Aseptic necrosis
  Atrophy—disease or disuse
  Blastomycosis
  Carcinoma
  Coccidioidomycosis
  Degenerative arthritis
  Ewing's tumor (children)
  Fibrosarcoma
  Giant cell sarcoma
  Gout
  Hemangioma
  Hodgkin's disease
  Hyperparathyroidism
  Leprosy
  Metastasis (osteolytic)
  Multiple myeloma
  Neuroblastoma
  New bone (fibrosis)
  Osteitis fibrosa cystica
  Osteoporosis/osteomalacia
  Radiation necrosis
  Solitary myeloma

RESPIRATORY SYSTEM

Additive (hard to penetrate)
  Actinomycosis
  Arrested tuberculosis (calcification)
  Atelectasis
  Bronchiectasis
  Edema
  Empyema
  Encapsulated abscess
  Hydropneumothorax
  Malignancy
  Miliary tuberculosis
  Pleural effusion
  Pneumoconiosis
    Anthracosis
    Asbestosis
    Calcinosis
    Siderosis
    Silicosis
  Pneumonia
  Syphilis
  Thoracoplasty
Destructive (easy to penetrate)
  Early lung abscess
  Emphysema
  Pneumothorax

CIRCULATORY SYSTEM

Additive (hard to penetrate)
  Aortic aneurysm
  Ascites
  Cirrhosis of liver
  Enlarged heart

SOFT TISSUE

Additive (hard to penetrate)
  Edema
Destructive (easy to penetrate)
  Emaciation

From Thompson TT: Cahoon's formulating x-ray techniques, ed 9, Durham, NC, Duke University Press, 1979.

may require an increased technique, whereas severe atrophy may require a decreased technique. Unless the radiographer has access to previous films with recorded techniques, a standard technique chart should be used to determine the initial exposures. Any necessary adjustments can then be made on subsequent films. Table 1-1 lists the changes in penetrability expected in advanced stages of various disease processes.

Certain diseases suppress the normal immune response. Immunocompromised patients (such as individuals with advanced leukemia) may require special care to prevent them from acquiring a disease from the radiographer. They may have to be placed in protective isolation (sometimes referred to as "reverse" isolation), and the radiographer may be required to mask, gown, and glove before approach-ing the patient. Conversely, diseases such as AIDS and hepatitis require blood and body fluid protection for the radiographer. It is essential that the radiographer wear rubber gloves when touching any area of the patient that may have been contaminated with blood or body fluids. When examining a patient with AIDS who has a productive cough, the radiographer must wear a mask and possibly protective eye goggles if there is a need to be extremely close to a patient's face. It is important to remember that many patients being radiographed have not been diagnosed and thus all patients should be treated as though they may have a communicable disease. Therefore proper precautions should be taken whenever you are exposed to any type of body secretion or blood.

Disease

Pathology is the study of diseases that can cause abnormalities in the structure or function of various organ systems. In essence, a disease is the pattern of response of the body to some form of injury. Diseases may be hereditary or may result from a broad spectrum of traumatic, infectious, vascular, or metabolic processes. They may reflect alterations of cell growth, as in tumors, or even be caused by physicians and their treatment (iatrogenic). In some cases the underlying cause is unknown and the disease is termed "idiopathic."

This chapter will discuss several basic reactions of the body that are the underlying mechanisms for the radiographic manifestations of most pathologic conditions. These processes include inflammation, edema, ischemia and infarction, hemorrhage, and alterations of cell growth leading to the development of neoplasms (tumors). In addition, this chapter will deal with hereditary diseases and their radiographic appearances, as well as immune reactions and the acquired immunodeficiency syndrome (AIDS).

INFLAMMATION

Acute inflammation is the initial response of body tissues to local injury. Among the various types of injury are blunt or penetrating trauma, infectious organisms, and irritating chemical substances. Regardless of the underlying cause, the inflammatory response consists of four overlapping events that occur sequentially:

1. Alterations in blood flow and vascular permeability
2. Migration of circulating white blood cells to the interstitium of the injured tissue
3. Phagocytosis and enzymatic digestion of dead cells and tissue elements
4. Repair of injury by regeneration of normal parenchymal cells or proliferation of granulation tissue and eventual scar formation

The earliest bodily response to local injury is dilation of arterioles, capillaries, and venules leading to a dramatic increase in blood flow in and around the injury site. This **hyperemia** produces the heat and redness associated with inflammation. As hyperemia develops, the venules and capillaries become abnormally **permeable,** allowing passage of a protein-rich plasma across vessel walls into the interstitium. This inflammatory **exudate** in the tissues produces the swelling associated with inflammation and puts pressure on sensitive nerve endings, which causes pain. The protein-rich exudate of inflammation must be differentiated from a **transudate,** a low-protein fluid such as the pulmonary edema that develops in congestive heart failure.

Very early in the inflammatory response, leukocytes (white blood cells, especially neutrophils and macrophages) of the circulating blood migrate to the area of injury. These white blood cells cross the capillary walls into the injured tissues, where they engulf and enzymatically digest infecting organisms and cellular debris, a process called **phagocytosis.**

The removal of necrotic debris and any injurious agents such as bacteria makes possible the repair of the injury that triggered the inflammatory response. In many tissues, such as the lung after pneumococcal pneumonia, regeneration of parenchymal cells permits reconstitution of entirely normal anatomy and function. However, some tissues, such as the heart after myocardial infarction, cannot heal by regeneration. The area of destroyed tissue is replaced by **granulation tissue** and eventually by a fibrous **scar.** Granulation tissue refers to a combination of young, budding capillaries and actively proliferating fibroblasts, which produce connective tissue fibers (collagen) that replace the dead tissue. Eventually, the strong connective tissue contracts to produce a fibrous scar. In the abdomen, such **fibrous adhesions** can narrow loops of intestine and result in an obstruction. The accumulation of excessive amounts of collagen (more common in blacks) may produce a protruding, tumorlike scar known as a **keloid.** Unfortunately, surgery to remove a keloid is usually ineffective because the subsequent incision tends to heal in the same way.

Many injuries heal by a combination of regeneration and scar tissue formation. An example is the response of the liver to repeated and persistent alcoholic injury that results in cirrhosis, in which irregular lobules of regenerated liver cells are crisscrossed and surrounded by bands of scar tissue.

The five clinical signs of acute inflammation are: rubor (redness), calor (heat), tumor (swelling), dolor (pain), and loss of function. The local heat and redness result from increased blood flow in the microcirculation at the site of injury. The swelling and pain are the result of exudate causing an increase in interstitial fluid and pressure on nerve endings.

Acute inflammation can also lead to systemic manifestations. Fever is especially common in inflammatory states associated with the spread of organisms into the bloodstream. There is also an increase in the number of circulating white blood cells (leukocytosis).

Some bacterial organisms (such as staphylococci and streptococci) produce **toxins** that damage the tissues and incite an inflammatory response. **Pyo-**genic bacteria lead to the production of a thick, yellow fluid called **pus,** which contains dead white blood cells, inflammatory exudate, and bacteria. An inflammation associated with pus formation is termed **suppurative.** When implanted beneath the skin or in a solid organ, a pyogenic infection produces an **abscess,** a localized collection of pus. All pyogens, wherever they become implanted, are capable of invading blood vessels to produce **bacteremia,** with the potential involvement of other organs and tissues in the body.

A **granulomatous** inflammation is a distinct pattern seen in relatively few diseases, including tuberculosis, syphilis, and sarcoidosis. A **granuloma** is a localized area of chronic inflammation, often with central necrosis. It is characterized by the accumulation of macrophages, some of which fuse to form multinucleated giant cells.

EDEMA

Edema is the accumulation of abnormal amounts of fluid in the intercellular tissue spaces or body cavities. It can be localized, as in an inflammatory reaction, or generalized, with marked swelling of subcutaneous tissues throughout the body **(anasarca).** Localized edema may result from inflammation with the escape of protein-rich intravascular fluid into the extravascular tissue or a local obstruction to lymphatic drainage as in **filariasis,** in which a parasitic worm causes lymphatic obstruction and localized edema termed **elephantiasis.** Generalized edema occurs most frequently in patients with congestive heart failure, cirrhosis of the liver, and certain forms of renal disease. Generalized edema is usually most prominent in dependent portions of the body because of the effects of gravity. Thus ambulatory patients tend to accumulate fluid in tissues around the ankles and lower legs, whereas in patients who are lying down, the edema fluid is most prominent in the back and sacral areas and the lung.

Extravascular fluid can also accumulate in serous cavities to produce pleural and pericardial effusions and peritoneal ascites.

Edema may produce minimal clinical symptoms or be potentially fatal. If localized to the subcutaneous tissues, large amounts of edema may cause minimal functional impairment. In contrast, pulmonary edema, pericardial effusion, or edematous swelling of the brain may have dire consequences.

ISCHEMIA AND INFARCTION

Ischemia refers to interference with the blood supply to an organ or part of an organ that deprives its cells and tissues of oxygen and nutrients. Ischemia may be caused by narrowing of arterial structures, as in atherosclerosis, or by thrombotic or embolic occlusion. Depending on several factors, occlusion of an artery or vein may have little or no effect on the involved tissue, or it may cause death of the tissue and even the individual. A major determinant is the availability of an alternative or newly acquired route of blood supply (collateral vessels). Other factors include the rate of development of the occlusion, the vulnerability of the tissue to hypoxia, and the oxygen-carrying capacity of the blood. Slowly developing occlusions are less likely to cause death of tissue because they provide an opportunity for the development of alternative pathways of flow. Ganglion cells of the nervous system and myocardial muscle cells undergo irreversible damage if deprived of their blood supply for 3 to 5 minutes. Anemic or cyanotic patients tolerate arterial insufficiency less well than do normal individuals, and thus occlusion of even a small vessel in such an individual may lead to death of tissue.

An **infarct** is a localized area of ischemic necrosis (death) within a tissue or organ produced by occlusion of either its arterial supply or its venous drainage. The two most common clinical forms of infarction are myocardial and pulmonary. Almost all infarcts result from thrombotic or embolic occlusion. Infrequent causes include twisting of an organ (volvulus), compression of the blood supply of a loop of bowel in a hernia sac, or trapping of a viscus under a peritoneal adhesion.

Severe arterial disease of the lower extremities may result in necrosis of several toes or a large segment of the foot, a condition called **gangrene.**

Infarctions tend to be especially severe because they are more common in patients least able to withstand them. Thus infarcts tend to occur in elderly individuals with advanced atherosclerosis or impaired cardiac function. The postoperative and post-delivery periods are also times in which infarctions often occur.

HEMORRHAGE

The term **hemorrhage** implies rupture of a blood vessel. Rupture of a large artery or vein is almost always caused by some form of injury, such as trauma, atherosclerosis, or inflammatory or neoplastic erosion of the vessel wall. Hemorrhage may be external, or blood may be trapped within body tissues, resulting in an accumulation termed a **hematoma.** The accumulation of blood in a body cavity results in hemothorax, hemopericardium, hemoperitoneum, or hemarthrosis (blood in a joint). Min-

imal hemorrhages into the skin, mucous membranes, or serosal surfaces are called **petechiae;** slightly larger hemorrhages are termed **purpura.** A large (greater than 1 to 2 cm) subcutaneous hematoma, or "bruise," is called an **ecchymosis**.

The significance of hemorrhage depends on the volume of blood loss, the rate of loss, and the site of hemorrhage. Sudden losses of up to 20% of the blood volume or slow losses of even larger amounts may have little clinical significance. The site of the hemorrhage is critical. For example, an amount of bleeding that would have little clinical significance in the subcutaneous tissues may cause death when located in a vital portion of the brain. Large amounts of external bleeding lead to the chronic loss of iron from the body and anemia. In contrast, internal hemorrhages into body cavities, joints, or tissues permit the iron to be recaptured for the synthesis of hemoglobin and the development of normal red blood cells.

ALTERATIONS OF CELL GROWTH

Changes in the number and size of cells, their differentiation, and their arrangement may develop in response to physiologic stimuli. **Atrophy** refers to a reduction in the size and/or number of cells in an organ or tissue, with a corresponding decrease in function. It must be distinguished from **hypoplasia** and **aplasia,** in which failure of normal development accounts for small size. An example is the **disuse atrophy** after immobilization of a limb by a plaster cast. There is a dramatic reduction in muscle mass of the encased limb. Because the cast also removes the stress and strain from the enclosed bone that normally stimulates new bone formation, normal bone resorption continues unchecked and loss of calcified bone can be seen on radiographs. In this situation, there is rapid recovery from the atrophic appearance when the cast is removed and normal function is resumed. Pathologic, irreversible atrophy may be caused by loss of innervation or hormonal stimulation or by decreased blood supply. For example, stenosis of a renal artery may cause atrophy of the kidney with shrinkage of individual nephrons and loss of interstitial tissue.

Hypertrophy refers to an increase in the size of cells of a tissue or organ in response to a demand for increased function. This must be distinguished from **hyperplasia,** an increase in the number of cells in a tissue or organ. Hypertrophy occurs most often in cells that cannot multiply, especially those in myocardial and peripheral striated muscle. Myocardial hypertrophy is necessary to maintain cardiac output despite increased peripheral resistance in patients with arterial hypertension or aortic valve disease. Loss of a normal kidney is followed by hypertrophy of the kidney on the opposite side in an attempt to continue adequate renal function. Examples of hyperplasia include proliferation of granulation tissue in the repair of injury and the increased cellularity of bone marrow in patients with hemolytic anemia or after hemorrhage. Hyperplasia of the adrenal cortex is a response to increased ACTH secretion; hyperplasia of the thyroid gland occurs with increased thyrotropic hormone secretion by the pituitary gland.

Dysplasia is a loss in the uniformity of individual cells and their architectural orientation. It is typically associated with prolonged chronic irritation or inflammation. Removal of the irritant may result in a return to normal, but often the tissue change persists and may evolve into a totally abnormal growth pattern. Thus dysplasia is generally considered at least potentially premalignant—a borderline lesion that may heal or progress to cancer.

NEOPLASIA

Neoplasia literally means "new growth" and refers to an abnormal proliferation of cells that are no longer controlled by factors that govern the growth of normal cells. Neoplastic cells act as parasites, competing with normal cells and tissues for their metabolic needs. Thus tumor cells may flourish while the patient becomes weak and emaciated, a condition termed **cachexia.**

Neoplasms are commonly referred to as "tumors;" indeed, the study of neoplasms is called **oncology,** which derives from the Greek word *oncos* meaning tumor. Although the word **tumor** originally referred to any swelling that could also be produced by edema or hemorrhage into a tissue, the word is now used almost exclusively to refer to a neoplasm.

Neoplasms are divided into benign and malignant categories based on a judgment of their potential clinical behavior. **Benign** tumors closely resemble their cells of origin in structure and function. They remain localized, do not spread to other sites, and thus can usually be surgically removed with survival of the patient. Nevertheless, some benign tumors can have severe consequences because of their position or hormonal secretion. For example, a benign pituitary tumor can cause pressure atrophy and destruction of the surrounding gland, and a benign tumor of the islets of Langerhans in the pancreas can produce excessive amounts of insulin resulting in possible fatal low levels of blood glucose. Other potentially dangerous benign tumors include those arising in the brain or spinal cord and tumors of the

trachea or esophagus that may occlude the air supply or make it impossible to swallow.

Malignant neoplasms invade and destroy adjacent structures and spread to distant sites (metastasize) to cause death. They tend to be poorly differentiated so that it may be impossible to determine the organ from which they arise. Malignant tumors are collectively referred to as **cancers.** This term is derived from the Latin word for crab, possibly because the fingerlike projections they extend into underlying tissue resemble crablike claws.

All tumors, both benign and malignant, have two basic components: (1) the parenchyma, made up of proliferating neoplastic cells, and (2) the supporting stroma, made up of connective tissue, blood vessels, and possibly lymphatic vessels. The parenchyma of the neoplasm largely determines its biologic behavior and is the component from which the tumor derives its name.

Most benign tumors are composed of parenchymal cells that closely resemble the tissue of origin. They are named by adding the suffix "oma" to the cell type from which the tumor arose. For example, benign tumors of fibrous tissue are termed fibromas, whereas benign cartilaginous tumors are chondromas. The term **adenoma** is the term for benign epithelial neoplasms that grow in glandlike patterns. Benign tumors that form large cystic masses are called **cystadenomas. Lipomas** are soft fatty tumors, **myomas** are tumors of muscle, and **angiomas** are tumors composed of blood vessels. An epithelial tumor that grows as a projecting mass on the skin or from an inner mucous membrane (like the gastrointestinal tract) is termed a **papilloma,** or **polyp.**

Malignant neoplasms of epithelial cell origin are called **carcinomas,** from the Greek word *karkinos* meaning crab. Carcinomas affect epithelial tissues, skin, and mucous membranes lining body cavities. Malignancies of glandular tissues such as the breast, liver, and pancreas, as well as the cells lining the gastrointestinal tract are called **adenocarcinomas. Squamous cell carcinoma** denotes a cancer in which the tumor cells resemble stratified squamous epithelium, as in the lung and head and neck regions. At times, the tumor grows in such a bizarre pattern that it is termed "undifferentiated" or "anaplastic" (without form).

Sarcomas are malignant tumors arising from connective tissues such as bone, muscle, and cartilage. Although less common than carcinomas, sarcomas tend to spread more rapidly and are highly malignant.

There is substantial evidence that most tumors arise from a single cell (monoclonal origin). The rate of growth generally correlates inversely with the level of parenchymal differentiation. Thus, well-differentiated tumors tend to grow slowly, whereas bizarre, undifferentiated neoplasms have a rapid growth rate.

Although the cause of cancer is still unknown, many possible causative factors (carcinogens) have been implicated. Chemical carcinogens may cause structural alteration of the DNA molecule (mutation) that may lead to the development of a neoplasm. Examples of chemical carcinogens include air or water pollution, cigarette smoke, asbestos, and a variety of other substances used in industry, food, cosmetics, and plastics. The development of specific types of cancer in certain families suggests some genetic predisposition. Excessive exposure to ultraviolet light (sunshine) may lead to the development of skin cancer. Survivors of the atom bomb who received huge doses of radiation have demonstrated a high incidence of leukemia. A greater-than-expected rate of leukemia was also seen in individuals working with x-radiation before the need for proper protection was appreciated.

The study of experimental animal tumors has offered convincing evidence that neoplastic transformation can be induced by DNA and RNA viruses. Viruses that invade normal cells may alter their genetic material, leading to the abnormal cell divisions and rapid growth observed in malignant tumors.

The clinical symptoms of cancer vary with the site of malignancy. Bleeding in the stools, a change in bowel activity (intermittent constipation and diarrhea), or intestinal obstruction suggest gastrointestinal malignancy. Difficulty in swallowing (dysphagia) or loss of appetite (anorexia), especially if accompanied by rapid weight loss, suggests a neoplasm in the esophagus or stomach. Hematuria may be a sign of kidney or bladder cancer, whereas difficulties in urination (urgency, burning sensations, inability to start the stream of urine) in an older man may be a sign of prostate tumor. Hemoptysis (coughing up blood) or a persistent cough or hoarseness suggests a neoplasm in the respiratory tract. Severe anemia may develop from internal bleeding or from malfunction of the bone marrow caused by growth of a malignant lesion in the skeleton. It should be stressed that these clinical symptoms may also be caused by benign disease. Nevertheless, since they may signal an underlying malignancy, these symptoms should be carefully investigated to exclude the presence of cancer.

Pain frequently is not an early sign of cancer. Unfortunately, pain often is only appreciated when the malignancy has spread too extensively to be curable. Secondary infections are common and an increasing cause of death. Most cancer patients are immuno-logically compromised, either because of their original disease or as a result of radiation or chemotherapy. In addition to typical bacterial and viral infections, immunocompromised patients with malignancy are especially susceptible to unusual **opportunistic** infections such as *Pneumocystis carinii* pneumonia and **cytomegalovirus.**

Some cancers that are still at a curable stage can be detected by screening procedures. Routine mammography may identify nonpalpable breast cancer; a Pap smear may show otherwise unsuspected cancer of the cervix. Surgical removal of these small tumors without metastatic spread offers an excellent prognosis.

Malignant neoplasms disseminate to distant sites by one of three pathways: (1) seeding within body cavities, (2) lymphatic spread, and (3) hematogenous spread.

Seeding (diffuse spread) of cancers occurs when neoplasms invade a natural body cavity. For example, a tumor of the gastrointestinal tract may penetrate the wall of the gut, permitting its metastases to enter the peritoneal cavity and implant at distant sites. A similar sequence may occur with lung cancers in the pleural cavity and neoplasms of the central nervous system (medulloblastoma, ependymoma) that spread from the cerebral ventricles by means of the cerebrospinal fluid to reimplant on the meningeal surfaces within the brain or in the spinal cord.

Lymphatic spread is the major metastatic route of carcinomas, especially those of the lung and breast. The pattern of lymph node involvement depends on the site of the primary neoplasm and the natural lymphatic pathways of drainage of that region. Carcinomas of the lung metastasize first to the regional bronchial lymph nodes and then to the tracheobronchial and hilar nodes. Carcinoma of the breast usually arises in the upper outer quadrant and first spreads to the axillary nodes. Medial breast lesions may drain through the chest wall to nodes along the internal mammary artery.

Hematogenous spread of cancer is a complex process involving several steps. Tumor cells invade and penetrate blood vessels and are released as neoplastic emboli into the circulation. These emboli of tumor cells are trapped in small vascular channels of distant organs, where they invade the wall of the arresting vessel and infiltrate and multiply in the adjacent tissue. The localization of hematogenous metastases tends to be determined by the vascular connections and anatomic relations between the primary neoplasm and the metastatic sites. For example, carcinomas arising in abdominal organs such as the gastrointestinal tract tend to metastasize to the liver because of the flow of portal vein blood to that organ. Cancers arising in midline organs close to the vertebral column (e.g., prostate, thyroid) tend to embolize through the paravertebral venous plexus to seed the vertebral column. Neoplasms in organs drained by the inferior and superior vena cava, such as the kidney, tend to metastasize to the lung. However, there are several well-defined patterns of metastatic spread that are not easily explained by vascular-anatomic relationships. Some examples include the tendency for carcinoma of the lung to involve the adrenal glands, simultaneous metastatic deposits in the brain and adrenal glands, and pituitary metastases occurring from breast carcinomas.

The **grading** of a malignant tumor assesses its aggressiveness, or degree of malignancy. The grade of a tumor usually suggests its biologic behavior and may predict its responsiveness to certain therapeutic agents. **Staging** refers to the extensiveness of a tumor at its primary site and the presence or absence of metastases to lymph nodes and distant organs such as the liver, lungs, and skeleton. The staging of a tumor is often critical to the choice of appropriate therapy. Well-localized tumors without evidence of metastases may be surgically removed. Fast-growing, undifferentiated tumors such as Hodgkin's disease may respond best to **radiation therapy. Hormonal therapy** is used to treat cancer of the prostate, either by removing the sources of male gonadal hormones that stimulate tumor growth or by the administration of the female gonadal hormone estrogen that inhibits it. **Chemotherapy** is the use of one or a combination of cytotoxic substances that kill neoplastic cells but also may injure many normal cells and result in significant complications.

HEREDITARY DISEASES

Hereditary diseases are passed from one generation to the next through the genetic information contained in the nucleus of each cell. They reflect an abnormality in the DNA (deoxyribonucleic acid), which is the blueprint for protein synthesis within the cell. In many hereditary diseases, there is an error in a single protein molecule that can lead to enzyme defects; defects in membrane receptors and transport systems; alterations in the structure, function, or quantity of nonenzyme proteins; and unusual reactions to drugs.

The most common hereditary abnormality is an enzyme deficiency. This leads to a metabolic block that results in a decreased amount of a substance needed for normal function or an accumulation of a metabolic intermediate that may cause injury. An example of the first mechanism is albinism, the absence of pigmentation resulting from an enzymatic deficiency that prevents the synthesis of the pigment melanin. An example of the second mechanism is phenylketonuria, in which absence of an enzyme leads to the accumulation of toxic levels of the amino acid phenylalanine.

A defect in the structure of the globin molecule leads to the development of the hemoglobinopathies such as sickle cell disease and thalassemia. An example of a genetically determined adverse reaction to drugs is glucose 6-phosphate dehydrogenase deficiency, in which an insufficient amount of the enzyme results in a severe hemolytic anemia in patients receiving a common antimalarial drug.

Despite our extensive knowledge of the biochemical basis of many genetic disorders, there are a large number of conditions for which the underlying mechanism is unknown. This list includes cystic fibrosis, neurofibromatosis, retinoblastoma, familial colonic polyposis, and Huntington's disease.

Each human cell contains 46 chromosomes divided into 23 pairs. The chromosomes, in turn, contain thousands of genes, each of which is responsible for the synthesis of a single protein. Forty-four of the chromosomes are called **autosomes;** the other two are the X and Y chromosomes that determine the sex of the person. A combination of XY chromosomes results in a male, whereas an XX configuration results in a female.

Half of each person's chromosomes are inherited from each parent. If the genes inherited from each parent are the same for a particular trait, the person is called **homozygous.** If the genes are different (e.g., one for brown eyes and one for blue eyes), the person is **heterozygous.** Genes that always produce an effect regardless of whether the person is homozygous or heterozygous are called **dominant;** genes that only manifest themselves when the person is homozygous for the trait are termed **recessive**. In determining eye color, brown is dominant, whereas blue is recessive. It must be remembered that although a recessive trait must have been contributed by both parents, it is possible that neither parent demonstrated that trait. For example, two parents each with one gene for brown eyes and one gene for blue eyes would show the dominant brown coloration, although they could each contribute a blue-eye gene to their offspring, who would manifest the recessive blue-eye trait.

In some traits, genes are **codominant** so that both are expressed. An example is the AB blood type, in which the gene for factor A is inherited from one parent and that for factor B is inherited from the other.

Mutations are alterations in the DNA structure

that may become permanent hereditary changes if they affect the gonadal cells. Mutations may result from radiation, chemicals, or viruses. They may have minimal effect and be virtually undetectable or be so serious that they are incompatible with life and cause the death of a fetus and spontaneous abortion.

Autosomal dominant disorders are transmitted from one generation to the next. Both males and females are affected, and both can transmit the condition. When an affected person marries an unaffected individual, half the children (on the average) will have the disease. The clinical manifestations of autosomal dominant disorders can be modified by reduced penetrance and variable expressivity. Reduced penetrance means that not everyone who has the gene will demonstrate the trait; variable expressivity refers to the fact that a dominant gene may be manifest somewhat differently among several individuals (e.g., polydactyly may be expressed in the toes or in the fingers as one or more extra digits). Examples of autosomal dominant disorders include achondroplasia, neurofibromatosis, Marfan's syndrome, and familial hypercholesterolemia.

Autosomal recessive disorders result only when a person is homozygous for the defective gene. The trait does not usually affect the parents, although siblings may show the disease. On average, siblings have a one in four chance of being affected; two out of four will be carriers, and one will be normal. Recessive genes appear more frequently in a family, and close intermarriage (as between first cousins) increases the risk of the particular disease. Unlike autosomal dominant diseases, the expression of the defect tends to be uniform in autosomal recessive diseases and the age of onset is frequently early in life. Examples of autosomal recessive disorders include phenylketonuria, cystic fibrosis, galactosemia, glycogen and lipid storage diseases, Tay-Sachs disease, and sickle cell anemia.

Sex-linked disorders generally result from defective genes on the X chromosome, since the Y chromosome is small and carries very few genes. Most of these conditions are transmitted by heterozygous carrier females virtually only to sons, who have only the single, affected X chromosome. Sons of a heterozygous woman have a one in two chance of receiving the mutant gene. An affected male does not transmit the disorder to sons, but all his daughters are carriers. In rare cases a female may have the sex-linked disease if she is homozygous for the recessive gene. Virtually all sex-linked disorders are recessive. The most common example of a sex-linked disorder is color blindness. Other conditions include glucose 6-phosphate dehydrogenase deficiency and some types of hemophilia and muscular dystrophy.

RADIOGRAPHIC MANIFESTATIONS OF HEREDITARY DISEASES

Down's syndrome (mongolism)

Down's syndrome is the most common of the trisomy disorders that are caused by the presence of an extra autosomal chromosome that results in an individual having three strands of a certain chromosome (number 21) instead of the normal two. It is usually diagnosed from birth because of the characteristic clinical appearance—mental deficiency, short stature, poor muscle tone, short neck, and a straight skin crease that extends across the palm of the hand. The typical facial appearance includes widely set eyes, short and flat nose, and coarse tongue that often protrudes through a partially open mouth.

The major skeletal abnormality in infancy is in the pelvis, where there is a decrease in the acetabular and iliac angles with hypoplasia and marked lateral flaring of the iliac wings (Figure 1-1). Other common skeletal abnormalities include shortening of the mid-

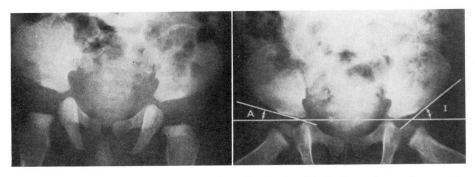

Figure 1-1 Down's syndrome. Two examples of typical pelvis in Down's syndrome, showing flared iliac wings and diminished acetabular (A) and iliac (I) angles. *(From James AE, Merz P, Janower ML, et al: Clin Radiol 22:417-433, 1971.)*

dle phalanx of the fifth finger, squaring of the vertebral bodies (superoinferior length becoming equal to or greater than the anteroposterior measurement), hypoplasia of the nasal sinuses, and delayed closure of the cranial sutures.

Congenital heart disease, especially septal defects, occurs in about 40% of patients with Down's syndrome. There is also a greater-than-normal incidence of duodenal obstruction (duodenal atresia or annular pancreas) and Hirschsprung's disease, as well as a substantially increased likelihood of developing leukemia.

Turner's syndrome

Turner's syndrome (gonadal dysgenesis) is characterized by primary amenorrhea (no ovulation or menstruation), sexual infantilism, short stature, and bilateral tiny gonads. Although the patient appears to be female, she has only one X chromosome.

A characteristic, but nonspecific, skeletal abnormality is shortening of the fourth metacarpal and sometimes also the fifth metacarpal (Figure 1-2).

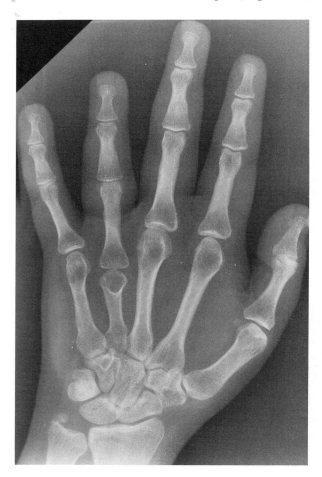

Figure 1-2 Turner's syndrome. Frontal projection of hand shows short fourth metacarpal.

This produces a positive metacarpal sign, in which a line drawn tangential to the distal ends of the heads of the fifth and fourth metacarpals passes through the head of the third metacarpal (indicating the disproportionate shortening of the fourth and fifth metacarpals), rather than extending distal to the head of the third metacarpal as in a normal person.

Various urinary tract anomalies, especially horseshoe kidney and other types of malrotation, are often seen in patients with gonadal dysgenesis. Coarctation of the aorta is the most common cardiovascular anomaly. Because coarctation of the aorta most often affects men, its appearance in a woman should suggest the possibility of underlying gonadal dysgenesis.

Klinefelter's syndrome

Klinefelter's syndrome is a disorder characterized by small testes that fail to mature or produce sperm. The fundamental defect is the presence in a male of two or more X chromosomes. At puberty, the breasts enlarge, and a female distribution of hair develops. The affected individual is tall, mentally deficient, and sterile.

Radiographically, the skeletal changes are both less common and less marked than in patients with Turner's syndrome, its female counterpart. A positive metacarpal sign is seen in fewer than 25% of the patients. Hypogonadism may lead to delayed epiphyseal fusion and retarded bone maturation.

Phenylketonuria (PKU)

Phenylketonuria is an inborn error of metabolism in which an enzyme deficiency results in the impaired conversion of phenylalanine to tyrosine. If the condition is not diagnosed and treated early, the patient usually suffers profound retardation, hyperactivity, and seizures, all related to brain atrophy that can be demonstrated as dilation of the ventricles and sulci on computed tomography (CT) or magnetic resonance imaging (MRI). Because of an inadequate amount of tyrosine, there is impaired production of the pigment melanin, and the patient is very light in color.

Homocystinuria

Homocystinuria is an inborn error of the metabolism of the amino acid methionine that causes a defect in the structure of collagen or elastin. The most frequent and striking radiographic feature of homocystinuria is osteoporosis of the spine, which is often associated with biconcave deformities of the vertebral bodies (Figure 1-3). Osteoporosis with cortical thinning is also common in the long bones. Patients with homocystinuria have a tendency to develop arterial and venous thrombosis, and premature occlusive vascular disease is the major cause of death.

Alkaptonuria and ochronosis

Alkaptonuria is a rare inborn error of metabolism in which an enzyme deficiency leads to an abnormal accumulation of homogentisic acid in the blood and urine. The urine is either very dark on voiding or becomes black after standing or being alkalinized. The disorder often goes unrecognized until middle life, when deposition of the black pigment of oxidized homogentisic acid in cartilage and other connective tissue produces a distinctive form of degenerative arthritis (ochronosis). The pathognomonic radiographic finding is dense laminated calcification of multiple intervertebral disks (Figure 1-4) that begins in the lumbar spine and may extend to involve the dorsal and cervical regions.

Cystinuria

Cystinuria is an inborn error of amino acid transport characterized by impaired tubular absorption and excessive urinary excretion of several amino acids. Large amounts of cystine in the urine predispose to the formation of renal, ureteral, and bladder stones. Pure cystine stones are not radiopaque and can only be demonstrated on excretory urography, where they appear as filling defects in the urinary tract. Stones containing the calcium salts of cystine are radiopaque and can be detected on plain abdominal radiographs.

Glycogen storage diseases

The glycogen storage diseases are a group of genetic disorders involving the pathways for the storage of carbohydrates as glycogen (in the liver) and for its use in maintaining blood sugar and providing energy. An excess amount of normal or abnormal glycogen infiltrates and enlarges multiple organs, especially the heart and liver (Figure 1-5).

Lipid storage diseases

See section on Gaucher's disease.

Marfan's syndrome

Marfan's syndrome is an inherited generalized disorder of connective tissue with ocular, skeletal, and cardiovascular manifestations. Most patients are tall

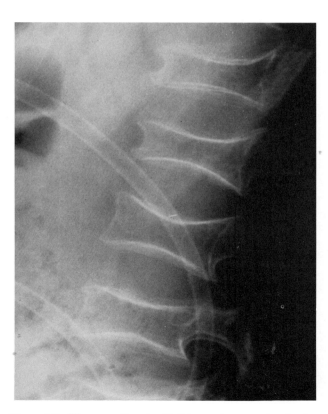

Figure 1-3 Homocystinuria. Striking osteoporosis of spine is associated with biconcave deformities of vertebral bodies. *(From Thomas PS and Carson NAJ: Ann Radiol 21:95, 1978.)*

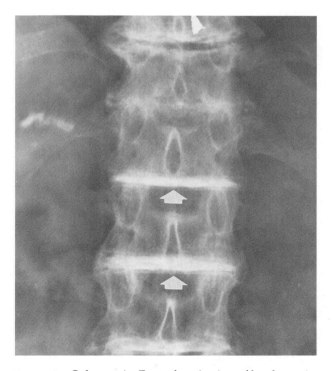

Figure 1-4 Ochronosis. Frontal projection of lumbar spine shows dense laminated calcification of multiple intervertebral disks *(arrows).*

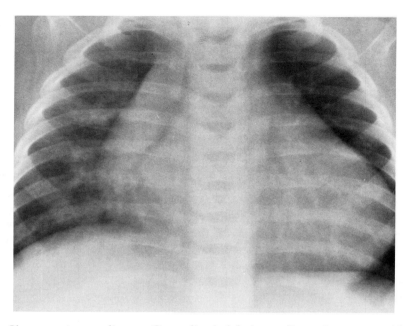

Figure 1-5 Glycogen storage disease. Generalized globular cardiac enlargement with left ventricular prominence.

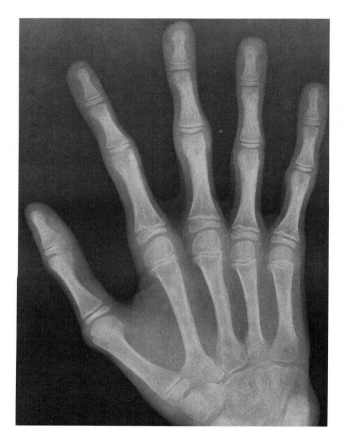

Figure 1-6 Arachnodactyly in Marfan's syndrome. Metacarpals and phalanges are unusually long and slender.

and slender and appear emaciated because of the decrease in subcutaneous fat. A typical feature of Marfan's syndrome is bilateral dislocation of the lens of the eye caused by weakness of its supporting tissues. A laxity of ligaments about the joints leads to loose-jointedness or double-jointedness, recurrent dislocations, and flat feet. The major radiographic abnormality is elongation and thinning of the tubular bones (Figure 1-6), most pronounced in the hands and feet and seen clinically as arachnodactyly (spiderlike digits). Almost all patients with Marfan's syndrome have abnormalities of the cardiovascular system. Necrosis of the medial portion of the aortic wall causes progressive dilation of the ascending aorta that produces a bulging of the upper right portion of the cardiac silhouette (Figure 1-7) and an unusual prominence of the pulmonary outflow tract as it is displaced by the dilated aorta. Dissecting aneurysm is a serious complication that may kill the patient in early life.

Osteogenesis imperfecta

See page 67.

Achondroplasia

See page 67.

DISORDERS OF IMMUNITY

The immune reaction of the body provides a powerful defense against invading organisms by recogniz-

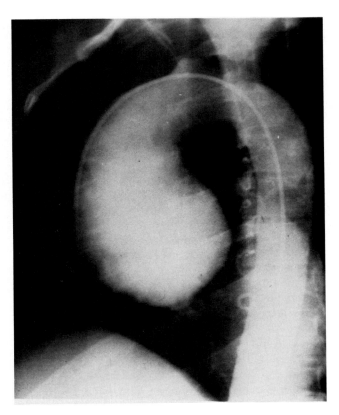

Figure 1-7 Marfan's syndrome. Arteriogram show enormous dilation of aneurysmal ascending aorta *(From Oven-fors CO and Godwin JD: In Eisenberg RL and Amberg JR, editors: Critical diagnostic pathways in radiology: an algorithmic approach, Philadelphia, JB Lippincott, 1981.)*

ing foreign substances (antigens), such as bacteria, viruses, fungi, and toxins, and producing antibodies to counteract them. The antibody binds together with the antigen to make the antigen harmless. Once antibodies have been produced, a person becomes **immune** to the antigen.

Antibodies, or **immunoglobulins,** are formed in lymphoid tissue, primarily in the lymph nodes, thymus gland, and spleen. Although an infant is born with some immunity, most immunity is acquired either naturally by exposure to a disease or artificially by immunization. There are two types of artificial immunity, active and passive. In **active immunity,** a person forms antibodies to counteract an antigen in the form of a vaccine or toxoid. A **vaccine** consists of a low dose of dead or deactivated bacteria or viruses. Although these organisms cannot cause disease, they are foreign proteins containing antigens that stimulate the body to produce antibodies against them. A **toxoid** is a chemically altered **toxin,** the poisonous material produced by a pathogenic

organism. As with a vaccine, the toxin cannot cause disease but does trigger the development of antibodies to it. Examples of active immunity are the vaccines given to prevent smallpox, polio, measles, tetanus, and diphtheria. Active immunity persists for a long time, although a relatively long time is required to build up immunity and a booster shot is frequently given for a stronger effect.

Passive immunity refers to the administration of a dose of preformed antibodies from immune serum of an animal, usually a horse. This type of immunity acts immediately but lasts for a relatively short time. It is used in situations when a person is exposed to a serious disease (hepatitis, rabies, tetanus) but has no immunity against it and thus requires an immediate supply of antibodies to prevent a possibly fatal infection.

There are several fundamental mechanisms of immunologic responses to antigens. The first type is a rapidly occurring reaction in which antigens are attacked by antibodies previously bound to the surface of mast cells. The mast cells release **histamine,** which causes a local increase in vascular permeability and smooth muscle contraction. Disorders resulting from localized reactions of this type (which probably have a genetically determined predisposition) include hay fever, asthma, and gastrointestinal allergies. Generalized, or systemic, **anaphylactic** reactions are characterized by hypotension and vascular collapse (shock) with urticaria (hives), bronchiolar spasm, and laryngeal edema. This reaction is the cause of acute death in patients who are hypersensitive ("allergic") to the sting of bees, wasps, and other insects and to medications such as penicillin and the iodinated contrast materials used in radiology.

In the second (cytotoxic) type of immune reaction, the antigen is either a component of a cell or is attached to the wall of red blood cells, white blood cells, platelets, or vascular endothelial cells. The reaction with an antibody leads to cell destruction by lysis or phagocytosis. Examples of this type of immune reaction include the transfusion reaction following the administration of ABO-incompatible blood and erythroblastosis fetalis, the hemolytic anemia of the Rh positive newborn whose Rh negative mother has produced anti-Rh antibodies.

The third type of immune reaction is a delayed reaction that occurs in an individual previously sensitized to an antigen. As an example, the first time a person touches poison ivy there is no reaction. However, on the next exposure to poison ivy, antibodies are present to attack the antigen, and the patient develops the typical rash and irritation. A similar process is involved in the reaction to tuberculosis, leprosy, many fungal diseases, and other infections. It is also the principal component of rejection in organ transplants.

ACQUIRED IMMUNODEFICIENCY SYNDROME (AIDS)

The acquired immunodeficiency syndrome (AIDS), which most commonly affects young homosexual males and intravenous drug abusers, is characterized by a profound and sustained impairment of cellular immunity that results in recurrent or sequential opportunistic infections and a particularly aggressive form of Kaposi's sarcoma. AIDS has also been reported in a substantial number of hemophiliacs, recipients of transfusions, and a group of heterosexual, non–drug abusing Haitians.

AIDS predominantly involves the lungs, gastrointestinal tract, and central nervous system. Pulmonary infections are extremely common in patients with AIDS and are frequently caused by organisms that only rarely produce disease in individuals with normal immune systems. About 60% of AIDS victims develop one or more attacks of *Pneumocystis carinii* pneumonia, which is characterized by a sudden onset, a rapid progression to diffuse lung involvement, and a marked delay in resolution. The typical early radiographic finding of this protozoan infection is a hazy, perihilar granular infiltrate that spreads to the periphery and appears predominantly interstitial. In later stages the pattern progresses to patchy areas of air space consolidation with air bronchograms, indicating the alveolar nature of the pro-

cess (Figure 1-8). The radiographic appearance may closely resemble pulmonary edema or bacterial pneumonia. Because *Pneumocystis carinii* cannot be cultured and the disease it causes is usually fatal if untreated, an open-lung biopsy is often necessary if a sputum examination reveals no organisms in a patient suspected of having this disease.

Gastrointestinal manifestations of AIDS include a variety of sexually transmitted diseases involving the rectum and colon, infectious processes (such as shigellosis, amebiasis, candidiasis, and giardiasis), and alimentary tract dissemination (spread) of Kaposi's sarcoma. Kaposi's sarcoma is a systemic disease that characteristically affects the skin and causes an ulcerated hemorrhagic dermatitis. Metastases to the small bowel are relatively common and consist of multiple reddish or bluish red nodules that intrude into the lumen of the bowel (Figure 1-9). Similar lesions can develop throughout the gastrointestinal tract. Central ulceration of the metastases causes gastrointestinal bleeding and a characteristic radiographic appearance of multiple "bull's-eye" lesions simulating metastatic melanoma.

About 40% of all AIDS victims have neurologic symptoms, most commonly progressive dementia. Focal neurologic symptoms and signs are common in patients who develop mass lesions of the brain. The multiple manifestations of AIDS in the central

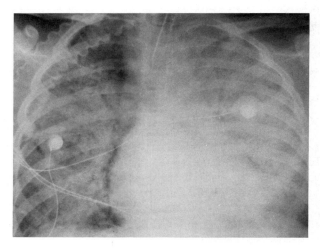

Figure 1-8 *Pneumocystis carinii* pneumonia. Diffuse bilateral airspace consolidation suggesting severe bacterial pneumonia or pulmonary edema.

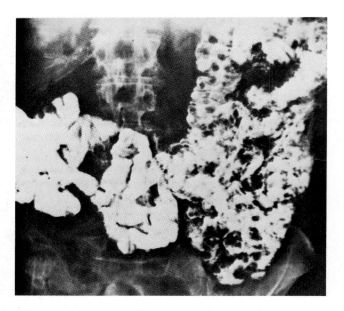

Figure 1-9 Kaposi's sarcoma. Small bowel study shows multiple intramural nodules (predominantly involving the jejunum) that distort the mucosal pattern and produce contour defects and intraluminal lucencies. *(From Bryk D, et al: Gastrointest Radiol 3:425, 1978.)*

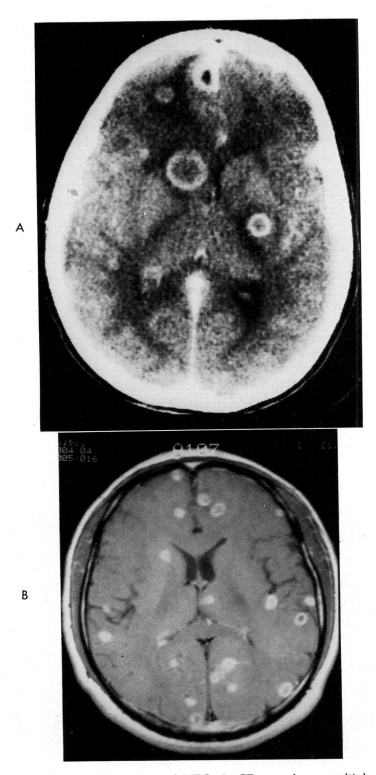

Figure 1-10 Neurologic manifestations of AIDS. **A,** CT scan shows multiple ring-enhancing lesions caused by cryptococcal brain abscesses. **B,** MR image after intravenous administration of contrast, demonstrating multiple enhancing abscesses caused by toxoplasmosis.

nervous system are best demonstrated on MRI, where they appear as areas of increased signal intensity on T2-weighted images. Atypical brain abscesses and meningeal infection often occur, most commonly as a result of toxoplasmosis, cryptococcosis, cytomegalovirus, and herpesvirus (Figure 1-10). Increasing evidence suggests that there also may be cerebral infections by the human immunodeficiency virus (HIV) itself. Patients with AIDS also have a high incidence of lymphoma involving the central nervous system.

Specialized Imaging Techniques

ULTRASOUND

Ultrasound (Figure 1-11) is a noninvasive imaging modality in which high-frequency sound waves that are produced by electrical stimulation of a specialized crystal are passed through the body (reduced in intensity) in relation to the acoustic properties of the tissues through which they travel. The crystal is mounted in a transducer, which also acts as a receiver to record echoes that are reflected back from the body whenever the sound wave strikes an interface between two tissues that have different acoustic impedances. A water-tissue interface produces strong reflections (echoes), whereas a solid tissue mass that contains only small differences in composition causes weak reflections. The display of the ultrasound image on a television monitor shows both the intensity level of the echoes and the position in the body from which they arose. Ultrasound images may be displayed as static gray-scale scans or as multiple images that permit movement to be viewed in "real-time."

In general, fluid-filled structures have intense echoes at their borders, no internal echoes, and good through transmission of the sound waves. Solid structures produce internal echoes of variable intensity. Since the solid structure tends to attenuate the sound waves, the posterior margin is less sharply defined than the anterior margin, and only a portion of the beam is transmitted.

The major advantage of ultrasound is its safety. To date, there is no evidence of any adverse effect on human tissues at the intensity level currently used for diagnostic procedures. Therefore ultrasound is the modality of choice for examination of children and pregnant women, in whom there is potential danger from the radiation exposure of other imaging studies. It is by far the best technique for evaluating fetal age, congenital anomalies, and complications of pregnancy. Ultrasound is used extensively to evaluate the intraperitoneal and retroperitoneal structures (with the exception of internal lesions of the gastrointestinal tract), to detect abdominal and pelvic abscesses, to diagnose obstruction of the biliary and urinary tracts, and to assess the patency of major blood vessels. Ultrasound may be used as a quick, inexpensive procedure to evaluate postoperative complications, although it may be difficult to perform in these patients because of

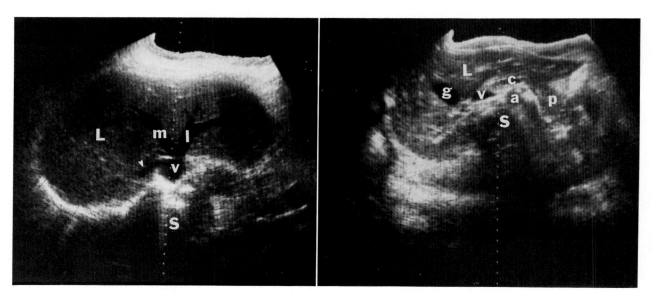

Figure 1-11 Normal abdominal ultrasound images. **A,** Upper portion of liver. **B,** Lower portion of liver. *L,* Liver; *g,* gallbladder; *a,* aorta; *v,* inferior vena cava; *p,* tail of pancreas; *S,* spine; *l,* left hepatic vein; *m,* middle hepatic vein; *arrowhead,* right hepatic vein.

overlying dressings, retention sutures, drains, and open wounds that may prevent the transducer from being in direct contact with the skin. In children with open fontanelles, ultrasound can be used to examine intracranial structures. Other more recent uses of ultrasound include breast imaging (to differentiate solid from cystic masses), prostate imaging (to detect and accurately stage neoplasms), and Doppler studies (to evaluate narrowing or obstruction of blood vessels). An exciting new field is the use of high-resolution, real-time ultrasound systems to assist surgeons during operative procedures. This technique has been applied to the neurosurgical localization of brain and spine neoplasms, evaluation of intraventricular shunt tube placement, localization of renal calculi, and surgical procedures involving the hepatobiliary system and pancreas.

The major limitation of ultrasound is the presence of acoustic barriers, such as air, bone, and barium. For example, air reflects essentially all of the ultrasound beam, so that structures beneath it cannot be imaged. This is a special problem when attempting to image the solid abdominal organs in a patient with adynamic ileus and is the major factor precluding the ultrasound examination of the thorax. For an ultrasound examination of the pelvis, the patient is usually given large amounts of fluid to fill the bladder, thus displacing the air-filled bowel from the region of interest.

COMPUTED TOMOGRAPHY

Computed tomography (CT) (Figure 1-12) is a radiographic technique for producing cross-sectional tomographic images by first scanning a "slice" of tissue from multiple angles with a narrow x-ray beam, then calculating a relative linear attenuation coefficient (amount of radiation absorbed in tissue for the various tissue elements in the section), and finally displaying the computed reconstruction as a gray-scale image on a television monitor. Unlike other imaging modalities (with the exception of the more recent magnetic resonance imaging), CT permits the radiographic differentiation among a variety of soft tissues. It is extremely sensitive to slight differences (1%) in tissue densities; for comparison, differences in tissue density of at least 5% are required for detection by conventional screen-film radiography. Thus in the head CT can differentiate between blood clots, white matter and gray matter, cerebrospinal fluid, cerebral edema, and neoplastic processes. The CT number reflects the attenuation

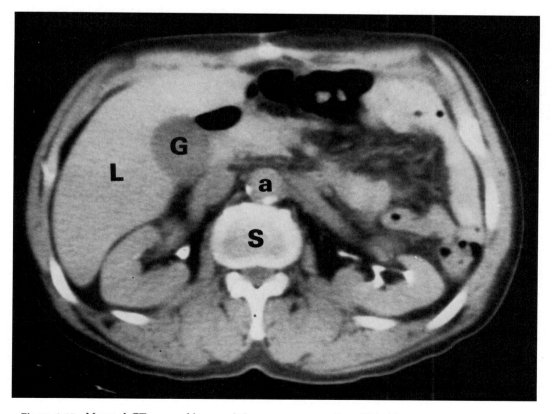

Figure 1-12 Normal CT scan of lower abdomen. *a*, aorta; *G*, gallbladder; *L*, liver; *S*, spine.

of a specific tissue relative to that of water, which is arbitrarily given a CT number of 0. The highest CT number is that of bone; the lowest is that of air. Fat has a CT number less than 0, whereas soft tissues have CT numbers higher than 0.

Technical improvements in CT instrumentation have greatly reduced the time required to produce a single slice (2 to 8 seconds), and this permits the CT evaluation of virtually any portion of the body. In most instances, some type of preliminary film is obtained (either a radiograph or a CT-generated image) for localization, the detection of potentially interfering high-density material (metallic clips, barium, electrodes), and correlation with the CT images. An overlying grid with numeric markers permits close correlation between the subsequent CT scans and the initial scout film.

The intravenous injection of iodinated contrast material is an integral part of many CT examinations. Scanning during or immediately after the administration of contrast material permits the differentiation of vascular from nonvascular solid structures.

Differences in the degree and the time course of contrast enhancement may permit the detection of neoplastic or infectious processes within normal parenchymal structures. Because of its relatively low CT number, fat can serve as a natural contrast material and can outline parenchymal organs. In patients with malignant lesions, the loss of adjacent fat planes is highly suspicious for tumor extension. For abdominal studies, especially those of the pancreas and retroperitoneum, dilute oral contrast material is frequently given to demonstrate the lumen of the gastrointestinal tract and permit the distinction between loops of bowel and solid abdominal structures.

MAGNETIC RESONANCE IMAGING

Magnetic resonance imaging (MRI) (Figure 1-13), once called nuclear magnetic resonance (NMR), has in a few short years become an important clinical tool for a variety of conditions. Although the physics of MRI is beyond the scope of this book, the tech-

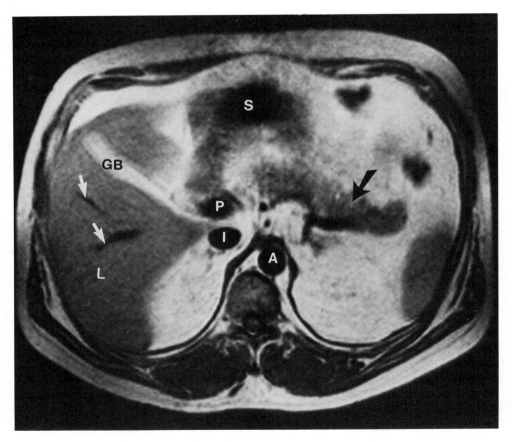

Figure 1-13 Normal MR image of upper abdomen. Transverse scan shows liver (*L*) and branches of portal veins (*white arrows*). Gallbladder (*GB*) has high intensity in this fasting person. Pancreas (*black arrow*) and stomach (*S*) are easily seen. Inferior vena cava (*I*), aorta (*A*), and main portal vein (*P*) are seen with signal void because they contain flowing blood.

nique basically consists of inducing transitions between energy states by causing certain atoms to absorb and transfer energy. This is accomplished by directing a radiofrequency pulse at a substance placed within a large magnetic field. Various measures of the time required for the material to return to a baseline energy state (relaxation time) can be translated by a complex computer program to a visual image on a television monitor. The two time constants associated with relaxation are T1 and T2 (explained below). To generate an MR image, the radiographer selects a pulse sequence, which represents a set of radiofrequency magnetic pulses and the time spacing between these pulses. The most commonly used pulse sequence is the spin echo. Other terminology used to describe the pulse sequences includes repetition time (TR) and echo delay time (TE). The TR is the time between the initiation of a pulse sequence and the beginning of the succeeding pulse sequence. The TE is the time between the generation of the radiofrequency pulse and the time at which the image is obtained.

MRI has many of the advantages offered by other imaging modalities without the associated disadvantages. Like ultrasound, MRI is nonionizing and capable of imaging in multiple planes. Unlike ultrasound, MRI depends less on the operator's skill or the habitus of the patient and can penetrate bone without significant decrease in intensity (attenuation) so that the underlying tissue can be clearly imaged. MRI provides excellent spatial resolution, equal to that of CT, and far better contrast resolution of soft tissue. The intravenous injection of contrast material is unnecessary with MRI because flowing blood produces a signal void that contrasts sharply with adjacent structures.

Unlike other imaging modalities that depend on information from one parameter (such as CT, which depends on electron density), MRI has the advantage that it derives information from multiple parameters such as hydrogen density and T1 and T2 relaxation times. Different imaging sequences demonstrate the effect of one or a combination of these parameters, allowing for a superb display of the differences between normal and abnormal tissues. In general, a pulse sequence using a short TR (500 to 700 msec) and short TE (20 to 30 msec) provides a T1-weighted image. A pulse sequence using a long TR (2000 to 2500 msec) and a long TE (60 to 80 msec) provides a T2-weighted image.

Although the degree of signal intensity of various substances on MR scans is complex and depends on multiple factors, some generalizations can be made. On T1-weighted images, substances causing high signal intensity (bright) include fat, subacute hemorrhage, highly proteinaceous material (e.g., mucus), and slow flowing blood. Water, as in cerebrospinal fluid or simple cysts, has a relatively low signal intensity and appears dark. Soft tissue has an intermediate level of signal.

On T2-weighted images, water has a high signal intensity (bright), whereas muscle and other soft tissues (including fat) tend to have low signal intensity and appear dark. Bone, calcium, and air appear very dark on all imaging sequences.

Although MRI has improved the sensitivity of detecting abnormal tissue, to date it has not had a significant effect on specificity. In the head, for example, infarction, edema, tumor, infection, and demyelinating disease all produce identical high signal intensity on T2-weighted images. Other disadvantages of MRI include a slower scanning time, leading to image degradation resulting from patient motion; the possibility of patient claustrophobia; and the contraindication to imaging patients with pacemakers (may prevent proper operation) or intracranial aneurysm clips (may slip and result in hemorrhage).

In the future, spectroscopic examinations using high magnetic fields and assessing various chemical elements may permit the sophisticated biochemical analysis of tissues in vivo. Improved hardware and software and the development of specific magnetic contrast agents should improve the specificity of this modality and make MRI the imaging procedure of choice for a broad spectrum of clinical findings.

QUESTIONS

1. The accumulation of abnormal amounts of fluid in the spaces between cells or in body cavities is termed ＿EDEMA＿.

2. ＿PHAGOCYTOSIS＿ is the process by which white blood cells surround and digest infectious organisms.

3. A tumorlike scar is referred to as a ＿KEDOID＿.
   keloid

4. Inflammation with pus formation is termed ＿SUPPERATIVE＿.

5. An interruption in the blood supply to an organ or body part is referred to as ＿ISCHEMIA＿.

6. A localized area of ischemic necrosis in an organ or tissue is termed an ＿INFARCT＿.

7. A swelling due to bleeding into an enclosed area is termed HEMATOMA.

8. A decrease in function of an organ or tissue, due to a reduction in the size and/or number of cells, is termed ATROPHY.

9. The term NEOPLASIA means new growth.

10. The term for benign epithelial neoplasms that have a gland-like pattern is ADENOMA.

11. __F__ Soft fatty tumors
12. __I__ Tumors composed of blood vessels
13. __Q__ Malignant neoplasms of epithelial cell origin
14. __B__ Tumors of muscle
15. __H__ Large cystic, benign tumor masses
16. __O__ Malignant tumors from connective tissues such as bone, muscle, and cartilage
17. __T__ Term meaning without form
18. __P__ Loss of appetite
19. __C__ Difficulty in swallowing
20. __G__ Coughing up blood
21. __D__ Major metastatic route of carcinomas

A. Cachexia
B. Myomas
C. Dysphagia
D. Lymphatic
E. Staging
F. Lipomas
G. Hemoptysis
H. Cystadenomas
I. Angiomas
J. Grading
K. Vaccine
L. Antigen
M. Polyp
N. Chemotherapy
O. Sarcomas
P. Anorexia
Q. Carcinomas
R. Pneumocystis pneumonia
S. Anaphylactic
T. Anaplastic

22. __J__ Assessing the aggressiveness of a malignant tumor
23. __E__ Refers to extensiveness of a tumor and whether or not it has metastasized
24. __N__ Use of cytotoxic substances that kill neoplastic cells and may cause injury to normal cells
25. __L__ Foreign substances produced by invading organisms
26. __K__ Consists of a low dose of dead or deactivated bacteria or viruses
27. __S__ Critical reaction that can cause death
28. __A__ Tumor cells grow well, patient becomes weak and emaciated
29. __R__ Opportunistic infection
30. __M__ Epithelial tumor that grows as a projecting mass arising on the skin or a mucous membrane

BIBLIOGRAPHY

General radiology
Eisenberg RL: Diagnostic imaging in internal medicine, New York, McGraw-Hill Book Co, 1985.
Eisenberg RL: Diagnostic imaging in surgery, New York, McGraw-Hill Book Co, 1986.
Juhl JH and Crummy AB: Essentials of radiologic imaging, Philadelphia, JB Lippincott Co, 1987.
Putman CE and Ravin CE: Textbook of diagnostic imaging, Philadelphia, WB Saunders Co, 1988.

Ultrasound
Mittelstaedt CA: Abdominal ultrasound, New York, Churchill-Livingstone, 1987.
Sarti DA: Diagnostic ultrasound: text and cases, Chicago, Yearbook Medical Publishers, 1987.

Computed tomography
Greenberg M and Greenberg BM: Essentials of body computed tomography. Philadelphia, WB Saunders Co, 1983.
Lee JKT, Sagel SS, and Stanley RJ: Computed body tomography with MRI correlation, New York, Raven Press, 1989.
Moss AA, Gamsu G, and Genant HK: Computed tomography of the body, Philadelphia, WB Saunders Co, 1983.

Magnetic resonance imaging
Higgins CB and Hricak H: Magnetic resonance imaging of the body, New York, Raven Press, 1987.
Stark DD and Bradley WG: Magnetic resonance imaging, St. Louis, The CV Mosby Co, 1988.

CHAPTER 2

Respiratory System

PREREQUISITE KNOWLEDGE

The student should have a basic knowledge of the anatomy and physiology of the respiratory system. In addition, proper learning and understanding of the material will be facilitated if the student has some clinical experience in chest radiography and film evaluation, including a concept of the changes in technique required to compensate for density differences produced by the underlying pathologic conditions.

GOALS

To acquaint the student radiographer with the pathophysiology and radiographic manifestations of all of the common and some of the unusual disorders of the respiratory system

OBJECTIVES

1. Describe the physiology of the respiratory system
2. Identify anatomic structures on both diagrams and radiographs of the respiratory system
3. Be able to define terminology relating to the respiratory system
4. Be able to describe the various pathologic conditions affecting the respiratory system, as well as their radiographic manifestations
5. Be familiar with the changes in technical factors required for obtaining optimal quality radiographs in patients with various underlying pathologic conditions

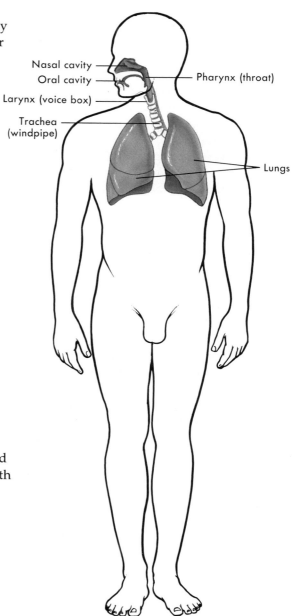

Nasal cavity
Oral cavity
Larynx (voice box)
Trachea (windpipe)
Pharynx (throat)
Lungs

RADIOGRAPHER NOTES

Proper positioning and the use of correct exposure factors are especially important in radiography of the respiratory system, so that the radiologist can detect the subtle changes in pulmonary and vascular structures necessary to make a precise diagnosis. Ideally, follow-up studies should be performed with the same exposure factors used in making the initial radiographs. In this way, any density changes can be attributed to true pathologic findings rather than to mere technical differences.

With the exception of those few pathologic conditions requiring expiration films, all chest radiography should be performed with the patient in full inspiration (inhalation). In an ideal film the upper 10 posterior ribs should be visualized above the diaphragm. Poor expansion of the lungs may cause a normal-sized heart to appear enlarged and makes it difficult to evaluate the lung bases. To obtain a full-inspiration radiograph, the patient should be instructed to take a deep breath, exhale, and inhale again (maximal inspiration), at which time the exposure should be made. This technique avoids the *Valsalva* effect, which is forced expiration against the closed glottis that increases the intrapulmonary pressure. The Valsalva effect results in compression and a marked decrease in size of the heart and adjacent blood vessels, and thus an inability to accurately evaluate heart size and pulmonary vascularity.

The patient must be precisely positioned for chest radiography to ensure symmetry of the lung fields and a true appearance of the heart and pulmonary vasculature. Whenever possible, all chest radiographs should be taken with the patient in the erect position. The only exception is the patient with a suspected pathologic condition that requires a lateral decubitus position. Although recumbent radiographs may be necessary in immobile or seriously ill patients, they are less than satisfactory because in this position the abdominal contents tend to prevent the diaphragm from descending low enough to permit visualization of well-expanded lung bases or fluid levels. A 72-inch focal-film distance should be used when possible to minimize magnification of the heart and mediastinal structures. Correct positioning with absence of rotation in the frontal projection can be demonstrated by symmetry of the ster-

noclavicular joints. The shoulders must be rolled forward (anteriorly) to remove the scapulas from overlying the lungs. In large-breasted women, it is often necessary to elevate and separate the breasts to allow good visualization of the lung bases. Nipple shadows of both men and women occasionally appear as soft-tissue masses. If the nature of these soft-tissue masses is unclear, it may be necessary to repeat the examination using small lead markers placed on the nipples. Collimation of the radiograph is required to reduce scattered radiation, although it is essential that both costophrenic angles be visualized.

Radiographs exhibiting a long scale of contrast are necessary to visualize the entire spectrum of densities within the thoracic cavity (mediastinum, heart, lung markings, pulmonary vasculature) and the surrounding bony thorax. Most authorities agree that a minimum of 120 kVp should be used with an appropriate ratio grid for all adult chest radiography. If it is necessary to decrease the overall density, this should be accomplished by reducing the mAs rather than the kVp. Decreasing the kVp tends to enhance the bony thorax, which may obscure vascular details and cause underpenetration of the mediastinal structures. In general the density and contrast should be such that the thoracic vertebrae and intervertebral disk spaces are faintly visible through the shadow of the mediastinum without obscuring the lung markings and pulmonary vascularity.

Short exposure times (10 msec or less) must be used in chest radiography because longer times may not eliminate the involuntary motion of the heart. Automatic exposure devices are generally recommended, and they help to ensure that follow-up studies will have a similar film density. An exception is the expiration (exhalation) chest radiograph, which should be exposed with a manual technique because the preset density of an automatic exposure device may cause excessive blackening of the lungs and thus obscure a small pneumothorax.

Compensatory filters are sometimes needed to overcome the broad range of different tissue densities within the chest. They are especially important to allow good visualization of the mediastinum without overexposing the lungs. The use of compensatory filters generally requires that the radiographic exposure be twice that used in the absence of additional filtration.

To demonstrate fluid levels, the patient should be in an erect position, and a horizontal x-ray beam must be used. Any angulation of the beam prevents a parallel entrance to the air-fluid interface. In some clinical situations (small pneumothorax, pleural thickening versus free pleural fluid) it is necessary to use a horizontal beam with the patient placed in the lateral decubitus position.

Certain pathologic conditions of the respiratory system require that the radiographer alter the routine technical factors. Some disorders produce in-

creased density that is harder to penetrate, whereas others decrease the density of the lungs so that they are easier to penetrate than normal. It is important to remember that these changes may vary for a single disease, since the chest structures may be easier or harder to penetrate, depending on the stage of the disease process. Unless the radiographer has access to previous films with recorded techniques, the initial exposures should be made using a standard technique chart. Adjustments and technical factors can then be made if necessary on subsequent films. Table 1-1 lists the changes in penetrability expected in advanced stages of various disease processes.

PHYSIOLOGY OF THE RESPIRATORY SYSTEM

The major role of the respiratory system is the oxygenation of blood and the removal of waste products of the body in the form of carbon dioxide. The trachea, bronchi, and bronchioles are tubular structures responsible for conducting air from the outside of the body into the lungs. The single trachea branches out into two bronchi (one to each lung), and then on to progressively smaller bronchioles, to produce a structure termed the "bronchial tree" because its appearance resembles an inverted tree. The tracheobronchial tree is lined with a mucous membrane (respiratory epithelium) containing numerous hairlike projections called cilia. During inspiration, the air is moistened and warmed as it passes to the lungs. The cilia act as miniature sweepers to prevent dust and foreign particles from reaching the lungs. Any damage to the respiratory epithelium and its cilia permits bacteria and viruses (entering with the inspired or inhaled air) to proliferate and produce an infection.

The vital gas exchange within the lung takes place within the alveoli, extremely thin-walled sacs surrounded by blood capillaries, which represent the true parenchyma of the lung. Oxygen in the inhaled air diffuses from the alveoli into the blood capillaries, where it attaches to hemoglobin molecules in red blood cells and is carried to the various tissues of the body. Carbon dioxide, a waste product of cellular metabolism, diffuses in the opposite direction from the blood capillaries into the alveoli and is thus re-

moved from the body during expiration (exhalation). Because individual alveoli are extremely small, chest radiographs can only demonstrate a cluster of alveoli and their tiny terminal bronchioles, which is the basic anatomic unit of the lung that is termed the acinus.

Respiration is controlled by a center in the medulla at the base of the brain. The respiratory center is regulated by the level of carbon dioxide in the blood. Even a slight increase in the amount of carbon dioxide in the blood increases the rate and depth of breathing, as when an individual exercises. The accumulation of waste gases that must be removed from the body (as well as the body's need for additional oxygen) causes the respiratory center to stimulate the muscles of respiration—the diaphragm and the intercostal muscles between the ribs. Contraction of the muscles of respiration causes the volume of the chest cavity to increase. This decreases the pressure within the lungs and forces air to move into the lungs through the tracheobronchial tree. As the respiratory muscles relax, the volume of the chest cavity decreases, and air is forced out of the lungs. Special muscles of expiration (abdominal and internal intercostal muscles) may be needed for difficult breathing or in patients with narrowed airways as in emphysema.

Unlike most other organs, the lung has two different blood supplies. The pulmonary circulation is a low-pressure, low-resistance system through which oxygen enters and carbon dioxide is removed. The bronchial circulation, which is a part of the high-pressure systemic circulation, supplies oxygenated blood to nourish (support) the lung tissue itself.

The lungs are encased by a double membrane consisting of two layers of pleura. The visceral pleura covers the lung, and the parietal pleura lines the inner chest wall (thoracic cavity). Although a potential space, the pleural cavity normally contains only a small amount of fluid to lubricate the surfaces to prevent friction as the lungs expand and contract. The airtight space between the lungs and the chest wall has a pressure a bit less than that in the lungs. This difference in pressure acts like a vacuum to prevent the lungs from collapsing. An inflammatory or neoplastic process that involves the pleura may produce fluid within the potential space (pleural effusion).

INFLAMMATORY DISORDERS

Pneumonia

Acute pneumonia is an inflammation of the lung that can be caused by a variety of organisms, most commonly bacteria and viruses. Regardless of the cause, pneumonias tend to produce one of three basic radiographic patterns.

Alveolar, or air-space, pneumonia, exemplified by pneumococcal pneumonia, is produced by an organism that causes an inflammatory exudate that replaces air in the alveoli so that the affected part of

the lung is no longer air containing but rather appears solid (Figure 2-1). The inflammation spreads from one alveolus to the next by way of communicating channels and may involve a whole lobe or even the entire lung. Consolidation of the lung parenchyma with little or no involvement of the airways produces the characteristic air-bronchogram sign (Figure 2-2). The sharp contrast between air within the bronchial tree and the surrounding airless lung parenchyma permits the normally invisible bronchial air column to become seen radiographically. The appearance of an air bronchogram requires the presence of air within the bronchial tree, implying that the bronchus is not completely occluded at its origin. An air bronchogram excludes a pleural or mediastinal lesion, since there are no bronchi in these regions. Because air in the alveoli is replaced by an equal or almost equal quantity of inflammatory exudate, and since the airways leading

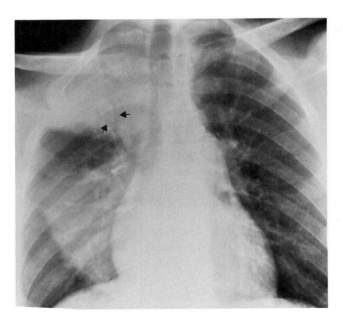

Figure 2-1 Alveolar pneumonia (pneumococcal). Homogeneous consolidation of right upper lobe and medial and posterior segments of right lower lobe. Note associated air bronchograms *(arrows).*

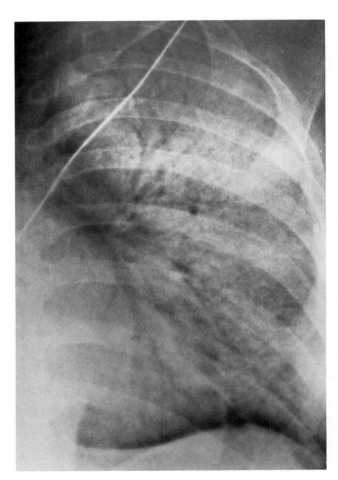

Figure 2-2 Air-bronchogram sign in pneumonia. Frontal chest radiograph demonstrates air within intrapulmonary bronchi in patient with diffuse alveolar pneumonia of left lung.

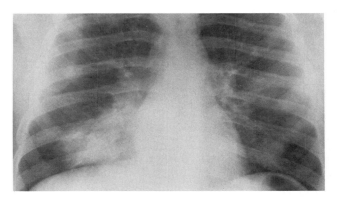

Figure 2-3 Bronchopneumonia (staphylococcal). Ill-defined consolidation at right base.

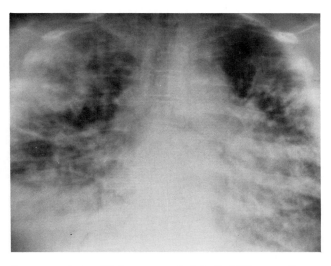

Figure 2-4 Interstitial pneumonia (viral). Diffuse peribronchial infiltrate with associated air-space consolidation obscures heart border (shaggy heart sign). Patchy alveolar infiltrate is present in right upper lung. *(From Eisenberg R: Atlas of signs in radiology, Philadelphia, JB Lippincott, 1984.)*

to the affected portions of the lung remain open, there is no evidence of volume loss in alveolar pneumonia.

Bronchopneumonia, typified by staphylococcal infection, is primarily an inflammation that originates in the airways and spreads to adjacent aveoli. Because alveolar spread in the peripheral air spaces is minimal, the inflammation tends to produce small patches of consolidation that may be seen throughout the lungs but are separated by an abundance of air-containing lung tissue (Figure 2-3). Bronchial inflammation causing airway obstruction leads to atelectasis with loss of lung volume; air bronchograms are absent.

Interstitial pneumonia is most commonly produced by viral and mycoplasmal infections. In this type of pneumonia the inflammatory process predominantly involves the walls of the alveoli and the interstitial supporting structures of the lung, producing a linear or reticular pattern (Figure 2-4). When seen on end, the thickened interstitium may appear as multiple small nodular densities.

Extensive inflammation of the lung can cause a mixed pattern of alveolar, bronchial, and interstitial pneumonia.

Aspiration pneumonia

The aspiration of esophageal or gastric contents into the lung can lead to the development of pneumonia. Aspiration of esophageal material can occur in patients with esophageal obstruction (tumor, stricture, achalasia), diverticula (Zenker's), or neuromuscular disturbances in swallowing. Aspiration of liquid gastric contents is most often related to general anesthesia, tracheostomy, coma, or trauma. Both types of aspiration cause multiple alveolar densities that may be distributed widely and diffusely throughout both lungs (Figure 2-5). Because the anatomic distribution of pulmonary changes is affected by gravity, the posterior segments of the upper and lower lobes are most commonly affected, especially in debilitated or bedridden patients. Early diagnosis of aspiration pneumonia and the prompt institution of corticosteroid and antibiotic therapy are essential to improve the otherwise grave prognosis in this condition.

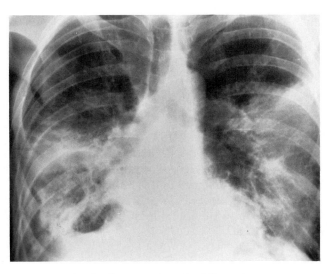

Figure 2-5 Aspiration pneumonia. Bilateral, nonsegmental air-space consolidation.

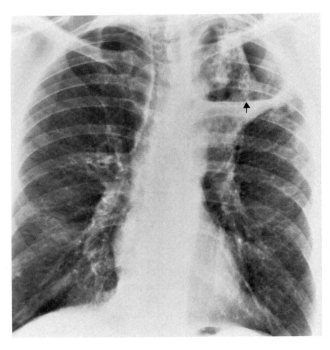

Figure 2-6 Lung abscess (bacterial pneumonia). Large, thick-walled left upper lobe abscess with air-fluid level *(arrow)* and associated infiltrate.

Lung abscess

Lung abscess is a necrotic area of pulmonary parenchyma containing purulent (puslike) material. A lung abscess may be a complication of bacterial pneumonia, bronchial obstruction, aspiration, a foreign body, or the hematogenous spread of organisms to the lungs either in a patient with diffuse bacteremia or as a result of septic emboli.

The earliest radiographic finding of lung abscess is a spherical density that characteristically has a dense center with a hazy, poorly defined periphery. If there is communication with the bronchial tree, the fluid contents of the cavity are partly replaced by air, producing a typical air-fluid level within the abscess (Figure 2-6). A cavitary lung abscess usually has a thickened wall with a shaggy, irregular inner margin.

Clinically, a patient with lung abscess has a fever and cough and produces copious amounts of foul-smelling sputum. An important complication of lung abscess is the development of a brain abscess, which is produced by infected material carried by the blood from the lung to the left side of the heart and then on to the brain.

Tuberculosis

Tuberculosis is caused by *Mycobacterium tuberculosis,* a rod-shaped bacterium with a protective waxy coat

that permits it to live outside the body for a long time. Tuberculosis spreads mainly by droplets in the air, which are produced in huge numbers by the coughing of an infected patient. Therefore it is essential that respiratory precautions be followed when radiographing patients with active disease. The organisms may be inhaled from sputum that has dried and been changed into dust. They are rapidly killed by direct sunlight but may survive a long time in the dark. Tuberculosis also may be acquired by drinking the milk of infected cows. However, routine pasteurization of milk has virtually eliminated this route of infection.

Unlike most bacteria, mycobacteria do not stain reliably by Gram's method. However, once the stain is taken up, the mycobacteria are difficult to decolorize by either acid or alcohol, and thus the organisms are often called "acid-fast" bacilli.

Tuberculosis is primarily a disease of the lungs, although it can spread to involve the gastrointestinal, genitourinary, and skeletal systems. In the initial tuberculous infection (primary lesion), a collection of inflammatory cells collects around a clump of tuberculosis bacilli to form a small mass (tubercle) that is visible to the naked eye. The outcome of this initial infection depends on the number of bacilli and the resistance of the infected tissue. If the resistance is good and the dose is small, the proliferation of fibrous tissue around the tumor limits the spread of infection and produces a mass of scar tissue. In the lung tuberculous scars are commonly found in the apices. They often contain calcium, which is deposited as healing occurs. If the dose of bacilli is larger or if the resistance of the patient is lowered, the disease tends to progress slowly. Within the center of the tubercle, inflammatory cells are killed by the bacilli so that the core becomes a necrotic, cheeselike mass (caseation). The caseous material may eventually become liquefied so that a cavity is formed. Coalescence of several small cavities can result in the formation of a large cavity, which may contain an air-fluid level. Rupture of blood vessels crossing a cavity causes bleeding and the coughing up of blood (hemoptysis). If the infection is overwhelming and resistance is minimal, there is diffuse destruction throughout the lung with the formation of huge cavities and often a fatal outcome.

Previous tuberculous infection can be detected by the tuberculin test, in which a purified protein derivative of the tuberculosis bacillus is injected into the skin and the injection site examined 2 to 3 days later. A visible and palpable swelling 10 mm or larger indicates that the individual has developed antibodies to a previous exposure to tuberculosis. If there is no such reaction, the individual has either not been exposed to the tuberculosis bacilli or is anergic (immunologically nonreacting). It is important to remember that the tuberculin test is not positive during an acute infection and for several weeks thereafter.

Primary pulmonary tuberculosis has traditionally been considered a disease of children and young adults. However, with the dramatic decrease in the prevalence of tuberculosis (especially in children and young adults), primary pulmonary disease can develop at any age.

There are four basic radiographic patterns of primary pulmonary tuberculosis. The infiltrate may be seen as a lobar or segmental air-space consolidation that is usually homogeneous, dense, and well defined (Figure 2-7). Associated enlargement of hilar or mediastinal lymph nodes is very common (Figure 2-8). Indeed, the combination of a focal parenchymal lesion and enlarged hilar or mediastinal nodes produces the classic primary complex (Ghon lesion), an appearance strongly suggestive of primary tuberculosis. Pleural effusion is common, especially in adults (Figure 2-9). Most primary tuberculous pleural effusions are unilateral and clear rapidly with

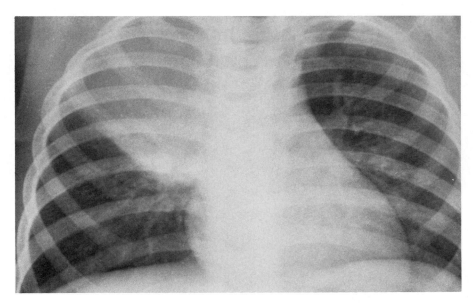

Figure 2-7 Primary tuberculosis. Consolidation of right upper lobe.

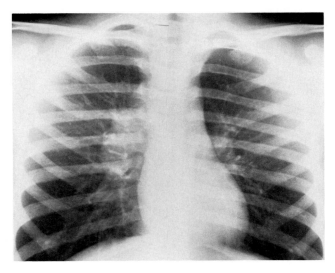

Figure 2-8 Primary tuberculosis. Enlargement of right hilar lymph nodes without discrete parenchymal infiltrate.

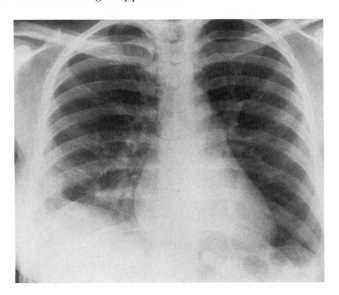

Figure 2-9 Primary tuberculosis. Unilateral right tuberculous pleural effusion without parenchymal or lymph node involvement.

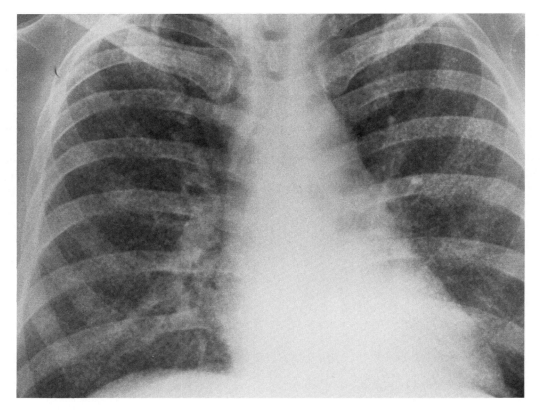

Figure 2-10 Miliary tuberculosis.

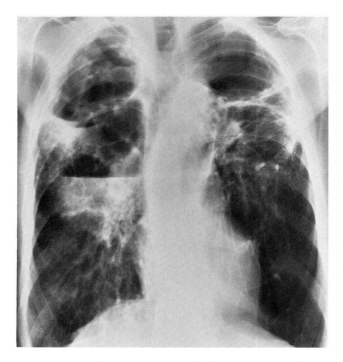

Figure 2-11 Tuberculosis. Multiple large cavities with air-fluid levels in both upper lobes. Note chronic fibrotic changes and upward retraction of hila.

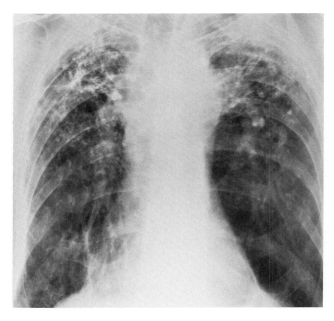

Figure 2-12 Secondary tuberculosis. Bilateral fibrocalcific changes at apices. Note upward retraction of hila.

treatment. Miliary tuberculosis refers to dissemination of the disease by way of the bloodstream. Radiographically, this produces innumerable fine discrete nodules distributed uniformly throughout both lungs (Figure 2-10).

Tuberculous pneumonia may resolve completely and leave a normal lung. However, if necrosis and caseation develop, some fibrous scarring occurs. Calcification may develop within both the parenchymal and the nodal lesions, and this may be the only residue of primary tuberculous infection on subsequent films. If the disease responds poorly to therapy and continues to progress (especially in patients with immunodeficiency or diabetes and in those receiving steroid therapy), the pneumonia may break down into multiple necrotic cavities or a single large abscess filled with caseous material (Figure 2-11).

Reactivation of organisms from previously dormant tubercles is termed a secondary lesion. At times, the tuberculosis bacillus may remain inactive for many years before a secondary lesion develops, often because of a decrease in the body's immune defense.

Secondary tuberculosis most commonly affects the upper lobes, especially the apical and posterior segments (Figure 12-12). It initially is seen as a nonspecific hazy, poorly marginated alveolar infiltrate that often radiates outward from the hilum. Necrosis and liquefaction commonly lead to the development of tuberculous cavities, which typically have thick walls with ill-defined inner margins. Secondary pulmonary tuberculosis heals slowly with extensive fibrosis. Contraction of the fibrous scars causes loss of volume of the involved segment or lobe and a decrease in the size of the hemithorax. The trachea and other mediastinal structures are retracted to the involved side; in upper lobe disease the hilum is elevated.

Because it is difficult to radiographically determine the activity of secondary tuberculosis, comparison with previous films is essential. An unchanged appearance of fibrosis and calcification on serial films is usually considered evidence of "healing" of the tuberculous process. Nevertheless, even densely calcified lesions can contain central areas of necrosis in which viable organisms can still be found even after long periods of apparent inactivity. Of course, new cavitation or an increasing amount of pulmonary infiltrate indicates active disease.

A tuberculoma is a sharply circumscribed parenchymal nodule, often containing viable tuberculosis bacilli, that can develop in either primary or secondary disease. Although the residual localized caseation may remain unchanged for a long period

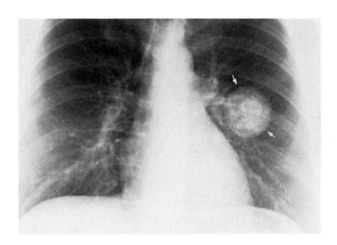

Figure 2-13 Calcified tuberculoma. Large soft-tissue mass in left lung *(arrows)* that contains dense central calcification.

or permanently, a tuberculoma is potentially dangerous because it may break down at any time and lead to dissemination of the disease. Radiographically, tuberculomas appear as single or multiple pulmonary nodules, usually 1 to 3 cm in diameter. They can occur in any part of the lung but are most common in the periphery and in the upper lobes. A central nidus of calcification (which may only be detectable on tomograms) strongly suggests that the lesion represents a tuberculoma (Figure 2-13). However, the lack of calcification is of no diagnostic value.

Histoplasmosis

Histoplasmosis, caused by the fungus *Histoplasma capsulatum*, is a common disease that often produces a radiographic appearance simulating that of tuberculosis.

The primary form of histoplasmosis is usually relatively benign and often passes unnoticed. Chest radiographs may demonstrate single or multiple areas of pulmonary infiltration that are most often in the lower lung and are frequently associated with hilar lymph node enlargement. Although this pattern simulates the primary complex of tuberculosis, pleural effusion rarely occurs with histoplasmosis. In children, striking hilar adenopathy, which may cause bronchial compression, may develop without radiographic evidence of parenchymal disease. Hilar lymph node calcification is common in adults. A frequent manifestation of pulmonary histoplasmosis is a solitary, sharply circumscribed, granulomatous nodule (histoplasmoma), which is usually less than 3 cm in diameter and is most often in a lower lobe. Central, rounded calcification within the mass (target lesion) is virtually pathognomonic of this disease

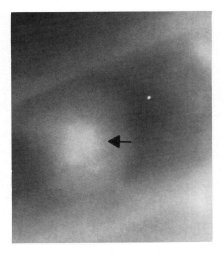

Figure 2-14 Histoplasmoma. Central calcification *(arrow)* in solitary pulmonary nodule.

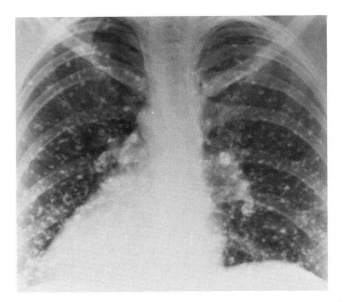

Figure 2-15 Histoplasmosis. Diffuse calcifications in lungs produce snowball pattern.

(Figure 2-14). Multiple soft-tissue nodules scattered throughout both lungs may simulate miliary tuberculosis. These shadows may clear completely or may fibrose and persist, often appearing on subsequent chest radiographs as widespread punctate calcifications (Figure 2-15).

The more chronic form of histoplasmosis is characterized by zones of parenchymal consolidation, often large and with a loss of lung volume, that usually develop in an upper lobe. Cavitation is common, and the radiographic appearance closely simulates reinfection tuberculosis.

Histoplasmosis can incite progressive fibrosis in the mediastinum. This can cause obstruction of the

superior vena cava, pulmonary arteries, and pulmonary veins, as well as severe narrowing of the esophagus.

Diffuse calcification in the liver, spleen, and lymph nodes is virtually diagnostic of histoplasmosis, especially in areas in which the disease is endemic (e.g., the Mississippi and Ohio valleys of the United States). These calcifications tend to be small, multiple, dense, and discrete, although occasionally they may appear as moderately large, solidly calcified granulomas.

Bronchiectasis

Bronchiectasis refers to permanent abnormal dilation of one or more large bronchi as a result of destruction of the elastic and muscular components of the bronchial wall. The origin of the destructive process is nearly always a bacterial infection, which may either be a severe necrotizing pneumonia or a result of a local or systemic abnormality that impairs the body's defense mechanisms and promotes bacterial growth. Since the advent of antibiotic therapy, the incidence of bronchiectasis has substantially decreased.

The patient with bronchiectasis typically has a chronic productive cough, often associated with recurrent episodes of acute pneumonia and hemoptysis. The disease usually involves the basal segments of the lower lobes and is bilateral in about half of the cases. Plain chest radiographs may show a coarseness and loss of definition of interstitial markings caused by peribronchial fibrosis and retained secretions (Figure 2-16). In more advanced disease, oval or circular cystic spaces can develop. These cystic dilations can be up to 2 cm in diameter and often contain air-fluid levels. In very severe disease, coarse interstitial fibrosis surrounding local areas of dilation can produce a honeycomb pattern.

Although plain radiographs may strongly suggest bronchiectasis, bronchography is necessary to fill the dilated cystic spaces with contrast material and to unequivocally establish the diagnosis. (Figure 2-17).

Croup

Croup is primarily a viral infection of young children that produces inflammatory obstructive swelling localized to the subglottic portion of the trachea. On frontal radiographs of the lower neck, there is a characteristic smooth, fusiform, tapered narrowing of the subglottic airway (Figure 2-18, *A*), unlike the broad shouldering seen normally (Figure 2-18, *B*).

Epiglottitis

Acute infections of the epiglottis, most commonly caused by *Haemophilus influenzae* in children, causes

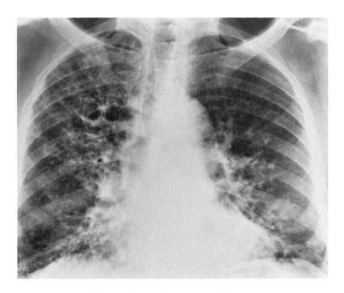

Figure 2-16 Chronic bronchiectasis. There is severe coarsening of interstitial markings involving bases and right upper lobe. Oval and circular cystic spaces, producing somewhat of a honeycomb pattern, are best seen in right upper lobe.

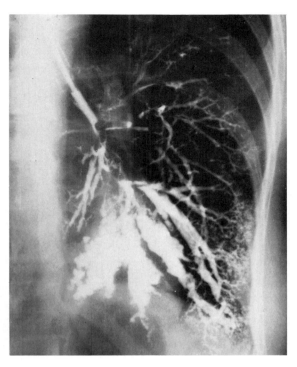

Figure 2-17 Chronic bronchiectasis. Bronchogram shows severe dilation of basal bronchi of left lower lobe. *(From Fraser RG and Pare JAP: Diagnosis of diseases of the chest, Philadelphia, WB Saunders Co, 1979.)*

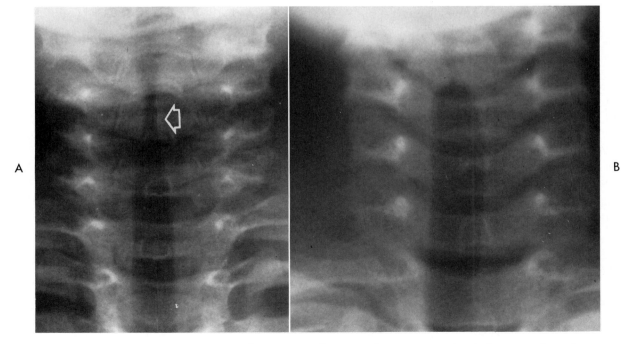

Figure 2-18 Croup. **A,** Arrow indicates smooth, tapered narrowing of subglottic portion of trachea (gothic arch sign). **B,** Normal trachea with broad shouldering in subglottic region.

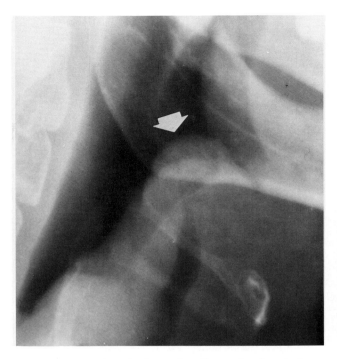

Figure 2-19 Epiglottitis. Lateral radiograph of neck demonstrates wide, rounded configuration of inflamed epiglottis *(arrow). (From Podgore JK and Bass JW: J Pediatr 88:154-155, 1976.)*

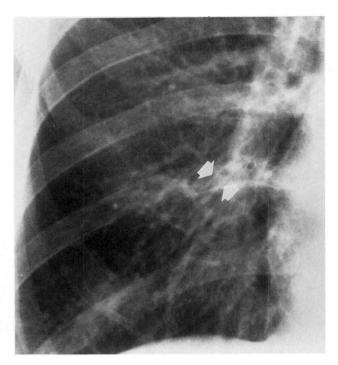

Figure 2-20 Chronic bronchitis. Coned view of right lower lung demonstrates coarse increase in interstitial markings. Arrows point to characteristic parallel line shadows ("tramlines") outside boundary of pulmonary hilum. *(From Eisenberg R: Atlas of signs in radiology, Philadelphia, JB Lippincott Co, 1984.)*

thickening of epiglottic tissue and surrounding pharyngeal structures. On lateral projections of the neck using soft tissue techniques, a rounded thickening of the epiglottic shadow gives it the configuration and approximate size of an adult's thumb (Figure 2-19), in contrast to the normal, narrow epiglottic shadow resembling an adult's little finger. The prompt recognition of acute epiglottitis is imperative because the condition may result in sudden complete airway obstruction.

DIFFUSE LUNG DISEASE

Chronic obstructive pulmonary disease

Chronic obstructive pulmonary disease (COPD) includes several conditions in which chronic obstruction of the airways leads to an ineffective exchange of respiratory gases and difficulty breathing. Chronic bronchitis is characterized by excessive tracheobronchial mucus production leading to the obstruction of small airways. Emphysema refers to the distention of distal air spaces as a result of the destruction of alveolar walls and the obstruction of small airways. Predisposing factors to chronic ob-

structive lung disease include cigarette smoking, infection, air pollution, and occupational exposure to harmful substances such as asbestos.

Chronic bronchitis

Chronic inflammation of the bronchi leads to severe coughing with the production of sputum. Bronchitis may be a complication of respiratory infection or be the result of long-term exposure to air pollution or cigarette smoking.

About half the patients with chronic bronchial disease demonstrate no changes on chest radiographs. The most common radiographic abnormality in chronic bronchitis is a generalized increase in bronchovascular markings (Figure 2-20), especially in the lower lungs ("dirty chest"). Thickening of bronchial walls and peribronchial inflammation can cause parallel or slightly tapered tubular line shadows ("tramlines") or appear as thickening of bronchial shadows when viewed end on. Eventually, excessive production of mucus and swelling of the bronchial mucosa may lead to narrowing of the airways and overinflation of the lungs (emphysema).

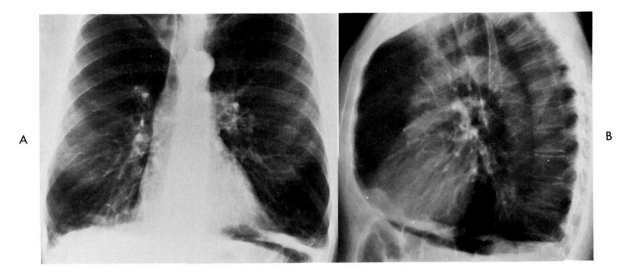

Figure 2-21 Emphysema. **A,** Frontal and, **B,** Lateral projections of chest demonstrate severe overinflation of lungs along with flattening and even a superiorly concave configuration of hemidiaphragms. There is also increased size and lucency of retrosternal air space, increase in AP diameter of chest, and reduction in number and caliber of peripheral pulmonary arteries.

Emphysema

Emphysema is a crippling and debilitating condition in which obstructive and destructive changes in small airways lead to a dramatic increase in the volume of air in the lungs. In many patients, the development of emphysema is closely associated with heavy cigarette smoking. Other predisposing factors are chronic bronchitis, air pollution, and long-term exposure to irritants of the respiratory tract.

Irritating smoke, fumes, and pollutants injure the fine hairs (cilia) of the respiratory mucosa, which can no longer sweep away foreign particles. This causes mucosal inflammation and the secretion of excess mucus that plugs up the air passages and leads to an increase in airway resistance. Collateral air drift permits the ventilation of lung parenchyma served by the obstructed airways. However, bronchial narrowing and loss of elasticity make it very difficult for the patient to exhale the stale air. The resulting air trapping and overinflation of the lung lead to alveolar distention and eventually to the rupture of alveolar septa. As the walls between alveoli are destroyed, these tiny air sacs become transformed into large air-filled spaces called bullae, which do not permit efficient transfer of oxygen into the bloodstream. As the lungs become less able to move air in and out, the heart is strained and even-

tually enlarges. The large air sacs (bullae) may rupture, leading to the entry of air into the pleural space (pneumothorax) and collapse of the lung (atelectasis).

The major radiographic signs of emphysema are related to pulmonary overinflation, alterations in the pulmonary vasculature, and bullae formation.

The hallmark of pulmonary overinflation is flattening of the domes of the diaphragm (Figure 2-21). Another important sign on lateral chest radiographs is increased size and lucency of the retrosternal air space, the distance between the posterior sternum and the anterior wall of the ascending aorta. There is also an increase in the anteroposterior (AP) diameter of the chest (barrel chest). Air trapping may be detected fluoroscopically as a decrease in the normal movement of the diaphragm during respiration.

The major vascular change in patients with emphysema is a reduction in the number and size of the peripheral arteries. As the pressure in the pulmonary arteries increases, the main and central pulmonary arteries become more prominent, which further accentuates the appearance of rapid tapering of peripheral vessels.

Bullae appear as air-containing cystic spaces whose walls are usually of hairline thickness. They range in size from 1 to 2 cm in diameter up to an

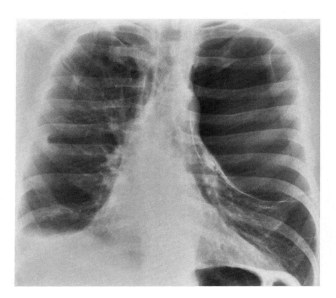

Figure 2-22 Giant emphysematous bulla. Air-containing mass fills most of left hemithorax.

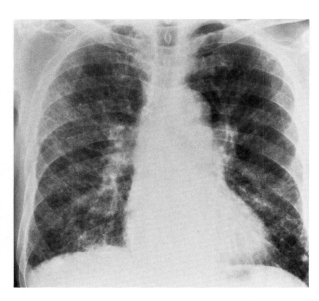

Figure 2-23 Asthma. Recurrent pulmonary infections have led to development of diffuse pulmonary fibrosis and prominence of interstitial markings in lungs.

entire hemithorax (Figure 2-22). These large, radiolucent, air-filled sacs are found predominantly at the apices or at the bases and may become so large that they cause respiratory insufficiency by compressing the remaining relatively normal lung.

A less common radiographic appearance of emphysema is the increased-markings pattern. Instead of being narrowed, the vascular markings in this condition are more prominent than normal and tend to be irregular and indistinct, producing a "dirty chest" appearance.

Emphysema can occasionally occur in young patients who have hereditary disorders of connective tissue (osteogenesis imperfecta). Striking lower lobe predominance develops in young patients who have a deficiency of the enzyme α-antitrypsin, which leads to destruction of elastic and connective tissue in the lungs.

In patients with advanced stages of pulmonary emphysema who have large amounts of air trapped in their lungs, it is necessary to reduce exposure factors for chest radiography.

Asthma

Asthma is a very common disease in which widespread narrowing of the airways develops because of an increased responsiveness of the tracheobronchial tree to various substances (allergens). Common allergens include house dust, pollen, molds, animal dander, certain fabrics, and various foods. The hypersensitivity reaction to one or more of these aller-gens leads to swelling of the mucous membranes of the bronchi, excess secretion of mucus, and spasm of the smooth muscle in the bronchial walls, all of which lead to severe narrowing of the airways. This makes breathing (especially expiration) difficult and results in the characteristic wheezing sound that is produced by air passing through the narrowed bronchial tubes.

Early in the course of the disease, chest radiographs obtained between acute episodes demonstrate no abnormalities. During an acute asthmatic attack, bronchial narrowing and difficulty in expiration lead to an increased volume of the hyperlucent lungs with flattening of the hemidiaphragms and an increase in the retrosternal air space. In contrast to emphysema, the pulmonary vascular markings in asthma are of normal size. In patients with chronic asthma, especially those with a history of repeated episodes of superinfection, thickening of bronchial walls can produce prominence of interstitial markings and the "dirty chest" appearance (Figure 2-23).

Pneumoconiosis

Prolonged occupational exposure to certain irritating dusts can cause severe pulmonary disease and a spectrum of radiographic findings. These inhaled dusts cause a chronic interstitial inflammation that leads to pulmonary fibrosis and a diffuse nonspecific radiographic pattern of linear streaks and nodules throughout the lungs. The most common of the

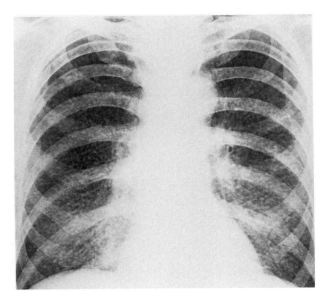

Figure 2-24 Silicosis. Calcification in miliary nodules scattered throughout both lungs.

pneumoconioses are silicosis, asbestosis, and coal worker's disease. Other causes include exposure to such dusts as tin, iron oxide, barium, and beryllium.

Silicosis

The inhalation of high concentrations of silicon dioxide primarily affects workers engaged in mining, foundry work, and sandblasting. Although acute silicosis can develop within 10 months of exposure in workers exposed to sandblasting in confined spaces, 15 to 20 years of long-term, relatively less intense exposure is required to produce radiographic changes.

intense exposure is required to produce radiographic changes.

The classic radiographic pattern in silicosis consists of multiple nodular shadows scattered throughout the lungs. These nodules are usually fairly well circumscribed and of uniform density and may become calcified (Figure 2-24). As the pulmonary nodules increase in size, they tend to coalesce and form conglomerates of irregular masses in excess of 1 cm in diameter (progressive massive fibrosis) (Figure 2-25). These masses are usually bilateral and relatively symmetric and are almost always restricted to the upper half of the lungs. Occasionally, a single large homogeneous mass in the perihilar area of one lung may closely simulate bronchogenic carcinoma. Hilar lymph node enlargement is common. The deposition of calcium salts in the periphery of enlarged lymph nodes produces the characteristic eggshell appearance (Figure 2-26), which is virtually pathognomonic of silicosis.

Asbestosis

Asbestosis may develop in improperly protected workers engaged in the manufacture of asbestos or in those handling building materials or insulation that is composed of asbestos. The radiographic hallmark of asbestosis is involvement of the pleura. Initially, pleural thickening appears as linear plaques of opacification, which are most often along the lower chest wall and diaphragm. A virtually pathognomonic appearance of asbestosis is calcification of pleural plaques, especially in the form of thin, cur-

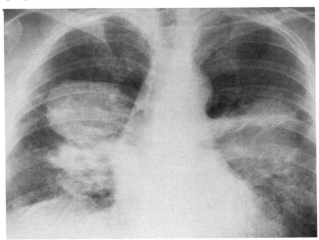

Figure 2-25 Progressive massive fibrosis in silicosis. Large, irregular nodules in both perihilar regions.

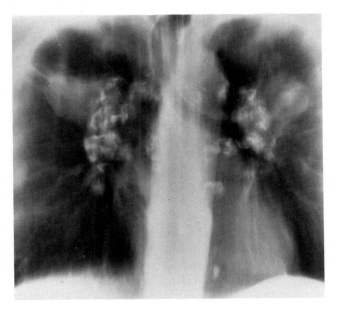

Figure 2-26 Silicosis. Chest tomogram demonstrates characteristic eggshell lymph node calcification associated with bilateral perihilar masses.

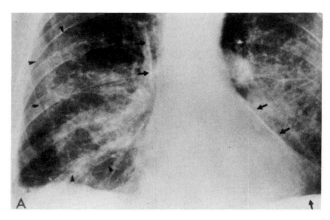

Figure 2-27 Asbestosis. Frontal film shows en face pleural calcifications on right *(arrowheads),* linear calcifications in profile in mediastinal reflection of pleura on right and in pericardium on left *(horizontal arrows),* and linear calcification in left diaphragmatic pleura *(vertical arrow). (From Sargent EN, Jacobson G, and Gordonson JS: Semin Roentgenol 12:287-297, 1977.)*

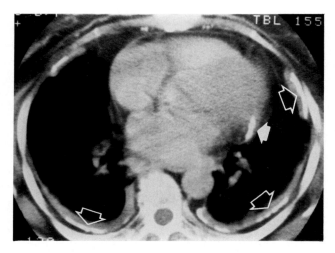

Figure 2-28 Asbestosis. CT scan shows calcified pleural plaques along lateral and posterior chest wall *(open arrows)* and adjacent to heart *(solid arrow).*

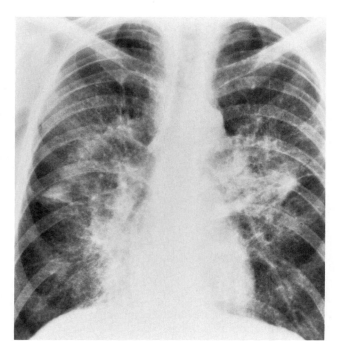

Figure 2-29 Coal worker's pneumoconiosis. Diffuse reticular pattern throughout both lungs associated with ill-defined masses of fibrous tissue in perihilar region that extend to right base.

vilinear densities conforming to the upper surfaces of the diaphragm bilaterally (Figure 2-27). This pleural calcification generally does not develop until at least 20 years after the first exposure to asbestos (Figure 2-28).

In the lungs round or irregular opacities produce a combined linear and nodular pattern that may obscure the heart border to produce the so-called shaggy heart. The major complication of asbestosis is the development of malignant neoplasms in the chest. Pleural mesothelioma is a highly malignant tumor that appears as an irregular scalloped or nodular density within the pleural space. It is frequently associated with a large pleural effusion that may obscure the underlying tumor. In addition to mesothelioma, bronchogenic carcinoma is also unusually common in patients with asbestosis, especially those who are cigarette smokers.

Coal worker's pneumoconiosis

Coal miners, especially those working with anthracite (hard coal), are susceptible to developing pneumoconiosis by inhaling high concentrations of coal dust. Initially, multiple small, irregular opacities produce a reticular pattern similar to that of silicosis (Figure 2-29). However, the nodules tend to be somewhat less well defined than those of silicosis and are of a granular density, unlike the homogeneous density of silicosis nodules. With advanced disease, the pattern of progressive massive fibrosis can develop. This appears as one or more masses of fibrous tissue with smooth, well-defined lateral borders that gradually migrate toward the hilum, leaving a zone of overinflated emphysematous lung between them and the chest wall. A single large homogeneous mass in the perihilar area of one lung may simulate bronchogenic carcinoma; the detection of the underlying background of pneumoconiosis is essential for the proper diagnosis.

VASCULAR DISEASES

Pulmonary embolism

Pulmonary embolism is a potentially fatal condition that is by far the most common pathologic process involving the lungs of hospitalized patients. In about 80% of patients with this disorder, the condition does not cause symptoms and is thus unrecognized because the emboli are too small or too few to occlude blood flow to a substantial portion of the lung. Even when symptomatic, pulmonary embolism may be difficult to diagnose. More than 95% of pulmonary emboli arise from thrombi that develop in the deep venous system of the lower extremities because of venous stasis. The remainder come from thrombi that occur in the right side of the heart or in brachial or cervical veins and are trapped by capillaries in the pulmonary artery circulation. Thrombi originating in the left side of the heart can embolize to the peripheral arterial circulation, where they are trapped in arterioles or capillaries before they can return in the venous blood to the heart and the pulmonary circulation. Most embolic occlusions occur in the lower lobes because of the preferential blood flow to these regions.

The physiologic consequences of embolic occlusion of the pulmonary arteries depend on the size of the embolic mass and the general state of the pulmonary circulation. In young persons with good cardiovascular function and adequate collateral circulation, the occlusion of a large central vessel may be associated with minimal, if any, functional impairment. In contrast, in patients with cardiovascular disease or severe debilitating illnesses, pulmonary vascular occlusion often leads to infarction.

Most patients with thromboembolism without infarction have a normal chest radiograph. Nevertheless, some subtle, yet distinctive, abnormalities on plain radiographs can strongly suggest the diagnosis. A large-vessel pulmonary embolism causes a focal reduction in blood volume without a substantial change in air or tissue volume. This leads to focal pulmonary oligemia and relative lucency of the involved portion of lung. Another sign of pulmonary embolism is enlargement of the ipsilateral main pulmonary artery caused by distention of the vessel by the bulk of the thrombus. This sign is of most value when serial radiographs demonstrate progressive enlargement of the affected vessel.

Pulmonary embolism with infarction appears radiographically as an area of lung consolidation. A highly characteristic, although somewhat uncommon, appearance of pulmonary infarction is the so-called Hampton's hump (Figure 2-30). This is a pleural-based, wedge-shaped density that has a rounded apex and is most commonly seen at the base of the lung, often in the costophrenic sulcus. In many instances an infarction merely produces a nonspecific parenchymal density that simulates acute pneumonia. A pleural effusion often develops.

Because the chest radiograph is usually either normal or nonspecific, the radionuclide lung scan is generally considered the most effective screening test for significant pulmonary embolism (Figure 2-31). On a perfusion scan that measures blood flow to the lungs, the area of lung distal to an embolus appears as a defect on the radionuclide scan. Unfortunately, false-positive scans may be recorded in portions of the lung that are poorly perfused because of impaired ventilation, even if no obstructing vascular lesion is present. Therefore ventilation lung scans are also performed to increase the diagnostic accuracy. The ventilation scan is usually relatively normal in patients with pulmonary embolism, whereas it generally demonstrates defects corresponding to areas of decreased perfusion in patients with chronic pulmonary disease.

Pulmonary arteriography is the definitive technique for evaluating the patient with suspected pulmonary embolism (Figure 2-32). However, it is associated with a small, although definite, risk of morbidity and mortality. The unequivocal arteriographic diagnosis of pulmonary embolism requires the demonstration of an abrupt occlusion (cutoff) of a pulmonary artery or a persistent intraluminal filling defect within it. More recently, MRI has been used to show a pulmonary embolus either as a moderate to high intensity signal within the black flow void of the normal pulmonary artery or as a generalized increased signal intensity caused by slow blood flow in an obstructed pulmonary vessel.

Septic embolism

Septic embolism refers to a shower of bacteria that enter the pulmonary circulation and are trapped within the lung. Septic emboli primarily arise from either the heart (bacterial endocarditis) or the peripheral veins (septic thrombophlebitis). Many patients have a history of intravenous drug abuse. Septic emboli are almost always multiple and appear radiographically as ill-defined, round or wedge-shaped opacities in the periphery of the lung. They often present a migratory pattern, first appearing in one area and then in another as the older lesions resolve. Cavitation frequently develops (Figure 2-33).

Pulmonary arteriovenous fistula

Pulmonary arteriovenous fistula is an abnormal vascular communication from a pulmonary artery to a

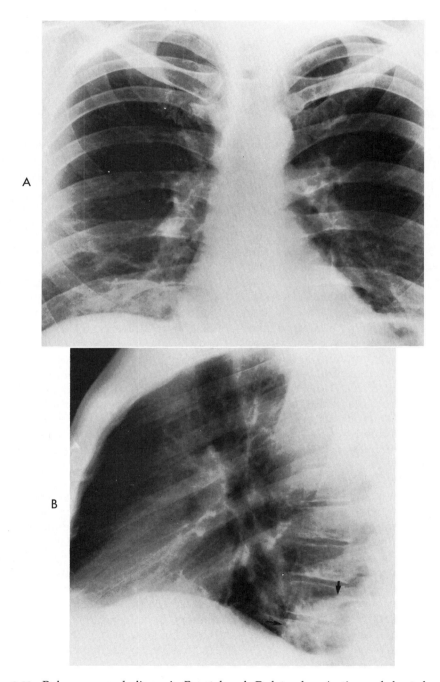

Figure 2-30 Pulmonary embolism. **A,** Frontal and, **B,** lateral projections of chest demonstrate fairly well-circumscribed shadow of homogenous density occupying posterior-based segment of right, lower lobe. On lateral projection pleural-based density has shape of truncated cone and is convex toward hilum (Hampton's hump; *arrows*). *(From Fraser RG and Pare JAP: Diagnosis of diseases of the chest, Philadelphia, WB Saunders Co, 1978.)*

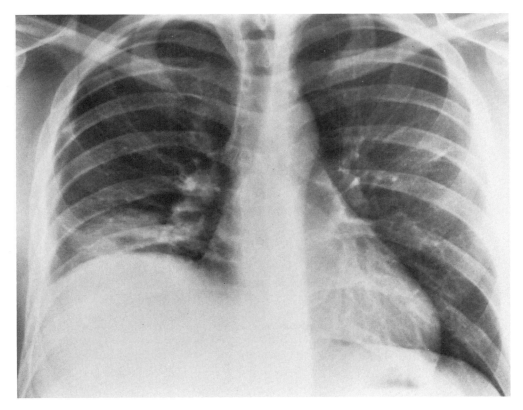

Figure 2-31 Pulmonary embolism. A plain chest radiograph demonstrates atelectasis at the right base, which is associated with elevation of the right hemidiaphragm that represents a large subpulmonic effusion.

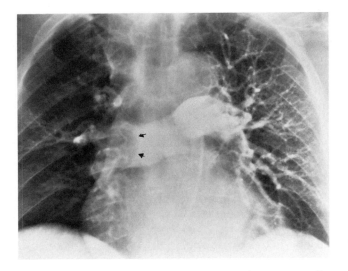

Figure 2-32 A pulmonary arteriogram shows virtually complete obstruction *(arrows)* of the right pulmonary artery.

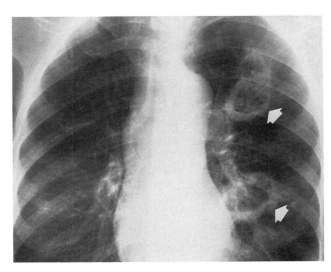

Figure 2-33 Septic pulmonary emboli. Large cavitary lesions *(arrows)* in left lung of intravenous drug abuser with septic thrombophlebitis.

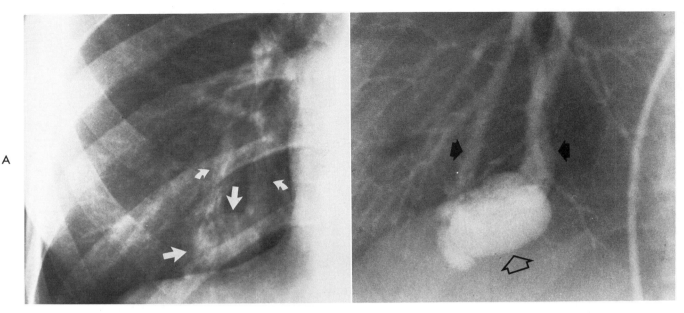

Figure 2-34 Pulmonary arteriovenous fistula. **A,** Film of right lung shows round soft-tissue mass *(straight arrows)* at base. Feeding and draining vessels *(curved arrows)* extend to lesion. **B,** Arteriogram clearly shows feeding artery and draining veins *(solid arrows)* associated with arteriovenous malformation *(open arrow)*.

pulmonary vein. Pulmonary arteriovenous fistulas are multiple in about one third of patients; up to two thirds of patients with these pulmonary malformations have similar arteriovenous communications elsewhere (hereditary hemorrhagic telangiectasia). Very large or multiple fistulas can cause so much shunting of blood from the pulmonary arteries to the pulmonary veins that the blood cannot be adequately oxygenated and cyanosis results.

A pulmonary arteriovenous fistula typically appears as a round or oval, lobulated soft-tissue mass that is most commonly situated in the lower lobes. A pathognomonic finding is the identification of a feeding artery and a draining vein (Figure 2-34, *A*). This may be difficult to demonstrate on plain radiographs and often requires tomography or arteriography (Figure 2-34, *B*). Pulmonary arteriography is required before surgical removal not only to confirm the diagnosis but also to detect smaller, unsuspected vascular malformations that cannot be identified on routine radiographs.

NEOPLASMS

Bronchial adenoma

Bronchial adenomas are neoplasms of low-grade malignancy that constitute about 1% of all bronchial neoplasms. They are at least as common in women as in men and are found in a younger age group than bronchogenic carcinoma. Hemoptysis and re-

curring pneumonia are the most common symptoms.

Because about 80% of bronchial adenomas are located centrally in major or segmental bronchi, bronchial obstruction with peripheral atelectasis and postobstructive pneumonitis is the most common radiographic finding. This characteristically produces a homogeneous increase in density corresponding exactly to a lobe or one or more segments, usually with a substantial loss of volume. If large enough, a central bronchial adenoma that has caused peripheral atelectasis and pneumonia may be identifiable as a discrete, lobulated, soft-tissue mass. If the tumor is too small to obstruct the lumen, the chest radiograph appears normal. Tomography may demonstrate the rounded tumor mass within an air-filled bronchus (Figure 2-35). Peripheral bronchial adenomas do not cause bronchial obstruction and appear as nonspecific solitary pulmonary nodules (Figure 2-36).

Bronchogenic carcinoma

Primary carcinoma of the lung arises from the mucosa of the bronchial tree. Although the precise cause is unknown, bronchogenic carcinoma is closely linked to smoking and to the inhalation of cancer-causing agents (carcinogens) such as air pollution, exhaust gases, and industrial fumes.

Bronchogenic carcinoma produces a broad spectrum of radiographic abnormalities that depend on

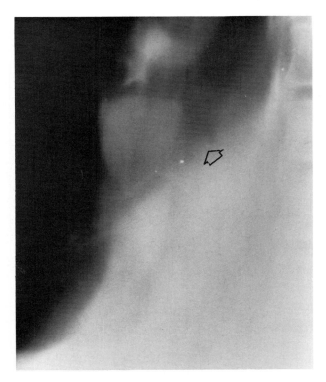

Figure 2-35 Central bronchial adenoma. Tomogram shows ill-defined mass causing high-grade obstruction of right lower lobe bronchus *(arrow)*.

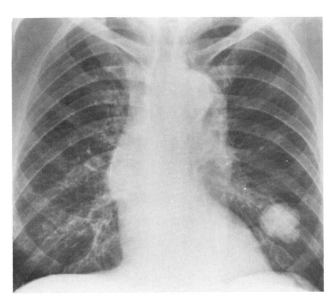

Figure 2-36 Peripheral bronchial adenoma. Nonspecific solitary pulmonary nodule at left base.

the site of the tumor and its relation to the bronchial tree. The tumor may appear as a discrete mass or be undetectable and identified only by virtue of secondary postobstructive changes caused by tumor within or compressing the bronchus.

The most common type of lung cancer is squamous carcinoma, which typically arises in the major central bronchi and causes gradual narrowing of the bronchial lumen. Adenocarcinomas usually arise in the periphery of the lung rather than in the larger central bronchi. Small cell (oat cell) carcinomas characteristically cause bulky enlargement of hilar lymph nodes that is often bilateral. The least common type of lung tumor is bronchiolar (alveolar cell) carcinoma, which has a spectrum of appearances varying from a well-circumscribed, peripheral solitary nodule to a poorly defined mass simulating pneumonia or multiple nodules scattered throughout both lungs.

A major form of bronchogenic carcinoma is the solitary pulmonary nodule within the lung parenchyma. This presents a diagnostic dilemma between malignancy and a benign process (tumor or granuloma). Although malignant tumors generally have ill-defined, irregular, or fuzzy borders (Figure 2-37)

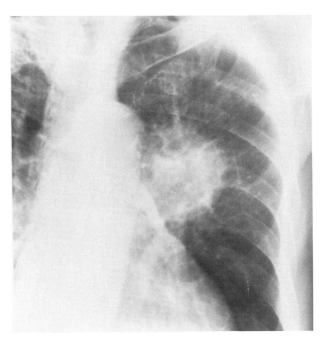

Figure 2-37 Malignant solitary pulmonary nodule (bronchogenic carcinoma). Note fuzzy, ill-defined margins.

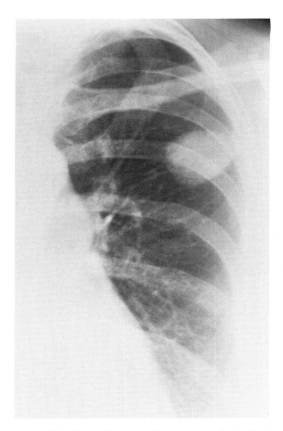

Figure 2-38 Benign solitary pulmonary nodule (tuberculoma). Note sharp, well-defined borders of this left upper lobe mass.

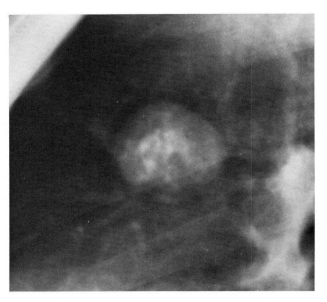

Figure 2-39 Benign solitary pulmonary nodule (tuberculoma). Note central calcification characteristic of benign lesion.

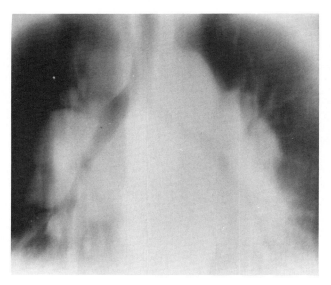

Figure 2-40 Bronchogenic carcinoma. Tomography demonstrates bilateral bulky hilar adenopathy typical of oat cell carcinoma.

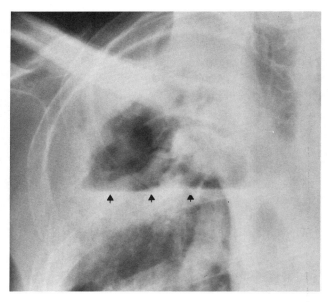

Figure 2-41 Bronchogenic carcinoma. Large cavitary right upper lobe mass with air-fluid level *(arrows)* and associated rib destruction.

in contrast to the sharp margins of benign lesions (Figure 2-38), there are many exceptions to this rule. The presence of central target or popcorn calcification is almost certain proof of an inflammatory cause (Figure 2-39). A comparison with previous films is essential because a nodule that is unchanged in size on radiographs made 2 or more years previously can be assumed to be benign. The growth rate of a solitary pulmonary nodule (doubling time) has been used to determine the likelihood of its being malignant. A pulmonary nodule that doubles in volume in less than 1 month or more than 18 months is usually benign. However, the overlapping of growth rates of benign and malignant lesions, particularly among rapidly growing nodules, makes the use of doubling time unreliable as an absolute indicator of malignancy. In the patient older than 35 to 40 years of age, a solitary pulmonary nodule should be resected unless it can be unequivocally demonstrated to be benign.

Airway obstruction by bronchogenic carcinoma may cause atelectasis of a segment of lung and often leads to postobstructive pneumonia that develops in the lung distal to the obstructed bronchus. An important sign differentiating postobstructive pneumonia from simple inflammatory disease is the absence of an air bronchogram in the former, since this sign can only be detected if there is an open airway leading to the area of consolidation.

Unilateral enlargement of the hilum, best appreciated on serial chest radiographs, may be the earliest sign of bronchogenic carcinoma. The enlarged hilum represents either a primary carcinoma arising in the major hilar bronchus or metastases to enlarged pulmonary lymph nodes from a small primary lesion elsewhere in the lung (Figure 2-40).

Cavitation is common in bronchogenic carcinoma. It most often involves upper lung lesions and represents central necrosis of the neoplasm. The cavities usually resemble acute lung abscesses and have thick walls with irregular, often nodular, inner surfaces (Figure 2-41).

Although the diagnosis of bronchogenic carcinoma may be made by detecting cancer cells in the sputum, a precise diagnosis usually requires biopsy of the tumor during bronchoscopy (direct visualization of the tracheobronchial tree using a tube inserted through the nose) or a needle biopsy in the radiology department under CT or fluoroscopic guidance.

The prognosis of bronchogenic carcinoma is poor, except when the tumor is in the form of a solitary pulmonary nodule that can be surgically removed. Direct lymphatic spread of a tumor can cause enlargement of hilar or mediastinal lymph nodes (Figure 2-42). Distant metastases most frequently involve the bones, where they cause osteolytic destruction. Metastases to the liver, brain, and adrenal glands commonly develop.

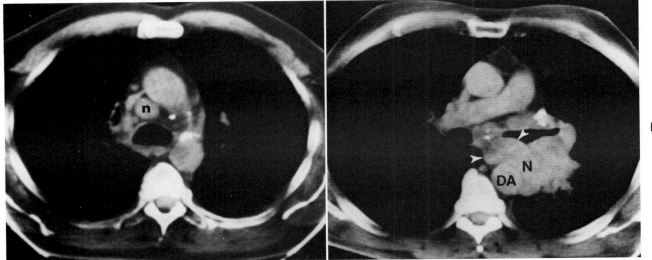

Figure 2-42 Spread of bronchogenic carcinoma to mediastinum. **A,** CT scan shows enlarged lymph node *(n)* in pretracheal region, consistent with unresectable mediastinal spread. **B,** In another patient, CT scan shows obliteration of fat plane around descending aorta *(DA)* by adjacent neoplasm *(N).* In addition, tumor extends deep into mediastinum *(arrowheads)* behind left main stem bronchus and in front of descending aorta. *(From Lee JKT, Sagel SS, and Stanley RJ, editors: Computed body tomography, New York, Raven, 1983.)*

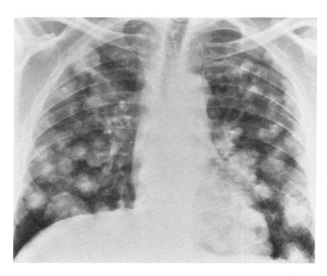

Figure 2-43 Hematogenous metastases. Multiple well-circumscribed nodules scattered diffusely throughout both lungs.

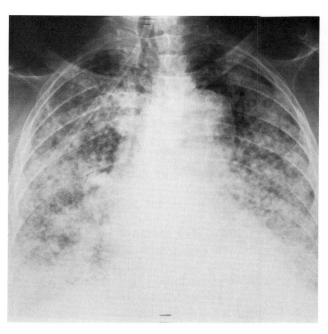

Figure 2-44 Metastatic thyroid carcinoma. Multiple fine miliary nodules scattered throughout both lungs.

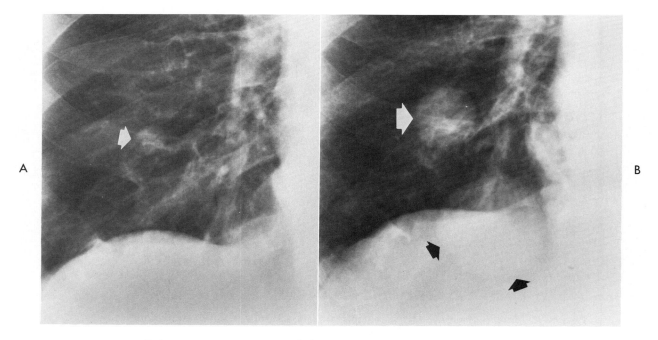

Figure 2-45 Pulmonary metastases. **A,** Solitary metastasis *(arrow)*. **B,** Repeat examination 5 months later shows rapid growth of previous solitary nodule *(white arrow)*. Second huge nodule *(black arrows)* was not appreciated on previous examination because it projected below right hemidiaphragm.

Pulmonary metastases

Up to one third of patients with cancer develop pulmonary metastases; in about half of these patients, the only demonstrable metastases are confined to the lungs. Pulmonary metastases may develop from hematogenous or lymphatic spread, most commonly from musculoskeletal sarcomas, myeloma, and carcinomas of the breast, urogenital tract, thyroid, and colon. Carcinomas of the breast, esophagus, or stomach may directly extend to involve the lungs. Primary lung lesions may metastasize by spread through the bronchial tree.

Hematogenous metastases typically appear radiographically as multiple, relatively well-circumscribed, round or oval nodules throughout the lungs (Figure 2-43). The pattern may vary from fine miliary nodules (Figure 2-44) produced by highly vascular tumors (kidney or thyroid gland carcinomas, sarcoma of bone, trophoblastic disease) to huge, well-defined masses (cannonball lesions) caused by metastatic sarcomas. Carcinoma of the thyroid gland typically causes a snowstorm of metastatic deposits yet remains unchanged for a prolonged period because of a very low grade of malignancy.

Solitary metastases, which occur in about 25% of cases, may be indistinguishable from primary bronchogenic carcinomas or benign granulomas (Figure 2-45). In such cases, CT may permit the detection of additional pulmonary masses that cannot be seen on standard chest radiographs.

Lymphangitic metastatic spread throughout the lungs most commonly is a complication of carcinoma of the breast, stomach, thyroid, pancreas, larynx, cervix, or prostate. The radiographic appearance consists of coarsened interstitial markings that are of irregular contour and poorly defined (Figure 2-46). They are most prominent in the lower lobes and may simulate interstitial pulmonary edema.

MISCELLANEOUS LUNG DISORDERS

Atelectasis

Atelectasis refers to a condition in which there is diminished air within the lung associated with reduced lung volume. It is most commonly the result of bronchial obstruction, which may be due to a neoplasm, foreign body (peanut, coin, or tooth), or mucous plug. Mucoid obstruction may be due to an excessive secretion in patients with chronic bronchitis or be a complication of abdominal surgery, in which mucus collects in the bronchi as a result of the irritative effect of anesthesia and coughing is decreased because of the pain of the abdominal wound. Atelectasis may also be due to compression of the lung by pneumothorax, pleural fluid, a tumor, a lung abscess, or a large emphysematous bulla. Regardless of the precise cause, air is unable to enter that part of the lung supplied by the obstructed bronchus. As the air already in the lung is absorbed into the bloodstream, the lung collapses.

The most common radiographic sign of atelectasis is a local increase in density caused by airless lung that may vary from thin platelike streaks (Figure 2-

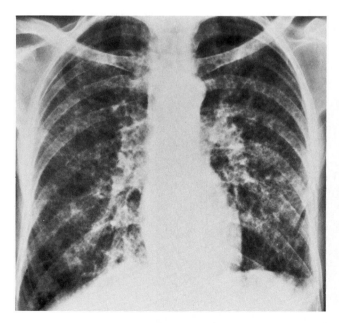

Figure 2-46 Lymphangitic metastases. Coarsened bronchovascular markings of irregular contour and poor definition in this patient with metastatic carcinoma of stomach.

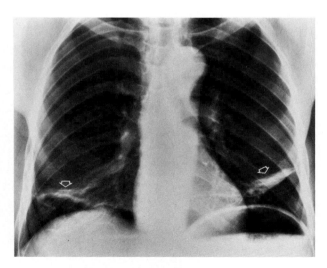

Figure 2-47 Platelike atelectasis. There are horizontal linear streaks of opacity *(arrows)* in lower portions of both lungs.

47) to lobar collapse (Figure 2-48). Indirect signs of atelectasis reflect an attempt by the remaining lung to compensate for the loss of the collapsed portion. These signs include elevation of the ipsilateral hemidiaphragm; displacement of the heart, mediastinum, and hilum toward the atelectatic segment; and compensatory overinflation of the remainder of the ipsilateral lung. An important direct sign of atelectasis is displacement of interlobar fissures, which shift and become bowed, conforming to the contour of the collapsed segment.

An important iatrogenic cause of atelectasis is the improper placement of an endotracheal tube below the level of the tracheal bifurcation. Because of geometric factors, the endotracheal tube tends to enter the right main stem bronchus, effectively blocking the left bronchial tree and causing collapse of part or all of the left lung (Figure 2-49).

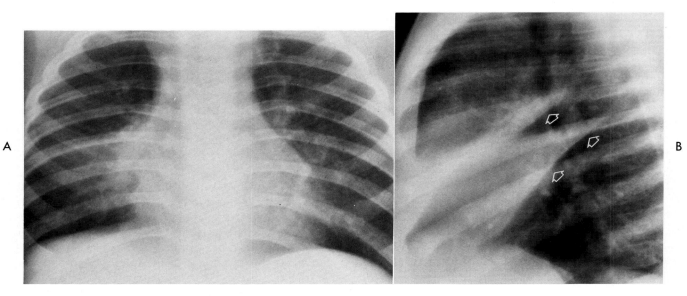

Figure 2-48 Right middle lobe and lingular collapse. **A,** Frontal chest radiograph demonstrates obliteration of right and left borders of heart. **B,** Lateral projection demonstrates collapse of right middle lobe and lingula *(arrows).*

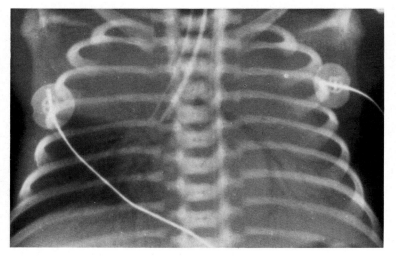

Figure 2-49 Malpositioned endotracheal tube. Excessively low position of endotracheal tube in bronchus intermedius causes collapse of right upper lobe and entire left lung.

Cystic fibrosis

Cystic fibrosis (mucoviscidosis) is a hereditary disease characterized by the secretion of excessively viscous mucus by all the exocrine glands.

In the lungs thick mucus secreted by the trachea and bronchi blocks the air passages and leads to focal areas of lung collapse. Recurrent pulmonary infections are common, since bacteria that are normally carried away by mucosal secretions adhere to the sticky mucus produced in this condition. Radiographically, cystic fibrosis causes generalized irregular thickening of linear markings throughout the lungs which, when combined with the almost invariable hyperinflation, produces an appearance similar to severe chronic lung disease in adults (Figure 2-50).

In the pancreas, blockage of the ducts by mucous plugs prevents pancreatic enzymes from entering the duodenum. This impairs the digestion of fat, resulting in failure of the child to gain weight and the production of large, bulky, foul-smelling stools. In about 10% of newborns with cystic fibrosis, the thick mucus causes obstruction of the small bowel (meconium ileus) (Figure 2-51). Bowel perforation with subsequent fatal peritonitis may occur.

Involvement of the sweat glands in cystic fibrosis causes the child to perspire excessively. This leads to a loss of large amounts of salt (sodium, potassium, and chloride), so that the patients are extremely sus-ceptible to heat exhaustion in hot weather. The presence of excessive chloride on the skin is the basis for the "sweat test," a simple and reliable test for cystic fibrosis.

Hyaline membrane disease

Hyaline membrane disease is one of the most common causes of respiratory distress in the newborn. It primarily occurs in premature infants, especially those who have diabetic mothers or who have been delivered by cesarean section. Hypoxia and increasing respiratory distress may not be immediately evident at birth but almost always appear within 6 hours of delivery.

The progressive underaeration of the lungs in hyaline membrane disease results from a lack of **surfactant**. This lipoprotein is normally produced by cells in the walls of the alveoli and is responsible for maintaining the surface tension within the alveoli that permits them to remain inflated.

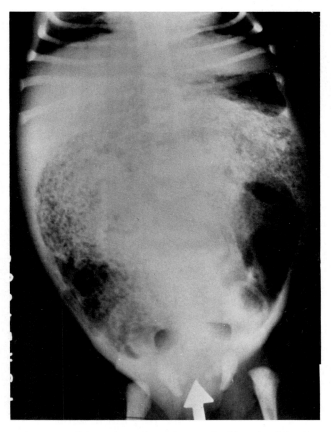

Figure 2-51 Meconium ileus in cystic fibrosis. Massive small bowel distention with profound soap-bubble effect of gas mixed with meconium. *(From Swischuk LE: Radiology of the newborn and young infant, Baltimore, Williams & Wilkins Co, 1980.)*

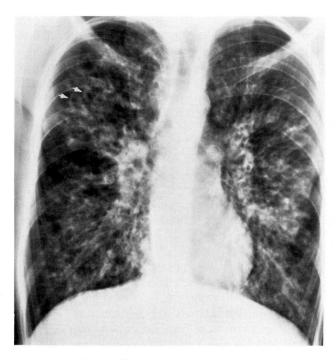

Figure 2-50 Cystic fibrosis. Multiple small cysts superimposed on diffuse, coarse, reticular pattern.

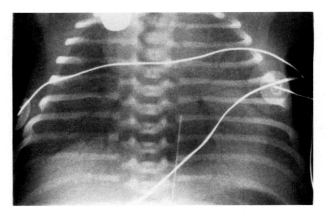

Figure 2-52 Hyaline membrane disease. Diffuse granular pattern of pulmonary parenchyma associated with air bronchograms *(arrows).*

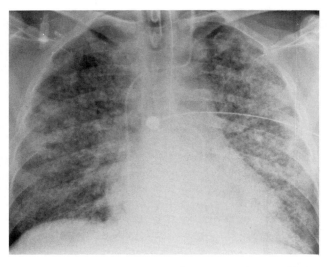

Figure 2-53 Acute respiratory distress syndrome. Ill-defined areas of alveolar consolidation scattered throughout both lungs.

In addition to pronounced underaeration, the radiographic hallmark of hyaline membrane disease is a finely granular appearance of the pulmonary parenchyma (Figure 2-52). A peripherally extending air bronchogram develops because the small airways dilate and stand out clearly against the atelectatic surrounding lung.

The treatment of hyaline membrane disease includes the use of positive pressure ventilators that pump air (often with high concentrations of oxygen) into the lungs through an endotracheal tube. The high ventilator pressure may cause leakage of air from overinflated alveoli or small terminal bronchioles, leading to interstitial emphysema, pneumothorax, and pneumopericardium, all of which further decrease the expansion of the lungs.

Adult respiratory distress syndrome

The term **adult respiratory distress syndrome** is used to describe a clinical picture of severe, unexpected, and life-threatening acute respiratory distress that develops in patients who have a variety of medical and surgical disorders but no major underlying lung disease. It occurs most commonly in patients with nonthoracic trauma who develop hypotension and shock and thus is often called "shock lung." Other conditions that may lead to the adult respiratory distress syndrome include severe pulmonary infection, aspiration or inhalation of toxins and irritants, and drug overdose. Regardless of the cause, there is a complete breakdown in the structure of the lung, leading to massive leakage of cells and fluid into the interstitial and alveolar spaces and severe hypoxemia caused by a marked respiratory impairment in the ability to oxygenate blood. Radiographically, there are patchy, ill-defined areas of alveolar consolidation scattered throughout both lungs (Figure 2-53). Unlike pulmonary edema caused by heart failure, in the adult respiratory distress syndrome the heart is usually of normal size, and there is no evidence of redistribution of blood flow to the upper zones.

The hypoxemia in adult respiratory distress syndrome may be fatal, even with intensive medical therapy. Continuous positive-pressure ventilation may cause air to enter the interstitium of the lung and lead to pneumothorax and pneumomediastinum. Diffuse interstitial and patchy air-space fibrosis may produce a coarse reticular pattern. If the patient recovers completely, the radiographic abnormalities may clear completely, and there may be only a mild decrease in pulmonary function.

Intrabronchial foreign bodies

The aspiration of solid foreign bodies into the tracheobronchial tree occurs almost exclusively in young children. Although some foreign bodies are radiopaque and easily detected on plain chest radiographs, most aspirated foreign bodies are nonopaque and can only be diagnosed by observing secondary signs in the lungs caused by partial or complete bronchial obstruction. The lower lobes are almost always involved, the right more often than the left.

The complete obstruction of a major bronchus leads to resorption of trapped air, alveolar collapse, and atelectasis of the involved segment or lobe. Extensive volume loss causes a shift of the heart and mediastinal structures toward the affected side along

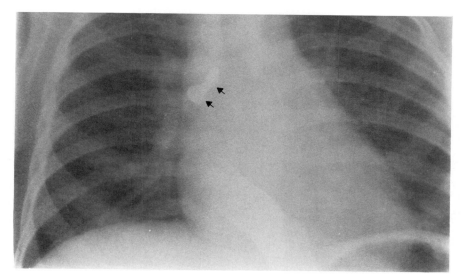

Figure 2-54 Intrabronchial foreign body. Nail *(arrows)* lies in right mainstem bronchus. *(From Cappitanio MA et al: The lateral decubitus film: an aid in determining air trapping in children, Radiology 103:460-461, 1972.)*

with elevation of the ipsilateral hemidiaphragm and narrowing of the intercostal spaces.

Partial bronchial obstruction may produce air trapping as a result of a check-valve phenomenon. Air freely passes the partial obstruction during inspiration but remains trapped distally as the bronchus contracts normally during expiration (Figure 2-54). Hyperaeration of the affected lobes causes a shift of the heart and mediastinum toward the normal, contralateral side. This finding is accentuated during forced expiration because the hyperaerated segment does not contract. This classic appearance of partial bronchial obstruction is dramatically demonstrated at fluoroscopy as the mediastinum shifts away from the affected side during deep expiration and returns toward the midline on full inspiration.

A malpositioned endotracheal tube can act as an intrabronchial foreign body. The tube tends to extend down the right main stem bronchus, causing hyperlucency of the right lung and obstructive atelectasis of the left lung.

Mediastinal emphysema (pneumomediastinum)

Air within the mediastinal space may appear spontaneously or be the result of chest trauma; perforation of the esophagus or tracheobronchial tree; or the spread of air along fascial planes from the neck, peritoneal cavity, or retroperitoneal space. Spontaneous pneumomediastinum usually results from a sudden rise in intra-alveolar pressure (e.g., severe coughing, vomiting, or straining) that causes alveolar rupture and the dissection of air along blood vessels in the interstitial space to the hilum and medi-

astinum. Air may also extend peripherally and rupture into the pleural space, causing an associated pneumothorax.

On frontal chest radiographs, air causes lateral displacement of the mediastinal pleura, which appears as a long linear opacity that is parallel to the heart border but separated from it by the air (Figure 2-55). On lateral projections, air typically collects behind the sternum, extending in streaks downward and anterior to the heart. Chest radiographs may

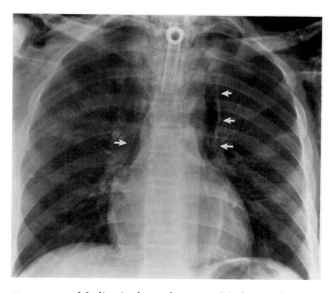

Figure 2-55 Mediastinal emphysema. Mediastinal pleura is displaced laterally and appears as long linear opacity *(arrows)* parallel to heart border but separated from it by gas.

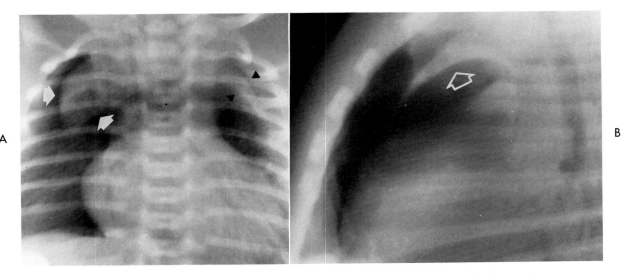

Figure 2-56 Mediastinal emphysema in infant. **A,** Elevation of both lobes of thymus by mediastinal air *(arrows)* produces angel-wings sign. **B,** Lateral projection shows mediastinal air lifting thymus off pericardium and great vessels *(arrows and arrowheads)*. *(From Eisenberg R: Altas of signs in radiology, Philadelphia, JB Lippincott Co, 1984.)*

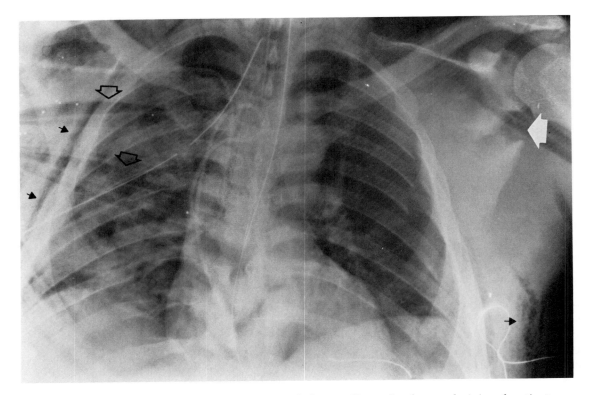

Figure 2-57 Subcutaneous emphysema. Frontal chest radiograph of severely injured patient shows streaks and bubbles of subcutaneous air *(black arrows)* in soft tissues along lateral borders of thorax, as well as broad lucencies outlining muscle bundles *(open arrows)* overlying anterior chest wall. Note fracture of left scapula *(white arrow)* and multiple rib fractures.

also demonstrate air outlining the pulmonary arterial trunk and aorta, as well as dissecting into the soft tissues of the neck.

In infants mediastinal air causes elevation of the thymus. Loculated air confined to one side produces an appearance similar to that of a windblown sail. Bilateral mediastinal air elevates both thymic lobes to produce an angel-wings configuration (Figure 2-56).

Subcutaneous emphysema

Subcutaneous emphysema is caused by penetrating or blunt injuries that disrupt the lung and parietal pleura so that air is forced into the tissues of the chest wall. The resulting radiographic appearance is bizarre, with streaks of lucency outlining muscle bundles (Figure 2-57).

DISORDERS OF THE PLEURA

Pneumothorax

Pneumothorax refers to the presence of air in the pleural cavity that results in a partial or complete collapse of the lung (Figure 2-58). It most commonly results from rupture of a subpleural bulla, either as a complication of emphysema or as a spontaneous event in an otherwise healthy young adult. Other causes of pneumothorax include trauma (stabbing, gunshot, or fractured rib), iatrogenic causes (after lung biopsy or the introduction of a chest tube for thoracentesis), and as a complication of neonatal hyaline membrane disease requiring prolonged assisted ventilation. Regardless of the cause, the increased air in the pleural cavity compresses the lung and causes it to collapse, resulting in the patient experiencing sudden, severe chest pain and difficulty breathing. A pneumothorax appears radiographically as a hyperlucent area in which all pulmonary markings are absent. The radiographic hallmark of pneumothorax is the demonstration of the visceral pleural line, which is outlined centrally by air within the lung and peripherally by air within the pleural space. A large pneumothorax can cause collapse of an entire lung. Chest radiographs for pneumothorax should be taken with the patient in the upright position, since it may be very difficult to identify this condition if the patient is supine. In addition to routine full-inspiration films, a PA (or AP) radiograph should be obtained with the lung in full expiration to identify small pneumothoraces

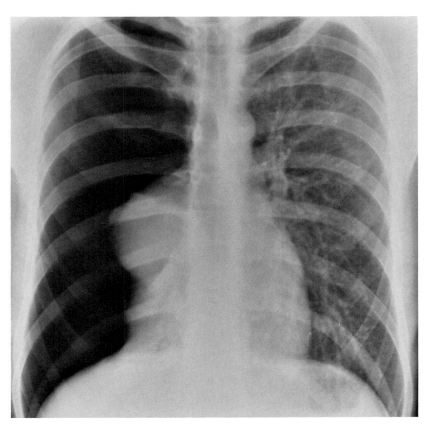

Figure 2-58 Spontaneous pneumothorax. Complete collapse of right lung.

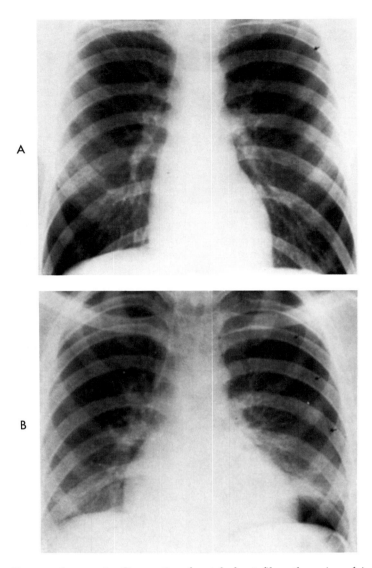

Figure 2-59 Pneumothorax. **A,** On routine frontal chest film, there is a faint rim of pleura *(arrows)* at left apex separated from thoracic wall by area containing air but no pulmonary vasculature. **B,** On expiratory film, left pneumothorax *(arrows)* is clearly seen. *(From Eisenberg RL: Diagnostic imaging in surgery, New York, 1987, McGraw-Hill Book Co.*

(Figure 2-59). This maneuver causes the lung to decrease in volume and become relatively denser, while the volume of air in the pleural space remains constant and is easier to detect. Another technique for demonstrating small pneumothoraces is a film obtained with a horizontal x-ray beam while the patient is in the lateral decubitus position. In this position, air rising to the highest point in the hemithorax is more clearly visible over the lateral chest wall than on erect views, in which a small amount of air in the apical region may be obscured by overlying bony densities. In obtaining any expiration ra-

diograph an automatic exposure device (AED) is *not* recommended, since the preset density may produce a film blackness capable of concealing a small pneumothorax. Using a manual technique, the exposure factor for an expiration radiograph should be about one third greater than that for an inspiration film.

Small pneumothoraces usually reabsorb spontaneously. Larger pneumothoraces may require chest tube drainage.

Tension pneumothorax is a medical emergency in which air continues to enter the pleural space but

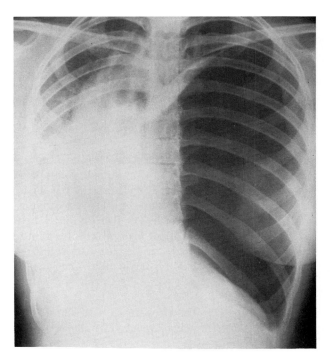

Figure 2-60 Tension pneumothorax. Left hemithorax is completely radiolucent and lacks vascular markings. There is dramatic shift of mediastinum to right. Left hemidiaphragm is markedly depressed and there is spreading of left ribs.

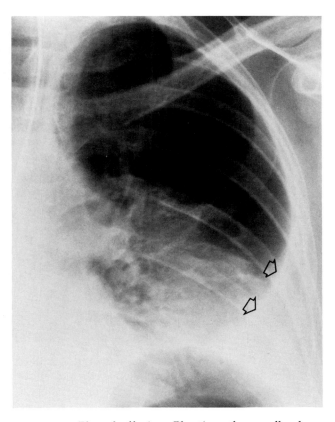

Figure 2-61 Pleural effusion. Blunting of normally sharp angle between diaphragm and rib cage *(arrows)* along with characteristic upward concave border (meniscus) of fluid level.

cannot leave it. The accumulation of air within the pleural space causes complete collapse of the lung on that side and depression of the hemidiaphragm (Figure 2-60). The heart and mediastinal structures are shifted toward the unaffected side, severely compromising cardiac output because the elevated intrathoracic pressure decreases venous return to the heart. If a tension pneumothorax is not treated promptly, the resulting circulatory collapse may be fatal.

Pleural effusion

The accumulation of fluid in the pleural space is a nonspecific finding that may be caused by a wide variety of pathologic processes. The most common causes include congestive heart failure, pulmonary embolism, infection (especially tuberculosis), pleurisy, neoplastic disease, and connective tissue disorders. Pleural effusion also can be the result of abdominal disease, such as recent surgery, ascites, subphrenic abscess, and pancreatitis.

The earliest radiographic finding in pleural effusion is blunting of the normally sharp angle between the diaphragm and the rib cage along with an upward concave border of the fluid level (meniscus)

(Figure 2-61). Because the costophrenic angles are deeper posteriorly than laterally, small pleural effusions are best seen posteriorly on the routine lateral projection. As much as 400 ml of pleural fluid may be present and still not produce blunting of the lateral costophrenic angles on erect frontal views of the chest. Larger amounts of pleural fluid produce a homogeneous whiteness that may obscure the diaphragm and adjacent borders of the heart. Massive effusions may compress the adjacent lung and even displace the heart and mediastinum to the opposite side (Figure 2-62).

Small pleural effusions may be difficult to distinguish from pleural thickening and fibrosis, which results from previous pleural inflammation and appears radiographically as a soft-tissue density along the lateral chest wall. The diagnosis of a small pleural effusion is best made using a horizontal x-ray beam with the patient in a lateral decubitus position with the affected side down. As little as 5 ml of pleural fluid can be seen layering out at a linear opacification along the dependent chest wall. At times, however,

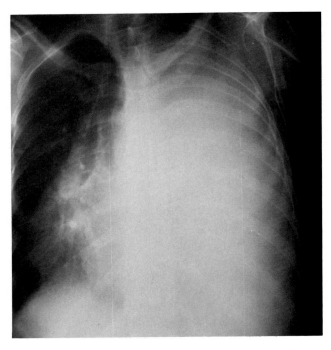

Figure 2-62 Pleural effusion causing shift of mediastinum. Left hemithorax is virtually opaque, and there is shift of mediastinal structures to right.

a collection of pleural fluid may be loculated (fixed in place by fibrous adhesions) and therefore will not layer out on decubitus views.

Pleural effusions may produce less common appearances on chest radiographs. A pleural fluid collection that has become fixed by inflammatory fibrosis may mimic a solid mass. At times, pleural fluid may collect below the inferior surface of the lung (subpulmonic effusion) and give the radiographic appearance of an elevated hemidiaphragm (Figure 2-63). In patients with congestive heart failure, an effusion may develop in an interlobar fissure to produce a round or oval density resembling a solitary pulmonary nodule. As the patient's heart condition improves, repeat examinations demonstrate decreased size or complete resolution of these "phantom tumors" (see Figure 6-10).

Empyema

Empyema refers to the presence of infected liquid or frank pus in the pleural space. Usually the result of the spread of an adjacent infection (bacterial pneumonia, subdiaphragmatic abscess, lung abscess, esophageal perforation), empyemas may also follow thoracic surgery, trauma, or instrumentation of the

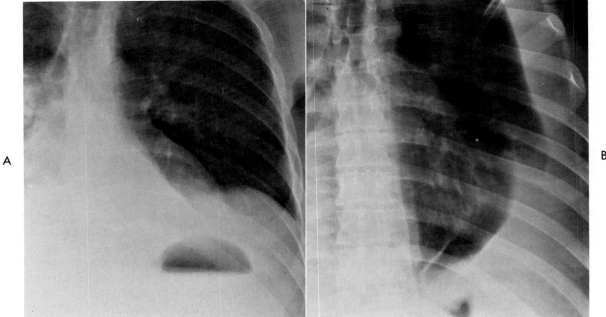

Figure 2-63 Pleural effusion. **A,** Frontal projection of chest demonstrates large distance between gastric air bubble and top of false left hemidiaphragm in this patient with large subpulmonic effusion. Note retrocardiac paraspinal density *(arrows)* that simulates left lower lobe infiltrate or atelectasis. **B,** Left lateral decubitus projection shows that retrocardiac density represents large amount of free pleural fluid. *(From Vix VA: Semin Roentgenol 12:277-286, 1977.)*

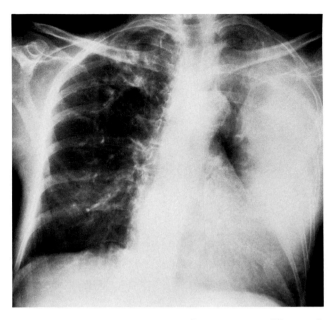

Figure 2-64 Empyema. Large soft tissue mass fills much of left hemothorax. *(From Eisenberg RL: Diagnostic imaging in surgery, New York, 1987, McGraw-Hill Book Co.*

pleural space. Since the development of antibiotics, empyemas are rare.

Radiographically, an empyema is initially indistinguishable from pleural effusion. As the empyema develops, it becomes loculated and appears as a discrete mass that may vary in size from a large lesion filling much of the hemithorax (Figure 2-64) to a small mass along the chest wall or in an interlobar fissure. Air within a free or loculated empyema causes an air-fluid level and indicates communication with a bronchus or the skin surface. Needle aspiration of an empyema may be performed using fluoroscopic guidance; if there is a loculated mass adjacent to the chest wall, ultrasound may be used to guide the aspiration needle.

MEDIASTINAL MASSES

Because various types of mediastinal masses tend to occur predominantly in specific locations, the mediastinum is often divided into anterior, middle, and posterior compartments. The anterior compartment extends from the sternum back to the trachea and the anterior border of the heart. The middle mediastinum contains the heart and great vessels, the central tracheobronchial tree and lymph nodes, and the phrenic nerves. The posterior compartment is composed of the space behind the pericardium.

Major lesions of the anterior mediastinum include thymomas (Figure 2-65), teratomas, thyroid masses, lipomas, and lymphoma. The middle mediastinum is involved with lymph node disorders (lymphoma,

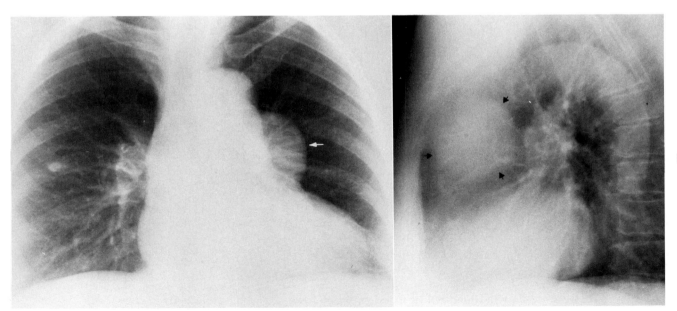

A   B

Figure 2-65 Anterior mediastinal mass. **A,** Frontal and, **B,** lateral projections of chest demonstrate large mass (thymoma) in anterior mediastinum *(arrows).*

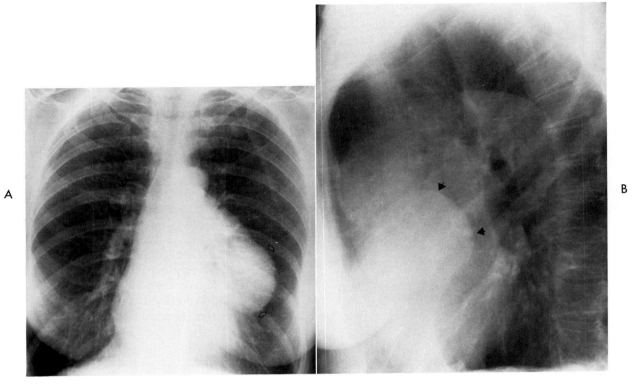

Figure 2-66 Middle mediastinal mass. **A,** Frontal and, **B,** lateral projections of chest demonstrate smooth-walled, spheric mediastinal mass *(arrows)* projecting into left lung and left hilum (bronchogenic cyst).

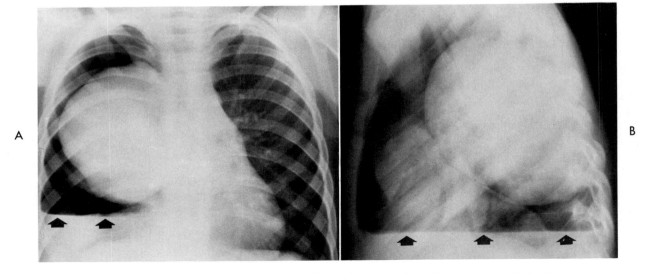

Figure 2-67 Posterior mediastinal mass. **A,** Frontal and, **B,** lateral projections of chest demonstrate large, oval, homogeneous mass in posterior mediastinum (neurenteric cyst). Note right hydropneumothorax *(arrows)* with long air-fluid level that developed as complication of diagnostic needle biopsy.

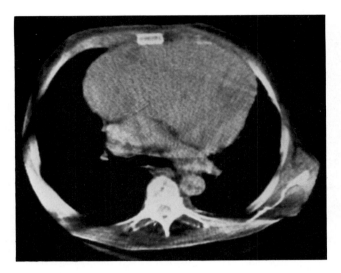

Figure 2-68 CT of anterior mediastinal mass. Enormous soft-tissue mass (thymoma) causes posterior displacement of other mediastinal structures. No difference in density can be seen between mass and heart behind it.

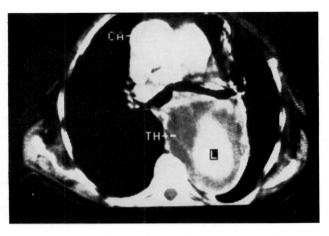

Figure 2-69 CT of posterior mediastinal mass. Contrast-enhanced scan at level just below carina shows large aneurysm of descending aorta. Large mural thrombus *(TH)* surrounds markedly dilated lumen of descending aorta *(L)*. Note also prominently dilated ascending aorta *(OA)*.

metastatic carcinoma, granulomatous processes), bronchogenic cysts (Figure 2-66), vascular anomalies, and various masses situated in the anterior costophrenic angle (pericardial cysts, foramen of Morgagni hernia). The posterior mediastinum is the site of neurogenic tumors, neurogenic cysts (Figure 2-67), aneurysms of the descending aorta, and extramedullary hematopoeisis.

The configuration of a mediastinal mass depends to a large degree on its consistency. Cystic masses are often compressed between blood vessels and the tracheobronchial tree, producing a multiloculated appearance. In contrast, solid masses tend to compress and displace adjacent structures.

About one third of patients with mediastinal masses are asymptomatic, and the lesion is detected on a routine chest radiograph. Chest pain, cough, dypsnea, and symptoms caused by compression or invasion of structures in the mediastinum (dysphagia, hoarseness as a result of recurrent laryngeal nerve involvement, superior vena caval obstruction) are highly suggestive of malignancy. In addition to plain chest radiographs, conventional tomography and contrast studies of the esophagus may be of value in defining the anatomic location and borders of the mass. CT of the chest after the intravenous injection of contrast material may help in distinguishing between vascular and nonvascular lesions, as well as in determining whether a lesion is cystic and thus most probably benign (Figures 2-68 and 2-69).

DISORDERS OF THE DIAPHRAGM

The diaphragm is the major muscle of respiration that separates the thoracic and abdominal cavities. Radiographically, the height of the diaphragm varies considerably with the phase of respiration. On full inspiration, the diaphragm is usually about the level of the tenth posterior intercostal space. On expiration, it may appear two or three intercostal spaces higher. The average range of diaphragmatic motion with respiration is 3 to 6 cm, but in patients with emphysema this may be substantially reduced. The level of the diaphragm falls as the patient moves from a supine to an upright position. In an erect patient, the dome of the diaphragm tends to be about half an interspace higher on the right than on the left. However, in about 10% of normal individuals the hemidiaphragms are at the same height, or the left is higher than the right.

Diaphragmatic paralysis

Elevation of one or both leaves of the diaphragm can be caused by paralysis resulting from any process that interferes with the normal function of the phrenic nerve. This may be due to accidental surgical transection of the phrenic nerve, involvement of the nerve by primary bronchogenic carcinoma or metastatic malignancy in the mediastinum, or a variety of intrinsic neurologic diseases (Figure 2-70). The radiographic hallmark of diaphragmatic paralysis is paradoxical movement of the diaphragm that is best

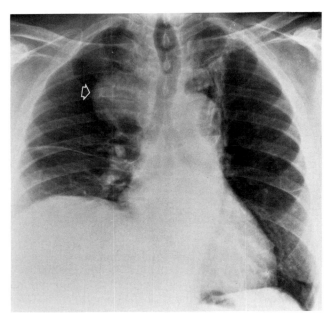

Figure 2-70 Paralysis of right hemidiaphragm due to involvement of phrenic nerve by primary carcinoma of lung *(arrow)*.

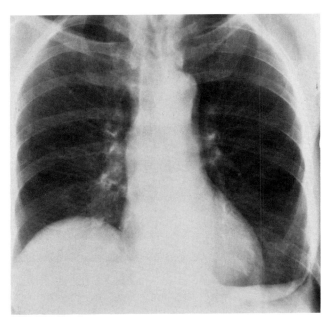

Figure 2-71 Eventration of right hemidiaphragm.

demonstrated at fluoroscopy by having the patient sniff. This rapid but shallow inspiration causes a quick downward thrust of a normal leaf of the diaphragm, whereas a paralyzed hemidiaphragm tends to rise with inspiration because of the increased intra-abdominal pressure. During expiration, the normal hemidiaphragm rises and the paralyzed one descends. The demonstration of a marked degree of paradoxical motion is a valuable aid in differentiating paralysis of the diaphragm from limited diaphragmatic motion resulting from intrathoracic or intra-abdominal disease.

Eventration of the diaphragm

Eventration of the diaphragm is a rare congenital abnormality in which one hemidiaphragm (very rarely both) is poorly developed and is too weak to permit the upward movement of abdominal contents into the thoracic cage. This leads to the radiographic appearance of a localized bulging or generalized elevation of the diaphragm (Figure 2-71). The condition is usually asymptomatic and is most common on the left. An eventration must be distinguished from a diaphragmatic hernia, through which abdominal contents are displaced into the chest. Oral administration of barium should permit the differentiation between the normal contours of the bowel below a diaphragmatic eventration and the crowding of these structures and narrowing of

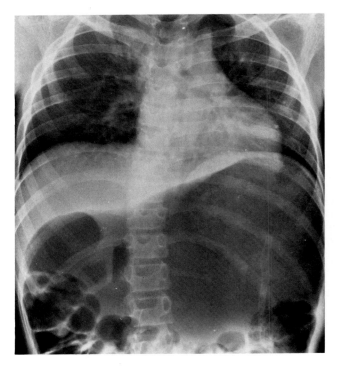

Figure 2-72 Diffuse elevation of both leaves of diaphragm caused by severe, acute gastric dilation.

their afferent and efferent limbs when trapped in a hernia sac.

Other causes of elevation of the diaphragm

Diffuse elevation of one or both leaves of the diaphragm can be caused by ascites, obesity, pregnancy, or any other process in which the intraabdominal volume is increased (Figure 2-72). Intraabdominal inflammatory diseases, such as subphrenic abscess, can lead to elevation of a hemidiaphragm with severe limitations of diaphragamatic motion. Cystic or tumor masses arising in the upper quadrants can cause localized or generalized bulging of the diaphragm. Acute intrathoracic processes (chest-wall injury, atelectasis, pulmonary embolism) can produce diaphragmatic elevation caused by splinting of the diaphragm. An apparent elevation of a hemidiaphragm may be caused by a subpulmonic pleural effusion, which can be correctly diagnosed on a chest radiograph performed with a horizontal x-ray beam and the patient in a lateral decubitus position.

QUESTIONS

1. Describe the proper breathing instructions to be given to a patient for chest radiography.

2. In what portion of the respiratory system does the vital gas exchange take place?

3. The covering of the lungs is termed the _____.

4. A necrotic area of pulmonary parenchyma containing purulent or puslike material is called a _____.

5. What radiographic procedure is often required to confirm the diagnosis of bronchiectasis when routine chest radiographs are inconclusive?

6. Flattening of the domes of the diaphragm, increased AP diameter of the chest, and increased lucency of the retrosternal air space suggests a diagnosis of _____.

7. The three most common pneumoconioses are _____, _____, and _____.

8. An abnormal vascular communication between a pulmonary artery and pulmonary vein is termed a _____.

9. _____ is a disease of newborns characterized by progressive underaeration of the lungs and a granular appearance.

10. What medical emergency has occurred when air continues to enter the pleural space and cannot escape, leading to complete collapse of a lung and shift of the heart and mediastinal structures?

11. Pus in the pleural space is called _____.

12. The major muscle of respiration is the _____.

13. Describe why a true horizontal beam is desirable when performing any chest radiograph.

14. The Valsalva maneuver can cause the heart and major blood vessels to:
    A. Appear enlarged   C. Appear elevated
    B. Appear smaller   D. Show no change

15. Place an "H" by those pathologic conditions that are harder to penetrate and an "E" by those that are easier to penetrate:
    _____ Pleural effusion   _____ Empyema
    _____ Miliary tubercu-   _____ Asbestosis
          losis   _____ Pneumonia
    _____ Emphysema   _____ Atelectasis
    _____ Lung abscess   _____ Brochiectasis
    _____ Pulmonary
          edema

16. Describe the pulmonary circulation of the lungs.

17. Describe the bronchial circulation of the lungs.

18. The lining of the thoracic cavity is called the _____.

19. A lung inflammation caused by bacteria or viruses is called a _____.

20. For technologist safety, it is important to remember that tuberculosis is spread mainly by _____, which produces infectious _____.

21. What medical term is used to describe the entry of air into the pleural space?

22. An increased volume of air in the lungs is seen in _____.

23. Inhalation of irritating dusts leading to chronic inflammation and pulmonary fibrosis is called _____.

24. Trapping of bacteria in the pulmonary circulation that occurs in patients with a history of intravenous drug abuse is called _____.

25. _____ is a hereditary disease in which thick mucus is secreted by all the exocrine glands.

26. Reduced air volume within a lung leading to collapse is termed _____.

27. Blunt or penetrating trauma to the chest can produce _____, which appears as streaks of air that outline muscles of the thorax and sometimes the neck.

28. Name the two positions that are sometimes used to demonstrate a pneumothorax that are different from the routine chest radiograph positions.

29. An abnormal connection between the esophagus and trachea is termed _____.

30. At what costal interspace does the diaphragm lie when the lungs are fully inflated?
    A. Eighth   C. Tenth
    B. Ninth   D. Eleventh

31. What radiographic position is sometimes helpful in diagnosing very small pleural effusions?

32. Air collecting behind the sternum and dissecting up into the soft tissues of the neck is called _____.

33. An accumulation of fluid in the pleural space, sometimes caused by heart failure or pulmonary embolus, is called:
    A. Empyema   C. Effusion
    B. Edema   D. Abscess

BIBLIOGRAPHY
Chest
Felson B: Chest roentgenology, Philadelphia, WB Saunders Co, 1971.
Heitzman ER: The lung: radiologic-pathologic correlations, St. Louis, The CV Mosby Co, 1984.
Paré JAP and Fraser RG: Synopsis of diseases of the chest, Philadelphia, WB Saunders Co, 1983.
Reed JC: Chest radiology: patterns and differential diagnoses, Chicago, Yearbook Medical Publishers, 1981.

CHAPTER 3

Skeletal System

PREREQUISITE KNOWLEDGE

The student should have a basic knowledge of the anatomy and physiology of the sketetal system. In addition, proper learning and understanding of the material will be facilitated if the student has some clinical experience in skeletal radiography and film evaluation, including a concept of the changes in technique required to compensate for density differences produced by the underlying pathologic conditions.

GOALS

To acquaint the student radiographer with the pathophysiology and radiographic manifestations of all of the common and some of the unusual disorders of the skeletal system

OBJECTIVES

1. Describe the physiology of the skeletal system
2. Identify anatomic structures on both diagrams and radiographs of the skeletal system
3. Be able to define terminology relating to the skeletal system
4. Be able to describe the various pathologic conditions affecting the skeletal system, as well as their radiographic manifestations
5. Be familiar with the changes in technical factors required for obtaining optimal quality radiographs in patients with various underlying pathologic conditions

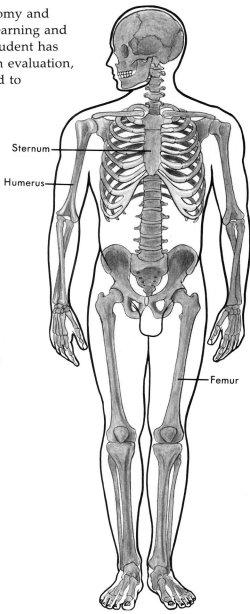

RADIOGRAPHER NOTES

Proper positioning, correct tube-part-film alignment, and the use of exposure factores designed to produce an optimal contrast level and visibility of detail are critical factors in radiography of the skeletal system. In patients with suspected fractures, two projections as close as possible to 90 degrees to each other must always be obtained. A variety of projections (oblique, tangential, coned-down) may be required to identify obscure fractures. At times, the poor condition of a patient may require ingenuity on the part of the radiographer to obtain diagnostic radiographs when routine positioning methods cannot be used.

Patients with bone tumors, arthritis, or recent trauma are frequently in severe pain and extremely frightened of being injured further or suffering more discomfort. It is essential that the patient be reassured of the radiographer's awareness of his or her pain or discomfort and that the radiographer will be as careful as possible. Remember that a radiographer can easily cause further injury to the patient if proper moving techniques are not used. At times, it may be necessary to perform cross-table or tube angulation projections to obtain the required films without having to move the patient. In such cases, the tube-part-film alignment is critical because variations of these relationships can obscure pathologic bone conditions or lead to errors in interpretation of the alignment of fracture fragments. The radiographic tube must be perpendicular to the image receptor and the body part to prevent image distortion.

Bone radiographs require a short scale of contrast to provide maximal visibility of detail. The periosteum, cortex, and internal bone structure (trabeculae) must be well demonstrated to detect the often subtle changes of fractures, demineralization, and bone destruction. For example, periosteal new bone formation may indicate underlying tumor, infection, or prior trauma, whereas minute juxta-articular erosions are often seen in arthritis. The scale of contrast must be such that the soft tissues and muscles also are well visualized. Soft-tissue swelling, calcifications, opaque foreign bodies, muscle wasting, and the presence of gas are all important radiographic findings.

It is recommended that lower to mid kVp ranges be used in all skeletal radiography. To achieve the necessary scale of contrast, the extremities should be examined using an exposure in the 40 to 69 kVp range, whereas a range of 70 to 80 kVp is recommended for studies of the spine, pelvis, thoracic cage, and shoulder. Appropriate ratio grids or Bucky devices should be used for all body parts 10 cm or greater.

Special techniques such as magnification or tomography may be necessary to detect subtle fractures or other pathologic bone conditions. For example, the navicular bone of the wrist typically requires the use of the magnification technique. For 2x linear or 4x area magnification, the part in question must be an equal distance from the radiographic tube and the image receptor. For 3x linear or 9x area magnification, the part must be twice as far from the image receptor as from the x-ray tube. Close collimation is extremely important to prevent undercutting the image. A radiographic tube with a fractional focal spot of 0.3 mm or less is mandatory, since larger focal spot sizes cause excessive distortion and an image that appears to have motion and lack detail as a result of excessive penumbra (blurring). Tomography may be required to make a definite diagnosis if the plain radiographs are equivocal or to precisely delineate the extent of bone involvement. For example, tomography is frequently needed in the evaluation of fractures of the tibial plateau and spine.

As a general rule, it is essential to prevent motion of the part of the body being radiographed. To accomplish this, the patient should be made as comfortable as possible, immobilization devices should be used when necessary, and the shortest possible exposure time should be used. However, a few portions of the skeletal system are better visualized using a motion technique. These include the sternum, lateral thoracic spine, transthoracic lateral projection of the upper humerus, and "wagging jaw" or Ottonello method for obtaining an AP projection of the cervical spine. For the first three, a breathing technique is used while the patient remains immobilized. A minimum exposure time of about 5 seconds and a very low milliamperage should be used. The patient is instructed to breathe rhythmically during the entire exposure to blur out overlying ribs and lung markings. In the Ottonello method, movement of the jaw blurs out the image of the mandible, which otherwise would superimpose the upper portion of the cervical spine.

Certain pathologic conditions of the skeletal system require that the radiographer alter the routine technical factors. Some disorders produce increased density (sclerosis, increased bone growth) that is harder to penetrate; others decrease the density of the bony structures (lytic bone destruction, loss of calcium from bone) so that they are easier to penetrate (Table 1-1). It is important to remember that the necessary technical changes may vary depending on the stage of the underlying condition.

PHYSIOLOGY OF THE SKELETAL SYSTEM

The skeletal system is primarily composed of two highly specialized connective tissues: bone and cartilage. Bone consists of an organic matrix in which inorganic salts (primarily calcium and phosphate) are deposited. The outer surfaces of bone are covered by a fibrous membrane termed the **periosteum**, except at joint surfaces where the bone is covered with articular cartilage that acts as a protective cushion. The periosteum contains a network of blood vessels from which nutrient arteries penetrate into the underlying bone. The main shaftlike portion is termed the **diaphysis**, and the ends of the bone are called **epiphyses**. The hollow, tubelike structure within the diaphysis is the **medullary**, or **marrow**, cavity, which is lined by an inner membrane termed the **endosteum**.

There are two major types of bone. The outer layer is composed of **compact bone**, which to the naked eye is dense and structureless. Under the microscope, the matrix of compact bone consists of complex structural units called haversian systems. **Cancellous (spongy) bone** is composed of a weblike arrangement of marrow-filled spaces separated by thin processes of bone called **trabeculae** that are visible to the naked eye. The relative amount of each type of bone depends on the degree of strength required and thus varies from bone to bone and in different portions of the same bone. For example, the shafts of long bones such as the femur and tibia have a thick outer layer of compact bone, whereas the layer of compact bone is relatively thin in irregular bones, such as vertebral bodies and facial bones, or short bones, such as the carpal and tarsal bones.

Most bones form from models composed of hyaline cartilage (enchondral ossification). In a typical long bone, a primary ossification center appears in the center of the cartilage precursor about the eighth week of intrauterine life, and bone formation extends so that the entire shaft is usually ossified before birth. Just before or after birth, secondary ossification centers appear in the epiphyses, the ends of developing long bones. Until the linear growth of bone is complete, the epiphysis remains separated from the diaphysis by a cartilaginous plate called the **epiphyseal cartilage**. The epiphyseal cartilage persists until the growth of the bone is complete. At that time, the epiphyseal plate ossifies, and the epiphysis and diaphysis fuse (various ages for specific bones).

The increase in length of a developing long bone occurs by growth of the epiphyseal cartilage followed by ossification. Bones grow in diameter by the combined action of two special types of cells called **osteoblasts** and **osteoclasts**. Osteoclasts enlarge the diameter of the medullary cavity by removing the bone of its walls. At the same time, osteoblasts from the periosteum produce new bone around its outer circumference. Osteoblasts and osteoclasts are continuously active in absorbing old bone and producing new bone. This constant process of remodeling occurs until the bone assumes its adult size and shape.

The radiographic determination of bone age is useful in evaluating physiologic age, growth potential, and prediction of adult stature. The most well-known and widely accepted method of determining skeletal bone age (skeletal maturation) is that of Greulich and Pyle in their radiographic atlas compiled from thousands of examinations of American children at different ages. This atlas contains standard radiographs for age and sex that permit an assessment of bone age based on the presence or absence of ossification centers and their configuration and the fusion of epiphyses in various portions of the hand and wrist.

Throughout life, bone formation (**ossification**) and bone destruction (**resorption**) continue to occur. They are in balance during the early and middle years of adulthood. After about age 40, however, bone loss at the inner or endosteal surface exceeds bone gain at the outer margins. Thus in long bones the thickness of compact bone in the diaphyses decreases, and the diameter of the medullary cavity increases. The bone eventually resembles a hollow shell and is less able to resist compressive and bending forces. This process may lead to collapse and loss of height of vertebral bodies and fractures of long bones after relatively mild injury.

Bones can also develop within a connective tissue membrane (**intramembranous ossification**). The clavicles and flat bones of the skull have no cartilaginous stage and begin to take shape when groups of primitive cells differentiate into osteoblasts, which secrete matrix material and collagenous fibrils. Deposition of complex calcium salts in the organic bone matrix produces rodlike trabeculae that join in a network of interconnecting spicules to form spongy or cancellous bone. Eventually, plates of compact or dense bone cover the core layer of spongy bone. Flat bones grow in size by the addition of osseous tissue to their outer surfaces (**appositional growth**). They cannot grow by expansion as is the case with enchondral bone growth.

Bones perform five basic functions. They serve as the supporting framework of the body and protect the vital organs (skull protecting the brain, rib cage protecting the heart and lungs). Bones serve as levers on which muscles can contract and shorten and thus produce movement at a joint. Red bone marrow within certain bones (spinal column, upper humerus and upper femur in the adult) is the major site of production of blood cells. Finally, bone serves as the major storehouse for calcium salts. The maintenance of a normal level of calcium, which is essential for survival, depends on a balance in the rates of calcium movement between the blood and bones.

CONGENITAL/HEREDITARY DISEASES OF BONE

Vertebral anomalies

A **transitional vertebra** is one that has characteristics of vertebrae on both sides of a major division of the spine. Transitional vertebrae most frequently occur at the lumbosacral junction and contain expanded transverse processes that may form actual unilateral or bilateral joints with the sacrum. When unilateral, this process often leads to degenerative change involving the opposite hip and the intervertebral disk space above it. At the thoracolumbar junction, the first lumbar vertebra may have rudimentary ribs articulating with the transverse processes. The seventh cervical vertebra may also have a rudimentary rib (Figure 3-1). This **cervical rib** may compress the brachial nerve plexus (causing pain or numbness in the upper extremity) or the subclavian artery (decreasing blood flow to the arm) and therefore require surgical removal.

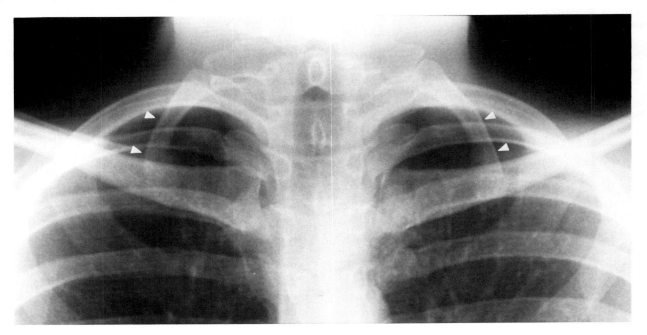

Figure 3-1   Bilateral cervical ribs (*arrowheads*).

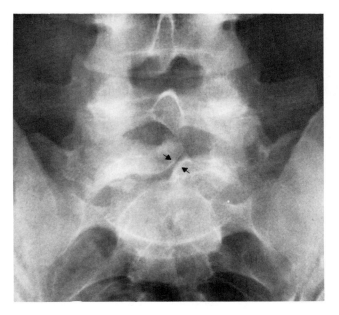

Figure 3-2 Spina bifida occulta (*arrows*).

Spina bifida

Spina bifida refers to a posterior defect of the spinal canal resulting from failure of the posterior elements to fuse properly. A mild, insignificant form is **spina bifida occulta**, in which there is a splitting of the bony neural canal at the L5 or S1 level (Figure 3-2). Large defects are associated with spinal cord abnormalities and may lead to a variety of muscular abnormalities and lack of bladder or bowel control. In many cases a slight dimpling of the skin or tuft of hair over the vertebral defect indicates the site of the lesion.

Large defects in the lumbar or cervical spine may be accompanied by herniation of the meninges (**meningocele**) or of the meninges and a portion of the spinal cord or nerve roots (**myelomeningocele**). Almost all patients with myelomeningocele have the Arnold-Chiari II malformation, with caudal displacement of posterior fossa structures into the cervical canal. Hydrocephalus is a frequent complication. These lesions are associated with large bony defects, absence of the laminae, and increased interpedicular distance (Figure 3-3). The herniated spinal contents are seen as a soft-tissue mass posterior to the spine.

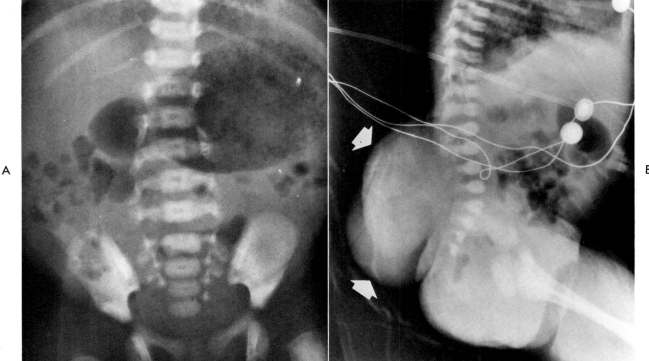

Figure 3-3 Meningomyelocele. **A,** Frontal projection of abdomen shows markedly increased interpedicular distance of lumbar vertebrae. **B,** In another patient lateral projection demonstrates large soft-tissue mass (*arrows*) situated posterior to spine. Note absence of posterior elements in lower lumbar and sacral regions.

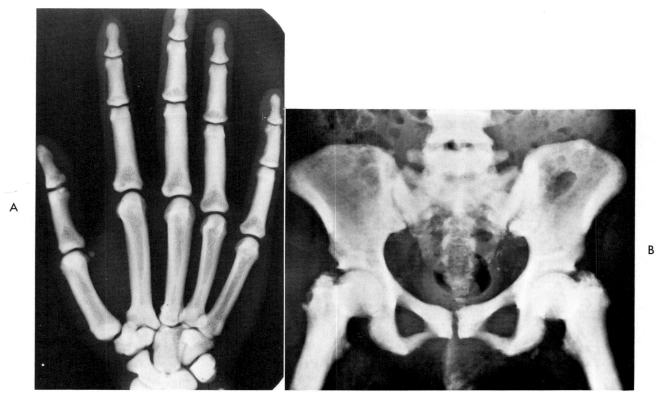

Figure 3-4 Osteopetrosis. **A,** Striking sclerosis of bones of hand and wrist. **B,** Generalized increased density of lower spine, pelvis, and hips.

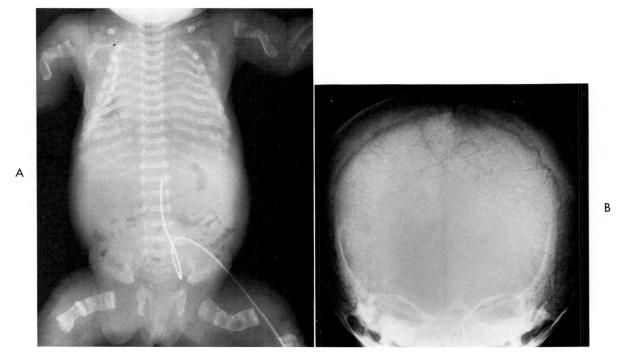

Figure 3-5 Osteogenesis imperfecta. **A,** Generalized flattening of vertebral bodies associated with fractures of multiple ribs and long bones in infant. **B,** Multiple wormian bones.

Myelography, CT, or MRI can demonstrate the presence of the spinal cord or nerve roots within the herniated sac. Prenatal real-time ultrasound can now demonstrate this serious malformation in utero.

Osteopetrosis

Osteopetrosis (marble bones) is a rare hereditary bone dysplasia in which failure of the resorptive mechanism of calcified cartilage interferes with its normal replacement by mature bone. This results in a symmetric, generalized increase in bone density (Figure 3-4). Osteopetrosis varies in severity and age of clinical presentation from a fulminant, often fatal condition involving the entire skeleton at birth or in utero to an essentially asymptomatic form that is an incidental radiographic finding.

Osteogenesis imperfecta

Osteogenesis imperfecta is an inherited generalized disorder of connective tissue characterized by multiple fractures and an unusual blue color of the normally white sclera of the eye. Patients with this condition suffer repeated fractures caused by the severe osteoporosis and the thin, defective cortices (Figure 3-5, *A*). The fractures often heal with exuberant cal-

lus formation (often so extensive as to simulate a malignant tumor) and may cause bizarre deformities. Ossification of the skull progresses slowly, leaving wide sutures and multiple juxtasutural accessory bones within a suture (wormian bones) that produce a mosaic appearance (Figure 3-5, *B*).

Achondroplasia

Achondroplasia is the most common form of dwarfism that results from diminished proliferation of cartilage in the growth plate (decreased enchondral bone formation). Because membranous bone formation is not affected, the individual has short limbs that contrast with the nearly normal length of the trunk. Other characteristic physical features include a large head with frontal bulging, saddle nose, a prognathous (jutting) jaw, and prominent buttocks that give the false impression of lumbar lordosis. Typical radiographic findings include progressive narrowing of the interpedicular distances from above downward, the opposite of normal, and scalloping of the posterior margins of the lumbar vertebral bodies (Figure 3-6).

METABOLIC BONE DISEASE

Osteoporosis

Osteoporosis is a generalized or localized deficiency of bone matrix in which the mass of bone per unit volume is decreased in amount but normal in composition. Bone is a living, constantly changing tissue, and normally there is a balance between the amount of old bone being removed and the amount of new bone replacing it. Osteoporosis is usually due to accelerated resorption of bone, although decreased bone formation may lead to osteoporosis in such entities as Cushing's syndrome, prolonged steroid administration, and disuse or immobilization osteoporosis as in a casted extremity (Figure 3-7). Loss of mineral salts causes osteoporotic bone to become more lucent than normal. This may be difficult to detect, since about 30% of the bone density must be lost before it can be demonstrated as a lucent area on routine radiographs. In patients with osteoporosis it is essential to use the lowest practical kVp. This technique provides the extremely short scale of contrast necessary to visualize the demineralized osteoporotic bones.

The major causes of generalized osteoporosis are aging and postmenopausal hormonal changes. As a person ages, the bones lose density and become more brittle, fracturing more easily and healing more slowly. Many elderly persons also are less active and have poor diets that are deficient in protein. In postmenopausal osteoporosis there is a deficiency in the

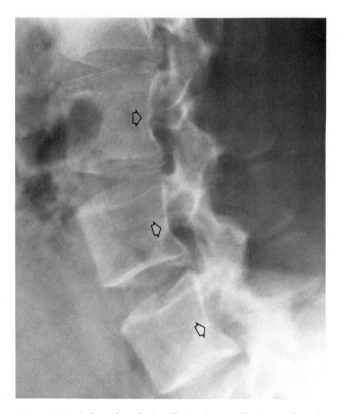

Figure 3-6 Achondroplasia. Posterior scalloping of multiple vertebral bodies (*arrows*).

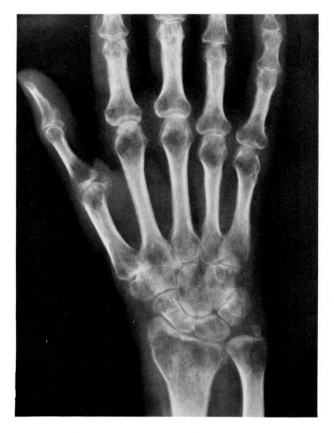

Figure 3-7 Disuse osteoporosis. Severe periarticular demineralization after prolonged immobilization of extremity.

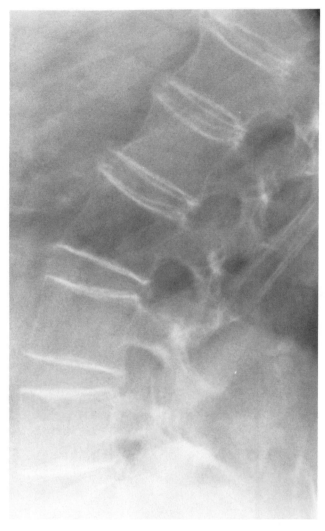

Figure 3-8 Osteoporosis of aging. Generalized demineralization of spine in postmenopausal woman. Cortex appears as thin line that is relatively dense and prominent (picture-frame pattern).

gonadal hormonal levels and decreased bone formation.

Regardless of the cause, the radiographic appearance is somewhat similar in all conditions producing osteoporosis. The most striking change is cortical thinning with irregularity and resorption of the endosteal (inner) surfaces (Figure 3-8). These findings are most evident in the spine and pelvis. As the bone density of a vertebral body decreases, the cortex appears as a thin line that is relatively dense and prominent, producing the typical picture-frame pattern. Because of the severe loss of bone density, anterior wedging or compression fractures of one or more vertebral bodies may result, most commonly in the middle and lower thoracic and upper lumbar areas. The intervertebral disk may expand into the weakened vertebral bodies and produce characteristic concave contours of the superior and inferior disk surfaces. In the skull the calvarium may show a spotty loss of density, and there is commonly deossification (bone loss) of the floor of the sella turcica and dorsum sellae.

Osteomalacia

Osteomalacia refers to insufficient mineralization of the adult skeleton. There is normally a balance between osteoid formation and mineralization. Osteomalacia is the result of either excessive osteoid formation or, more frequently, insufficient mineralization. Proper calcification of osteoid requires that adequate amounts of calcium and phosphorus be available at the mineralization sites. Failure of calcium and phosphorus deposition in bone matrix in osteomalacia may be due to an inadequate intake or failure of absorption of calcium, phosphorus, or vitamin D, which is necessary for intestinal absorption of calcium and phosphorus and may have a direct

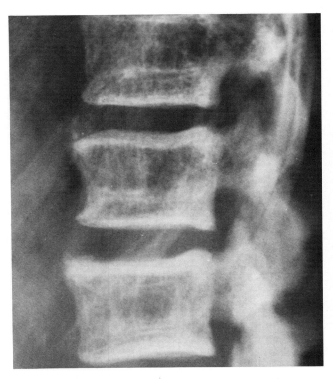

Figure 3-9 Osteomalacia. Striking prominence of cortices of vertebral bodies with increased trabeculation of spongy bone.

effect on bone. At times, the level of vitamin D is sufficient but the material is not used because of resistance to the action of the vitamin at end organs, such as the kidneys. Other non-nutritional causes of osteomalacia include chronic kidney failure and certain renal diseases in which calcium is lost in the urine and bone is broken down in an attempt to maintain a normal calcium level in the blood.

Regardless of the cause, osteomalacia appears radiographically as a loss of bone density owing to the presence of nonmineralized osteoid. Although the cortex is thinned, it may stand out more prominently than normal because of the uniform deossification of medullary bone (Figure 3-9). In contrast to osteoporosis, the cortical borders in osteomalacia are often indistinct. Fine-detail radiographs of the hands in patients with osteomalacia often demonstrate intracortical lines caused by local resorption or lack of mineralization, a finding not seen in osteoporosis.

Bones that are softened by osteomalacia may bend or give way as a result of weight-bearing. Bowing deformities primarily involve the pelvis, vertebral column, thorax, and proximal extremities. In the pelvis, there may be characteristic inward bending of the sidewalls with deepening of the acetabular cavities (protrusio acetabuli) (Figure 3-10).

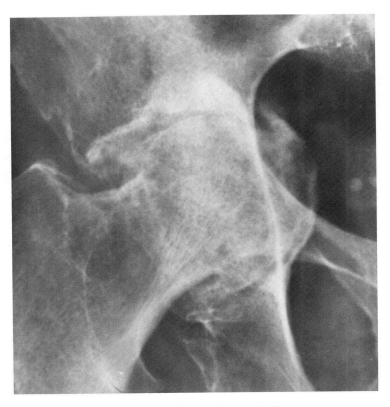

Figure 3-10 Protrusio acetabuli.

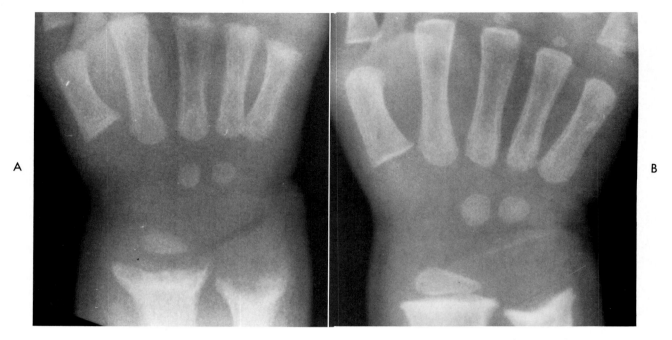

A   B

Figure 3-11 Rickets. **A,** Initial film of wrist shows characteristic cupping and fraying of metaphyseal ends of radius and ulna, with disappearance of normally sharp metaphyseal lines. **B,** After therapy with vitamin D, there is remineralization of metaphyseal ends of radius and ulna, increased sharpness of metaphyseal lines, and return of epiphyseal centers to normal density and sharpness of outline.

Rickets

Rickets is a systemic disease of infancy and childhood that is the equivalent of osteomalacia in the mature skeleton. In this condition, calcification of growing skeletal elements is defective because of a deficiency of vitamin D in the diet or a lack of exposure to ultraviolet radiation (sunshine), which converts the sterols in the skin into vitamin D. Rickets is most common in premature infants and usually develops between the ages of 6 months and 1 year.

The early radiographic changes in rickets are best seen in the fastest growing portions of bone, such as the sternal ends of the ribs, proximal ends of the tibia and humerus, and distal ends of the radius and ulna. An overgrowth of noncalcified osteoid tissue appears radiographically as a characteristic increased distance between the ossified portion of the epiphysis and the end of the shaft. In response to the pull of muscular and ligamentous attachments, the metaphyseal ends of the bone become cupped and frayed, and the normally sharp metaphyseal lines disappear (Figure 3-11). Lack of calcification leads to a delayed appearance of the epiphyseal ossification centers. Because of poor mineralization, bowing of weight-bearing bones (especially the tibia) develops once the infant begins to stand or walk. Extensive osteoid tissue in the sternal ends of the ribs produces a characteristic beading (rachitic rosary).

Softening of the vertebral bodies leads to the development of kyphosis. In females, narrowing of the pelvic inlet may make normal delivery impossible in later life.

Gout

Gout is a disorder of purine metabolism (a component of nucleic acids) in which an increase in the blood levels of uric acid leads to the deposition of uric acid crystals in the joints, cartilage, and kidney. Several inherited enzyme defects can cause overproduction of uric acid (primary gout). In secondary gout, hyperuricemia can be due to an overproduction of uric acid because of increased turnover of nucleic acids (metastatic carcinoma, myeloma, hemolytic anemia), drugs (chemotheraphy, thiazides used to treat hypertension), or a decrease in the excretion of uric acid because of kidney failure.

The primary manifestation of acute gout is an exquisitely painful arthritis that initially attacks a single joint, primarily the first metatarsophalangeal joint. Radiographic changes develop late in the disease and only after repeated attacks. Therefore negative radiographs do not exclude gout and thus are of no help in early diagnostic evaluation.

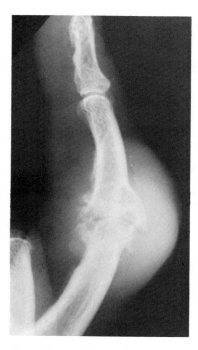

Figure 3-12 Gout. Severe joint effusion and periarticular swelling of proximal interphalangeal joint of finger. Note associated erosion of articular cartilage.

Deposition of nonopaque urate crystals in the joint synovial membrane and on the surface of articular cartilage incites an inflammatory reaction that produces the earliest radiographic signs of joint effusion and periarticular swelling (Figure 3-12). Clumps of urate crystals (tophi) form along the margins of the articular cortex and erode the underlying bone, producing small, sharply marginated, punched-out defects at the joint margins of the small bones of the hand and foot. These erosions often have the appearance of cystlike lesions with thin sclerotic margins and characteristic overhanging edges ("rat bite") (Figure 3-13). In advanced disease severe destructive lesions are associated with joint space narrowing and even fibrous ankylosis. Because patients are relatively free of symptoms between acute exacerbations of the disease, the bone density remains relatively normal, and diffuse osteoporosis is not part of the radiographic appearance.

Continued deposition of urate crystals in the periarticular tissues causes the development of characteristic large, lumpy soft-tissue swellings representing gouty tophi. In addition to the first metatarsophalangeal joints, other common sites of tophi

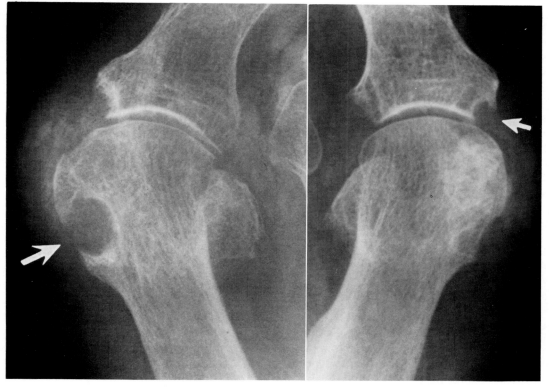

Figure 3-13 Two examples of typical rat-bite erosions about first metatarsophalangeal joint (arrows). Cystlike lesions have thin sclerotic margins and characteristic overhanging edges.

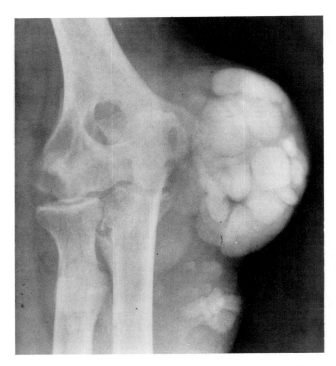

Figure 3-14 Gout. Massive deposition of calcium in long-standing tophaceous lesion about elbow.

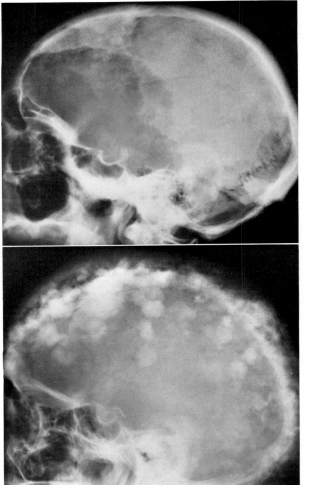

Figure 3-15 Paget's disease of skull. **A,** Radiograph obtained during destructive phase of disease demonstrates area of sharply demarcated radiolucency (osteoporosis circumscripta) that primarily involves frontal portion of calvarium. **B,** During reparative phase in another patient, irregular areas of sclerosis produce characteristic cotton-wool appearance of skull.

include the ear, the olecranon bursa, and the insertion of the Achilles tendon. Tophi consisting only of sodium urate are of soft-tissue density. Deposition of calcium in these urate collections causes the tophaceous periarticular masses to become radiopaque (Figure 3-14).

Although some renal dysfunction occurs in almost all patients with gouty arthritis, no radiographic abnormalities in the urinary tract can be demonstrated unless uric acid stones are formed. Pure uric acid stones are not radiopaque and can only be demonstrated on excretory urograms, where they appear as filling defects in the pelvocalyceal system or ureter. Stones containing the calcium salts of uric acid are radiopaque and can be detected on plain abdominal radiographs.

Paget's disease

Paget's disease (osteitis deformans) is one of the most common chronic diseases of the skeleton. Destruction of bone followed by a reparative process results in weakened, deformed, and thickened bony structures that tend to fracture easily. The disease is seen most commonly during middle life, affects men twice as often as women, and has been reported to occur in about 3% of all persons older than 40 years of age. Although the destructive phase often predominates initially, there is most frequently a combination of destruction and repair; in the pelvis and weight-bearing bones of the lower extremities, the reparative process may begin early and be the prominent feature. Often involving multiple bones, Paget's disease particularly affects the pelvis, femurs, skull, tibias, vertebrae, clavicles, and ribs.

In the skull Paget's disease begins as an area of sharply demarcated radiolucency (osteoporosis circumscripta) that represents the destructive phase of the disease (Figure 3-15, *A*). During the reparative process, the development of irregular islands of sclerosis and cortical thickening results in a mottled,

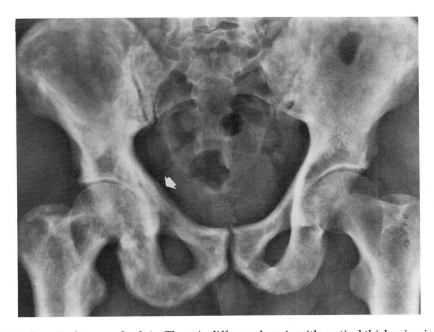

Figure 3-16 Paget's disease of pelvis. There is diffuse sclerosis with cortical thickening involving right femur and both iliac bones. Note characteristic thickening and coarsening of iliopectineal line (*arrow*) on involved right side.

cotton wool appearance (Figure 3-15, *B*). In the spine Paget's disease characteristically causes enlargement of the vertebral body. Increased trabeculation, which is most prominent at the periphery of the bone, produces a rim of thickened cortex and a picture-frame appearance. Uniform dense sclerosis of one or more vertebral bodies (ivory vertebra) may occur.

The pelvis is the most common and often the initial site of Paget's disease. A distinctive early sign is coarsening of the trabeculae along the iliac margins that produces thickening of the pelvic brim (Figure 3-16).

In the long bones the destructive phase almost invariably begins at one end of the bone and extends along the shaft for a variable distance before ending in a typical sharply demarcated, V-shaped configuration (blade of grass appearance). In the reparative stage the bone is enlarged, with an irregularly widened cortex and coarse, thickened trabeculae (Figure 3-17). Although dense, the bones are soft, and deformities are common.

Paget's disease may lead to severe clinical complications. The downward thrust of the heavy head on the softened bone of the spine may compress the brain stem and cause numerous cranial nerve deficits. Expansion and distortion of softened vertebral bodies, sometimes with pathologic fractures, may compress the spinal cord and produce nerve root deficits. Multiple microscopic arteriovenous malformations in pagetoid bone may result in high-output

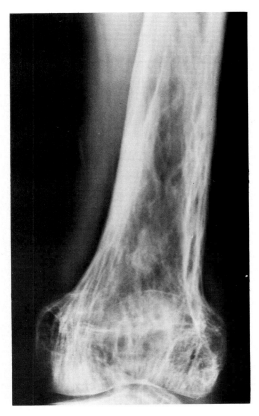

Figure 3-17 Paget's disease of knee. Characteristic cortical thickening, destruction of fine trabeculae, and accentuation of secondary trabeculae.

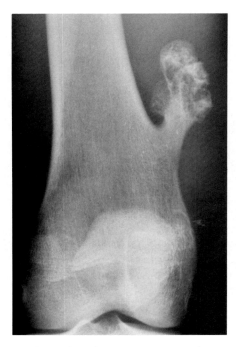

Figure 3-18 Osteochondroma. Long axis of tumor is parallel to that of femur and pointed away from knee joint.

cardiac failure. The most serious complication of Paget's disease is the development of osteosarcoma, which fortunately occurs in less than 1% of patients with this condition.

BENIGN BONE TUMORS

Osteochondroma (exostosis) is a benign projection of bone with a cartilaginous cap that arises in childhood or the teens, especially about the knee. The cortex of an osteochondroma blends with that of normal bone, and the long axis of the tumor characteristically is parallel to the parent bone and points away from the nearest joint (Figure 3-18).

Enchondromas are slow-growing benign cartilaginous tumors arising in the medullary canal. They are most frequently found in children and young adults and primarily involve the small bones of the hands and feet. Enchondromas are slow growing and often multiple. As the well-demarcated tumor grows, it expands bone locally, causing thinning and endosteal scalloping of the cortex that often leads to a pathologic fracture with minimal trauma (Figure 3-19). A characteristic finding of enchondroma is calcifications within the lucent matrix.

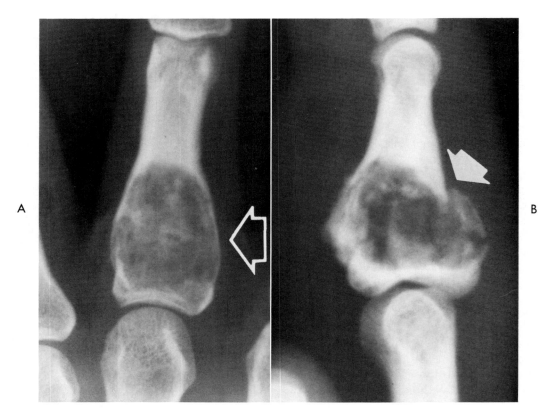

Figure 3-19 Enchondroma. **A**, Well-demarcated tumor (*arrow*) expands bone and thins cortex. **B**, Pathologic fracture (*arrow*).

Giant cell tumor typically arises at the end of the distal femur or proximal tibia of a young adult after epiphyseal closure. It begins as an eccentric lucent lesion in the metaphysis and characteristically extends to the immediate subarticular cortex of the bone but does not involve the joint (Figure 3-20). As the tumor expands toward the shaft, it produces the characteristic radiographic appearance of multiple large bubbles separated by thin strips of bone.

Osteomas most often arise in the outer table of the skull, the paranasal sinuses (especially frontal and ethmoid), and the mandible. They appear radiographically as well-circumscribed, extremely dense round lesions that are rarely larger than 2 cm in diameter (Figure 3-21).

Osteoid osteoma usually develops in teenagers or young adults and produces the classic clinical symptom of local pain that is worse at night and is dramatically relieved by aspirin. Most osteoid osteomas occur in the femur and tibia. The tumor typically is seen as a small, round or oval lucent center (nidus), less than 1 cm in diameter, that is surrounded by a large, dense sclerotic zone of cortical thickening

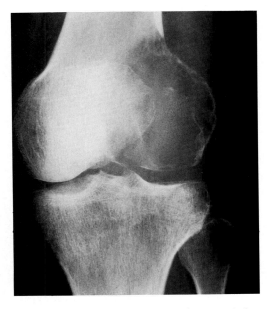

Figure 3-20 Giant cell tumor. Typical eccentric lucent lesion in distal femoral metaphysis extends to immediate subarticular cortex. Surrounding cortex, though thinned, remains intact.

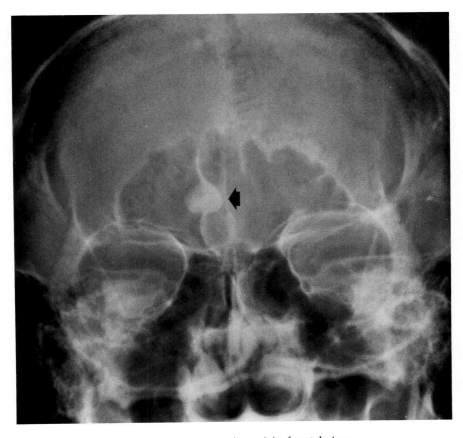

Figure 3-21 Osteoma (*arrow*) in frontal sinus.

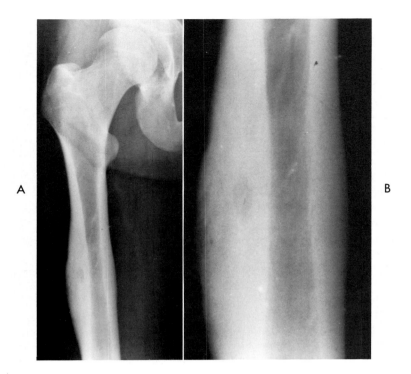

Figure 3-22   Osteoid osteoma. **A** Full and, **B**, coned projections of midshaft of femur demonstrate dense sclerotic zone of cortical thickening laterally, which contains small oval lucent nidus (*arrowhead*).

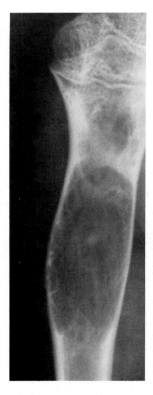

Figure 3-23   Simple bone cyst. This cyst in proximal humerus has oval configuration, with its long axis parallel to that of host bone.

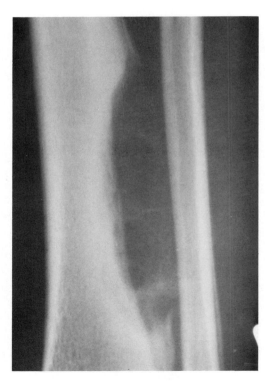

Figure 3-24   Aneurysmal bone cyst. Expansile, eccentric, cystic lesion of tibia with multiple fine internal septa. Because severely thinned cortex is difficult to detect, tumor resembles malignant process.

(Figure 3-22). Because this dense reaction may obscure the nidus on conventional radiographs, overpenetrated films or tomography (conventional or computed) may be necessary for its demonstration. Surgical excision of the nidus is essential for cure; it is not necessary to remove the reactive calcification, even though it may form the major part of the lesion.

A **simple bone cyst** is a true fluid-filled cyst with a wall of fibrous tissue. Although not a true neoplasm, a simple bone cyst may resemble one radiographically and clinically. Solitary bone cysts are asymptomatic and are discovered either incidentally or after pathologic fracture. It appears as an expansile lucent lesion that is sharply demarcated from adjacent normal bone and may have a thin rim of sclerosis around it. A simple bone cyst has an oval configuration, with its long axis parallel to that of the host bone (Figure 3-23).

An **aneurysmal bone cyst**, rather than being a true neoplasm or cyst, consists of numerous blood-filled arteriovenous communications. In long bones an aneurysmal bone cyst is an expansile, eccentric, cystlike lesion that causes marked ballooning of the thinned cortex (Figure 3-24). At times, the cortex may be so thin that it is invisible on plain radiographs, and thus this benign lesion may be mistaken for a malignant bone tumor.

Bone islands are solitary, sharply demarcated areas of dense compact bone that occur most commonly in the pelvis and upper femurs but may be seen in every bone except the skull (Figure 3-25). Although almost half the bone islands enlarge over a period of years and many show activity on radionuclide scans, bone islands are asymptomatic and completely benign and must be distinguished from osteoblastic metastases.

MALIGNANT BONE TUMORS

Osteogenic sarcoma generally occurs in the end of a long bone (especially about the knee). Most osteogenic sarcomas arise in persons between 10 and 25 years of age, although a smaller peak incidence is seen in older age groups in whom the tumor is superimposed on a pre-existing bone disorder, particularly Paget's disease. The usual initial complaints are local pain and swelling, sometimes followed by fever, weight loss, and secondary anemia. Pulmonary metastases develop early, and a plain chest radiograph should be obtained to exclude this unfavorable prognostic sign. If no metastases to the lung are detected by this modality, CT should be performed.

The typical radiographic appearance of osteogenic sarcoma is a mixed destructive and sclerotic lesion associated with a soft-tissue mass, irregular periosteal reaction, and reactive new bone formation (Figure 3-26, *A*). In the classic sunburst pattern, horizontal bony spicules extend in radiating fashion into the soft-tissue mass (Figure 3-26, *B*). A characteristic finding is elevation of the periosteum at the periphery of a lesion with subsequent new bone formation (Codman's triangle) (Figure 3-27).

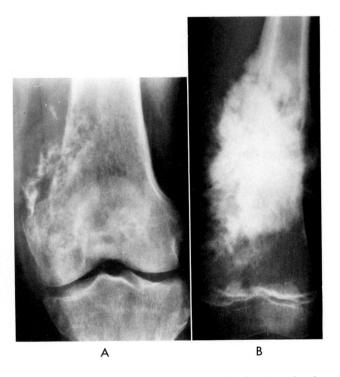

A B

Figure 3-26 Osteogenic sarcoma. **A**, Predominantly destructive lesion with irregular periosteal reaction. **B**, Classic sunburst pattern with bony spicules extending outward in radiating fashion.

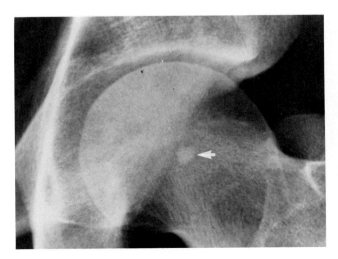

Figure 3-25 Bone island (*arrow*) in femoral head.

Chondrosarcoma is a malignant tumor of cartilaginous origin that may originate de novo or within a pre-existing cartilaginous lesion (osteochondroma, enchondroma). The tumor is about half as common as osteogenic sarcoma, develops at a later age (half the patients are older than 40 years of age), grows more slowly, and metastasizes later. In addition to the bone destruction seen with all malignant tumors, chondrosarcoma often contains punctate or amorphous calcification within its cartilaginous matrix (Figure 3-28).

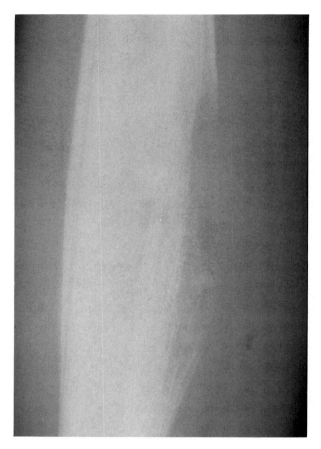

Figure 3-27 Codman's triangle. Thin periosteal elevation and subsequent new bone formation at periphery of this neoplastic lesion.

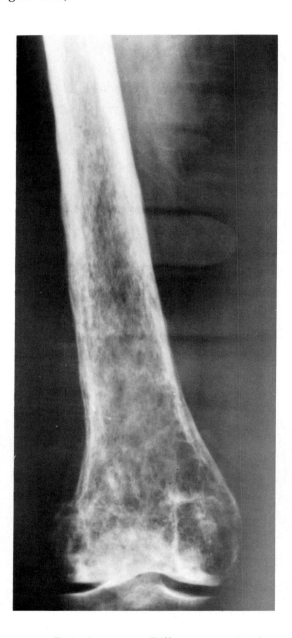

Figure 3-29 Ewing's sarcoma. Diffuse permeative destruction with mild periosteal response involving distal half of femur.

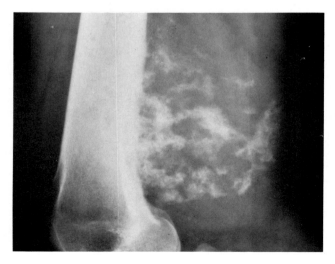

Figure 3-28 Chondrosarcoma. Prominent dense calcification in large neoplastic mass.

Ewing's sarcoma is a primary malignant tumor arising in the bone marrow. A tumor of children and young adults, Ewing's sarcoma has a peak incidence in the mid teens and is rare over the age of 30. The major clinical complaint is local pain, often of several months' duration, that persistently increases in severity and may be associated with a tender soft-tissue mass. Patients with this tumor characteristically have malaise and appear sick, often with fever and leukocytosis, suggesting osteomyelitis. The classic radiographic appearance of Ewing's sarcoma is an ill-defined permeative area of bone destruction that involves a large central portion of the shaft of a long bone and is associated with a fusiform layered periosteal reaction parallel to the shaft (Figure 3-29).

Multiple myeloma is a disseminated (widespread) malignancy of plasma cells that may be associated with bone destruction, bone marrow failure, hypercalcemia, renal failure, and recurrent infections. The disease primarily affects persons between 40 and 70 years of age. Typical laboratory findings include an abnormal spike of monoclonal immunoglobulin and the presence of Bence Jones protein in the urine. The classic radiographic appearance of multiple myeloma is multiple punched-out osteolytic lesions scattered throughout the skeletal system and best seen on lateral views of the skull (Figures 3-30 and 3-31). Because the bone destruction is due to the proliferation of plasma cells distributed throughout the bone marrow, the flat bones containing red marrow (vertebrae, skull, ribs, pelvis) are primarily affected. The appearance may be indistinguishable from that of a metastatic carcinoma, although the lytic defects in multiple myeloma tend to be more discrete and uniform in size.

Extensive plasma cell proliferation in the bone marrow with no tendency to form discrete tumor masses may produce generalized skeletal deossifications simulating postmenopausal osteoporosis. In the spine, decreased bone density and destructive changes in multiple myeloma are usually limited to the vertebral bodies, sparing the pedicles (lacking red marrow) that are frequently destroyed by metastatic disease. The severe loss of bone substance in the spine often results in multiple vertebral compression fractures (Figure 3-32). Because multiple myeloma causes little or no stimulation of new bone formation, radionuclide bone scans may be normal even with extensive skeletal infiltration.

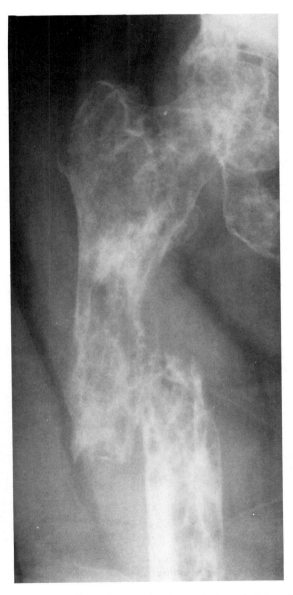

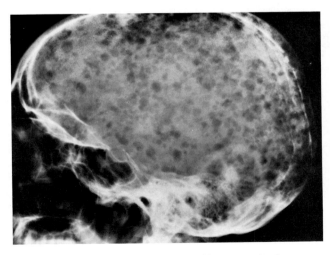

Figure 3-30 Multiple myeloma. Diffuse punched-out osteolytic lesions scattered throughout skull.

Figure 3-31 Diffuse destructive bone lesion that has led to pathologic fracture of femur.

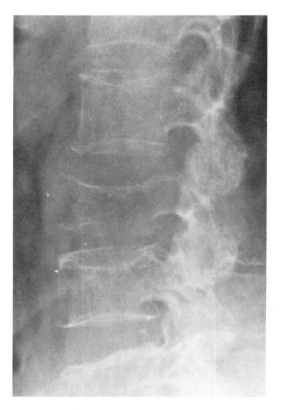

Figure 3-32 Multiple myeloma. Diffuse myelomatous infiltration causes generalized demineralization of vertebral bodies and compression fracture of L2.

CT and MRI can precisely define the location of a malignant bone tumor, as well as its extension into the medullary cavity and spread to surrounding structures (Figure 3-33).

BONE METASTASES

Metastases are the most common malignant bone tumors, spreading by means of the bloodstream or lymphatic vessels or by direct extension. The most common primary tumors are carcinomas of the breast, lung, prostate, kidney, and thyroid. Favorite sites of metastatic spread are bones containing red marrow, such as the spine, pelvis, ribs, skull, and the upper ends of the humerus and femur. Metastases distal to the knees and elbows are infrequent but do occur, especially with bronchogenic (lung) tumors.

The detection of skeletal metastases is critical in the management of patients with known or suspected neoplastic disease, both at the time of initial staging and during the period of continuing follow-up care. The presence of metastases may exclude some patients from the radical "curative" therapy that is offered to those without disseminated (widespread) disease, thus sparing them from fruitless, high-morbidity procedures for a nonremediable condition. The best screening examination for the detection of asymptomatic skeletal metastases is the

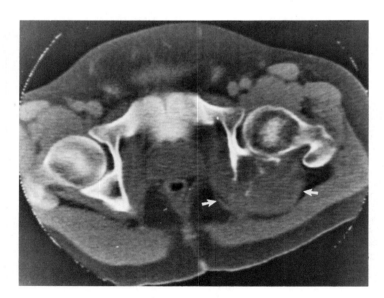

Figure 3-33 CT of osteogenic sarcoma. Scan through level of femoral heads shows destruction of left ischium that was seen on plain radiographs. In addition, CT scan demonstrates large soft-tissue mass (*arrows*) in area covered by gluteus maximus muscle and separated from rectum. Mass was not clinically palpable. *(From deSantos LA, Bernardino ME, and Murray JA: AJR 132:535-540, 1979.)*

radionuclide bone scan (Figure 3-34), which is unquestionably more sensitive than the radiographic "skeletal survey." Because almost half the mineral content of a bone must be lost before the loss is detectable on plain radiographs, the skeletal survey should be abandoned as a general screening examination for the detection of asymptomatic skeletal metastases. The only false-negative bone scans occur with aggressively osteolytic lesions, especially in patients with multiple myeloma. The role of plain radiographs in screening for metastases is to further evaluate focal abnormalities detected on radionuclide scanning, since a variety of lesions (e.g., infections, benign tumors, fibrous dysplasia, bone islands) can also give positive bone scans. Because the presence of multiple focal abnormalities is typical of metastatic disease, it is only necessary to radiographically examine a single lesion or area to confirm the diagnosis. In addition, because of the occasional false-negative bone scan, it is imperative that all *symptomatic* sites in patients with neoplastic disease be examined by plain radiographs unless the radionuclide bone scan unequivocally demonstrates diffuse metastatic disease.

Metastatic disease may produce a broad spectrum of radiographic appearances. Osteolytic metastases cause destruction without accompanying bone proliferation. They develop from tumor embolic deposits in the medullary canal and eventually extend to destroy cortical bone. The margins of the lucent lesions are irregular and poorly defined, rarely sharp and smooth. The most common primary lesions causing osteolytic metastases are carcinomas of the breast, kidney, and thyroid. Metastases from carcinomas of the kidney and thyroid typically produce a single large metastatic focus that may appear as an expansile trabeculated lesion ("blow-out") (Figure 3-35). Metastases from breast carcinoma are most often multiple when first detected.

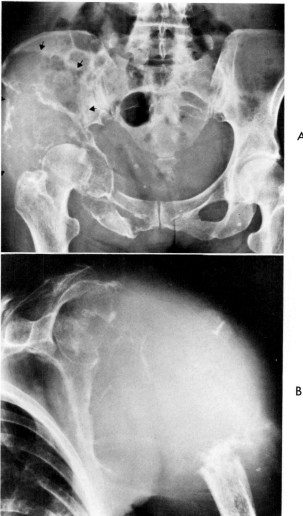

Figure 3-35 Blow-out metastases. **A**, Lytic expansile destruction of left ilium (*arrows*) in metastatic thyroid carcinoma. **B**, Osteolytic metastasis to humerus from carcinoma of kidney.

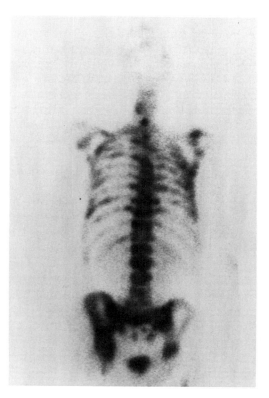

Figure 3-34 Screening radionuclide bone scan. Multiple focal areas of radionuclide uptake in axial skeleton, representing metastases from prostate carcinoma.

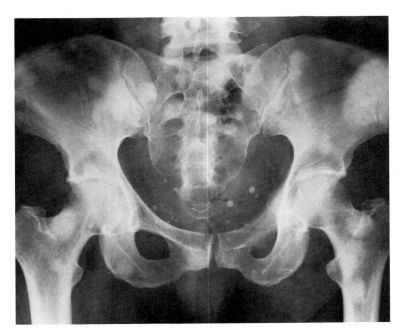

Figure 3-36   Osteoblastic metastases. Multiple areas of increased density involving pelvis and proximal femurs representing metastases from carcinoma of urinary bladder.

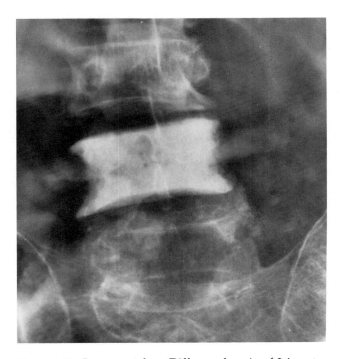

Figure 3-37   Ivory vertebra. Diffuse sclerosis of L4 vertebral body from metastatic carcinoma of prostate.

In the spine, osteolytic metastases tend to involve not only the vertebral bodies but also the pedicles and posterior arches. Destruction of one or more pedicles may be the earliest sign of metastatic disease and may help in differentiating this process from multiple myeloma, in which the pedicles are much less often involved. Because cartilage is resistant to invasion by metastases, preservation of the intervertebral disk space may help to distinguish metastases from an inflammatory process. Pathologic collapse of vertebral bodies frequently occurs in advanced disease.

Osteoblastic metastases are generally considered evidence of slow growth in a neoplasm that has allowed time for a proliferation of reactive bone. In men, osteoblastic metastases are usually a result of carcinoma of the prostate gland; carcinoma of the breast is the most common primary site of osteoblastic metastases in woman. These lesions initially appear as ill-defined areas of increased density that may progress to complete loss of normal bony architecture. They may vary from small, isolated round foci of sclerotic density to a diffuse sclerosis involving most or all of a bone (Figure 3-36). In the spine, this may produce the characteristic uniform density of an "ivory" vertebral body (Figure 3-37).

The combination of destruction and sclerosis in the mixed type of metastasis causes the affected bone to have a mottled appearance, with intermixed areas of lucency and increased density.

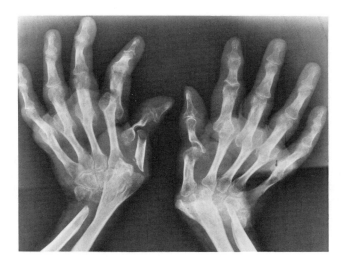

Figure 3-38 Mutilating rheumatoid arthritis. Severe, bilaterally symmetric destructive changes of hands and wrists with striking subluxations.

ARTHRITIS

Rheumatoid arthritis

Rheumatoid arthritis is a chronic systemic disease of unknown cause that primarily is seen as a non-suppurative (noninfectious) inflammatory arthritis of the small joints of the hands and feet. Women are affected about three times more frequently than men, and the average age of onset in adults is 40 years. Rheumatoid arthritis usually has an insidious origin and may either run a protracted and progressive course, leading to a crippling deformity of affected joints, or undergo spontaneous remissions of variable length. There is usually symmetric involvement of multiple joints, and the disease often progresses proximally toward the trunk until practically every joint in the body is involved.

Rheumatoid arthritis begins as an inflammation of the synovial membrane that lines the joints. The resulting mass of thickened granulation tissue (pannus) causes erosion of the articular cartilage and underlying bony cortex, fibrous scarring, and even the development of ankylosis (bony fusion across a joint). A combination of fusion of joint surfaces combined with inflammatory laxity of ligaments leads to the development of crippling deformities in the end-stage of the disease (Figure 3-38).

The earliest radiographic evidence of rheumatoid arthritis is fusiform periarticular soft-tissue swelling caused by joint effusion and hyperplastic synovial inflammation. Disuse and local hyperemia (increased blood flow) lead to periarticular osteoporosis that initially is confined to the portion of bone adjacent to the joint but may extend to involve the entire bone (Figure 3-39). Extension of the pannus

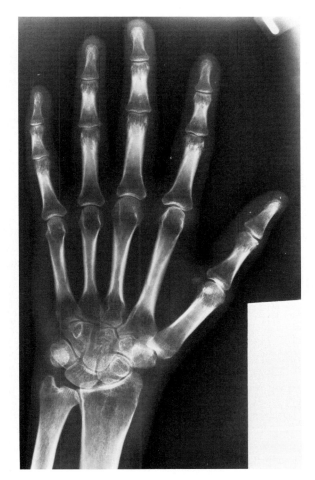

Figure 3-39 Rheumatoid arthritis. Striking periarticular osteoporosis. *(From Brown JC and Forrester DM: Arthritis. In Eisenberg RL and Amberg JR, editors: Critical diagnostic pathways in radiology, Philadelphia, JB Lippincott, 1981.)*

from the synovial reflections onto the bone causes characteristic small foci of destruction at the edges of the joint, where articular cartilage is absent. These typical marginal erosions have poorly defined edges without a sclerotic rim and sometimes may be seen only on oblique or magnification views. Destruction of articular cartilage causes narrowing of the joint space. The laying down of bony trabeculae across a narrow joint space may completely obliterate the joint cavity and produce solid bony ankylosis, which most frequently involves the bones of the wrist.

Ligamentous involvement produces a variety of contractures and subluxations and the common ulnar deviation of the hands. In the cervical spine, rheumatoid arthritis characteristically produces at-

lantoaxial subluxation (Figure 3-40), an increased distance between the anterior border of the odontoid and the superior border of the anterior arch of the atlas (normally less than 2.5 mm), which is caused by weakening of the transverse ligaments from synovial inflammation.

Rheumatoid nodules are soft-tissue masses that usually appear over the extensor surfaces on the ulnar aspect of the wrist or the olecranon but occasionally are seen over other body prominences, tendons, or pressure points. These characteristic nodules are seen in no other disease and develop in about 20% of patients with rheumatoid arthritis.

Rheumatoid variants

Ankylosing spondylitis, Reiter's syndrome, and psoriatic arthritis are variants of rheumatoid arthritis. **Ankylosing spondylitis** almost always begins in the sacroiliac joints, causing bilateral and usually symmetric involvement. Blurring of the articular margins and patchy sclerosis generally progress to narrowing of the joint space and may lead to complete fibrous and bony ankylosis (Figure 3-41). The disease typically progresses from the lumbar spine upward. Ossification in the paravertebral tissues and longitudinal spinal ligaments combines with extensive lateral bony bridges (syndesmophytes) between vertebral bodies to produce the characteristic "bamboo spine" of advanced disease. Limitation of activity leads to generalized skeletal osteoporosis and a tendency to fracture in response to the stress of minor trauma (Figure 3-42).

Reiter's syndrome is characterized by arthritis, urethritis, and conjunctivitis. It primarily affects

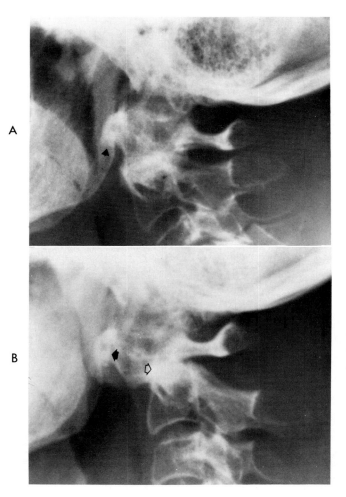

Figure 3-40 Subluxation of atlantoaxial joint in rheumatoid arthritis. **A**, Routine lateral film of cervical spine shows normal relation between anterior border of odontoid process and superior portion of anterior arch of atlas (*arrow*). **B**, With flexion, there is wide separation between anterior arch of atlas (*solid arrow*) and odontoid (*open arrow*).

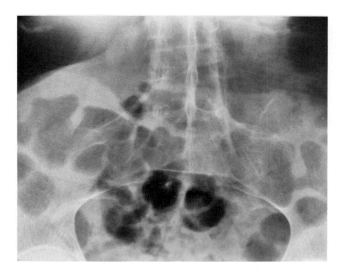

Figure 3-41 Ankylosing spondylitis. Bilateral, symmetric obliteration of sacroiliac joints and "bamboo spine."

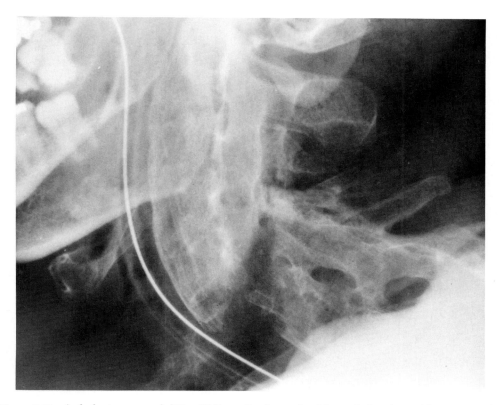

Figure 3-42 Ankylosing spondylitis. Oblique fracture of mid cervical spine with anterior dislocation of superior segment is seen in patient who fell while dancing and struck his head. Fracture extends through lateral mass and lamina.

young adult men and appears to be a postinfectious syndrome after certain types of venereal or gastrointestinal infections. Reiter's syndrome most frequently involves the sacroiliac joints, heel, and toes (Figure 3-43). Unlike ankylosing spondylitis, sacroiliac involvement is usually bilateral but asymmetric, and Reiter's syndrome tends to cause only minimal changes in the spine. Although the radiographic changes in peripheral joints often mimic rheumatoid arthritis, Reiter's syndrome tends to be asymmetric and primarily involves the feet rather than the hands (Figure 3-44).

Psoriatic arthritis refers to a rheumatoid-like destructive process involving peripheral joints that develops in patients with typical skin changes of psoriasis (Figure 3-45). Unlike rheumatoid arthritis, psoriatic arthritis predominantly involves the distal rather than the proximal interphalangeal joints of the hands and feet, produces asymmetric rather than symmetric destruction, and causes little or no periarticular osteoporosis. Characteristic findings include bony ankylosis of the interphalangeal joints of the hands and feet and resorption of the terminal tufts of the distal phalanges (Figure 3-46).

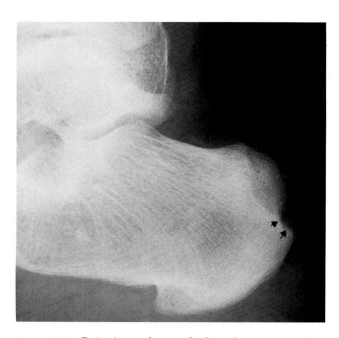

Figure 3-43 Reiter's syndrome. Striking bony erosion (*arrows*) at insertion of Achilles tendon on posterosuperior margin of calcaneus.

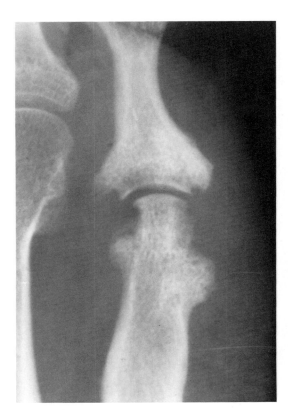

Figure 3-44 Reiter's syndrome. Erosive changes about metatarsophalangeal joint of fifth digit. Erosions involve juxta-articular region, leaving articular cortex intact.

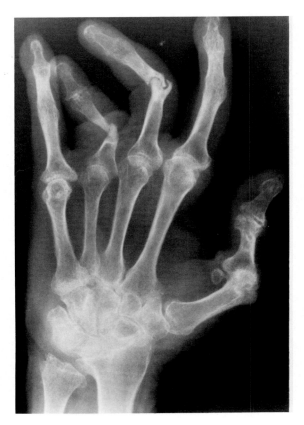

Figure 3-45 Psoriatic arthritis. Bizarre pattern of asymmetric bone destruction, subluxation, and ankylosis. Note particularly pencil-in-cup deformity of third proximal interphalangeal joint and bony ankylosis involving wrist and phalanges of second and fifth digits.

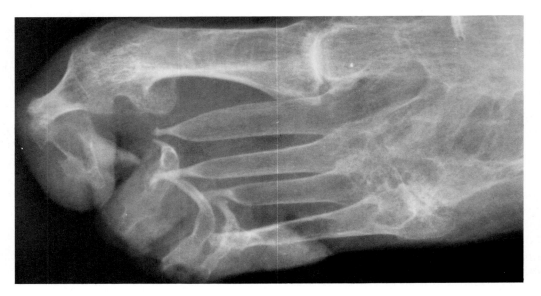

Figure 3-46 Psoriatic arthritis. Severe mutilating arthritis of foot and ankle. There is extreme pencil-like destruction of metatarsals and phalanges with ankylosis of almost all tarsal joints.

Osteoarthritis (degenerative joint disease)

Osteoarthritis is an extremely common generalized disorder that is characterized pathologically by loss of joint cartilage and reactive new bone formation. Part of the wear and tear of the aging process, degenerative joint disease tends to predominantly affect the weight-bearing joints (spine, hip, knee, ankle) and the interphalangeal joints of the fingers. A secondary form of degenerative joint disease may develop in a joint that has been repeatedly traumatized or subjected to abnormal stresses because of orthopedic deformities, or may be a result of a septic or inflammatory arthritis that destroys cartilage.

The earliest radiographic findings in degenerative joint disease are narrowing of the joint space, caused by thinning of the articular cartilage, and development of small bony spurs (osteophytes) along the margins of the articular edges of the bones. In contrast to the smooth, even narrowing of the joint space in rheumatoid arthritis, the joint space narrowing in degenerative joint disease is irregular and more pronounced in that part of the joint in which weight-bearing stress is greatest and degeneration of the articular cartilage is most marked. The articular ends of the bones become increasingly dense (periarticular sclerosis). Erosion of the articular cortex may produce typical irregular, cystlike lesions with sclerotic margins in the subchondral bone near the joint. Calcific or ossified loose bodies may de-

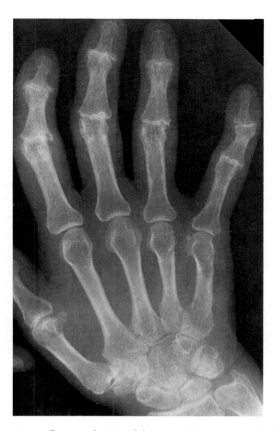

Figure 3-47 Osteoarthritis of fingers. Narrowing of interphalangeal joints with spurring and erosions.

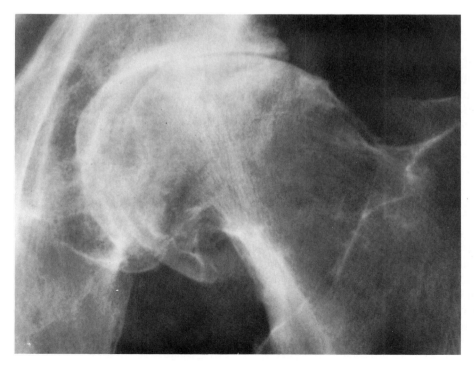

Figure 3-48 Osteoarthritis of hip.

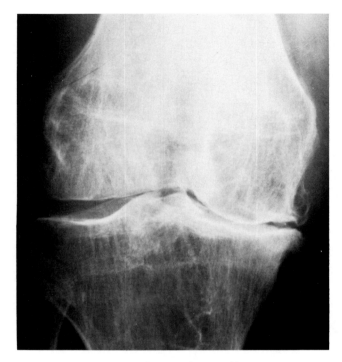

Figure 3-49   Osteoarthritis of knee.

velop, especially at the knee. With advanced disease, relaxation of the joint capsule and other ligamentous structures may lead to subluxation. Local osteoporosis does not occur unless pain causes prolonged disuse of the joint.

In the fingers degenerative joint disease primarily involves the distal interphalangeal joints (Figure 3-47). Marginal spurs produce well-defined bony protuberances that appear clinically as the palpable and visible knobby thickening of Heberden's nodes. In the hip the most prominent finding is asymmetric narrowing of the joint space that predominantly involves the superior and lateral aspects of the joint, where the stress of weight bearing is greatest (Figure 3-48). Joint space narrowing is also asymmetric in the knee, where it predominantly involves the medial femorotibial compartment (Figure 3-49).

Infectious arthritis

Pyogenic (pus-forming) organisms may gain entry into a joint by the hematogenous route, by direct extension from an adjacent focus of osteomyelitis, or from trauma to the joint (surgery, needling). The onset of bacterial arthritis is usually abrupt, with high fever, shaking chills, and one or a few severely tender and swollen joints.

Soft-tissue swelling is the first radiographic sign of acute bacterial arthritis. In children, fluid distention of the joint capsule may cause widening of

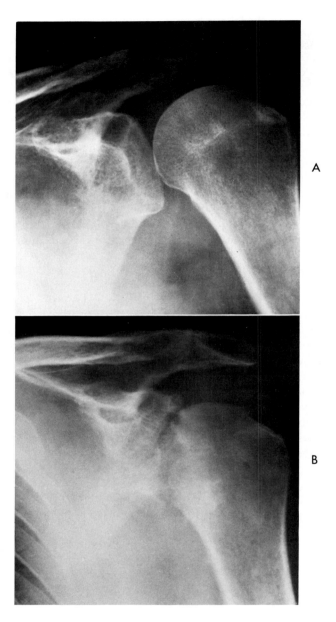

Figure 3-50   Acute staphylococcal arthritis. **A,** Several days after instrumentation of shoulder for joint pain, there is separation of humeral head from glenoid fossa caused by fluid in joint space. **B,** Six weeks later there is marked cartilage and bone destruction, with sclerosis on both sides of glenohumeral joint.

the joint space and actual subluxation, especially about the hip and shoulder. Periarticular edema displaces or obliterates adjacent tissue fat planes (Figure 3-50, *A*). Rapid destruction of articular cartilage causes joint space narrowing early in the course of the disease. The earliest bone changes, which tend to appear 8 to 10 days after the onset of symptoms, are small focal erosions in the articular cortex. Be-

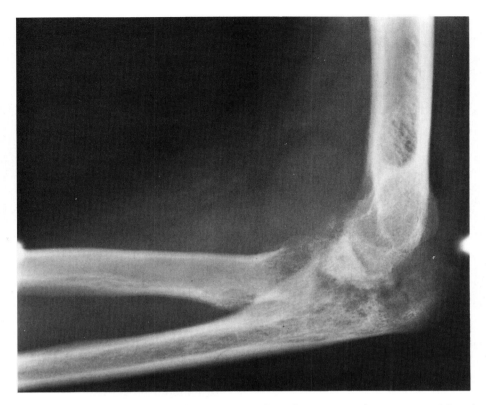

Figure 3-51 Tuberculous arthritis of elbow. Complete destruction of joint space. Note large chronic granulomatous mass in antecubital region. *(From Forrester DM, Brown JC, and Nesson JW: The radiology of joint disease. Philadelphia, WB Saunders, 1978.)*

cause of the delay in bone changes, detection of the characteristic soft-tissue abnormalities is essential for early diagnosis. Severe, untreated infections cause extensive destruction and a loss of the entire cortical outline (Figure 3-50, *B*). With healing, sclerotic bone reaction results in an irregular articular surface. If the articular cartilage has been completely destroyed, bony ankylosis usually follows.

Tuberculous arthritis is a chronic, indolent infection that has an insidious onset and a slowly progressive course (Figure 3-51). Usually involving only one joint, tuberculous arthritis primarily affects the spine, hips, and knees. Most patients have a focus of tuberculosis elsewhere in the body, most commonly the lungs.

A distinctive early radiographic feature of tuberculous arthritis is extensive juxta-articular osteoporosis that precedes bone destruction in contrast to bacterial arthritis, in which osteoporosis is a relatively late finding. Joint effusion leads to a nonspecific periarticular soft-tissue swelling. Cartilage and bone destruction occur relatively late in the course of tuberculous arthritis and tend to initially involve the periphery of the joint, sparing the maximal–

weight bearing surfaces that are destroyed in pyogenic arthritis. Therefore joint space narrowing occurs late in tuberculous arthritis in contrast to the early narrowing with bacterial infections. As in pyogenic arthritis, the earliest evidence of bone destruction is usually erosion at the margins of the articular ends of bone. With progressive disease there is ragged destruction of the articular cartilage and subchondral cortex and disorganization of the joint, often with preservation of necrotic fragments of bone (sequestra) that may involve apposing surfaces ("kissing sequestra").

Bursitis

Bursitis refers to an inflammation of the bursae, small fluid-filled sacs located near the joints that reduce friction on movement. The major radiographic manifestation of this condition is the deposition of calcification in adjacent tendons, which is a common cause of pain, limitation of motion, and disability about a joint. Calcific tendinitis most commonly involves the shoulder, and calcification may be demonstrated radiographically in about half the patients with persistent pain and disability in the shoulder

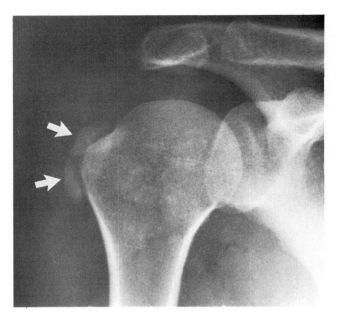

Figure 3-52 Calcific tendinitis. Frontal view of shoulder demonstrates amorphous calcium deposits (*arrows*) in supraspinatus tendon.

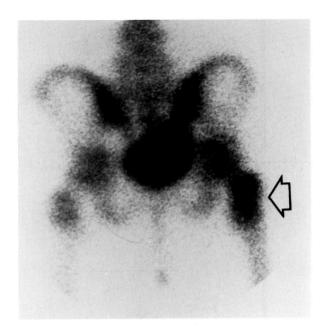

Figure 3-53 Osteomyelitis. Radionuclide bone scan (posterior projection) demonstrates increased uptake of radionuclide in trochanteric portion of right femur (*arrow*). Plain film of pelvis and hips obtained at same time showed no detectable abnormality.

region (Figure 3-52). However, calcification may also be detected in asymptomatic persons; conversely, severe clinical symptoms may occur without evidence of calcification. Calcific tendinitis appears as amorphous calcium deposits that most frequently occur about the shoulder in the supraspinatous tendon, where they are seen directly above the greater tuberosity of the humerus. The deposits vary greatly in size and shape, from thin curvilinear densities to large calcific masses.

OSTEOMYELITIS

Bacterial osteomyelitis

Osteomyelitis is an inflammation of the bone (osteitis) and bone marrow (myelitis) that is caused by a broad spectrum of infectious organisms that reach bone by hematogenous spread, by extension from an adjacent site of infection, or by direct introduction of organisms (trauma or surgery). Acute hematogenous osteomyelitis tends to involve bones with rich red marrow. In infants and children the metaphyses of long bones, especially the femur and tibia, are most often affected; staphylococci and streptococci are the most common organisms. In adults acute hematogenous osteomyelitis primarily occurs in the vertebrae and rarely involves the long bones. Although the incidence and severity of osteomyelitis

have decreased since the advent of antibiotics, this disease has recently become more prevalent as a complication of intravenous drug abuse. In diabetic patients and those with other types of vascular insufficiency, a soft-tissue infection may spread from a skin abscess or a decubitus ulcer, usually in the foot, to cause cellulitis and eventually osteomyelitis in adjacent bones.

Osteomyelitis begins as an abscess of the bone. Pus produced by the acute inflammation spreads down the medullary cavity and outward to the surface. Once the infectious process has reached the outer margin of the bone, it raises the periosteum from the bone and may spread along the surface for a considerable distance.

Because the earliest changes of osteomyelitis are usually not evident on plain radiographs until about 10 days after the onset of symptoms, radionuclide bone scanning is the most valuable imaging modality for the early diagnosis of osteomyelitis. Increased nuclide uptake, reflecting the inflammatory process and increased blood flow, is evident within hours of the onset of symtoms (Figure 3-53).

On plain radiographs the earliest evidence of osteomyelitis in a long bone is a localized, deep soft-tissue swelling adjacent to the metaphysis. The inflammation causes displacement or obliteration of the normal fat planes adjacent to and between the

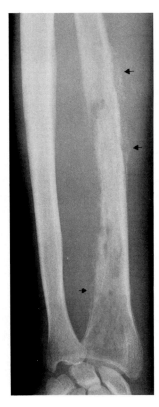

Figure 3-54 Osteomyelitis. Patchy pattern of bone destruction involves much of shaft of radius. Note early periosteal new bone formation (*arrows*).

deep muscle bundles, unlike skin infections, in which the initial swelling is superficial. The initial bony change is subtle areas of metaphyseal lucency reflecting resorption of necrotic bone. Soon, bone destruction becomes more prominent, producing a ragged, moth-eaten appearance (Figures 3-54 and 3-55). The more virulent the organism, the larger the area of destruction. Subperiosteal spread of inflammation elevates the periosteum and stimulates the laying down of layers of new bone parallel to the shaft. This results in a layered periosteal reaction that is characteristic of benign diseases, especially infection. Eventually, a large amount of new bone surrounds the cortex in a thick, irregular bony sleeve (involucrum). Disruption of cortical blood supply leads to bone necrosis. Segments of avascular dead bone (sequestra) remain as dense as normal bone and are clearly differentiated from the demineralized bone, infected granulation tissue, and pus about them (Figure 3-56).

After the acute infection has subsided, a pattern of chronic osteomyelitis develops. The bone appears thickened and sclerotic with an irregular outer margin. The cortex may become so dense that the medullary cavity is difficult to demonstrate. Reactivation of infection may appear as the recurrence of deep soft-tissue swelling, periosteal calcification, or the development of lytic abscess cavities within the bone. However, plain radiographs are often inade-

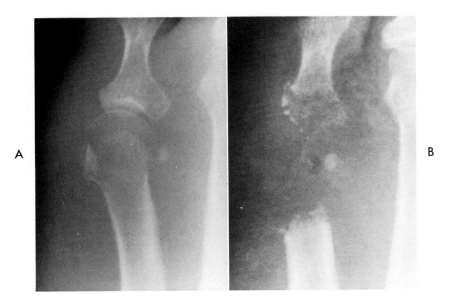

Figure 3-55 Staphylococcal osteomyelitis. **A,** Initial film of first metatarsophalangeal joint shows soft-tissue swelling and periarticular demineralization owing to increased blood flow to region. **B,** Several weeks later, there is severe bony destruction about metatarsophalangeal joint.

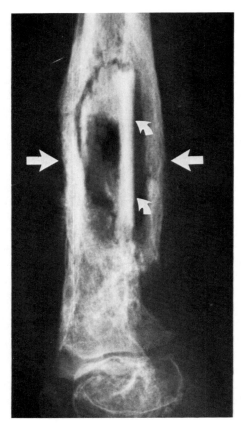

Figure 3-56 Chronic osteomyelitis. Involucrum (*straight arrows*) surrounds sequestrum (*curved arrows*).

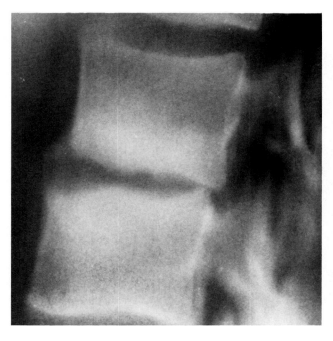

Figure 3-57 Bacterial vertebral osteomyelitis. Narrowing of intervertebral disk space with irregularity of end plates and reactive sclerosis.

quate to determine whether an active infection is present. Radionuclide scanning is much more sensitive and accurate in establishing a recurrence.

The earliest sign of vertebral osteomyelitis is subtle erosion of the subchondral bony plate with loss of the sharp cortical outline. This may progress to total destruction of the vertebral body associated with a paravertebral soft-tissue abscess (Figure 3-57). Unlike neoplastic processes, osteomyelitis usually affects the intervertebral disk space and often involves adjacent vertebrae. Depending on the site of disease, anterior extension of osteomyelitis may cause retropharyngeal abscess, mediastinitis, empyema, pericarditis, subdiaphragmatic abscess, psoas muscle abscess, or peritonitis; posterior extension of inflammatory tissue can compress the spinal cord or produce meningitis if the infection penetrates the dura to enter the subarachnoid space.

CT can be of value in the diagnosis of osteomyelitis, especially that involving the spine. This modality can precisely define the size of the surrounding soft-tissue mass, its relation to nearby vital structures (aorta, spinal cord), and the presence of abscess cavities requiring surgical drainage.

Tuberculous osteomyelitis

Tuberculous osteomyelitis most commonly involves the thoracic and lumbar spine. The infection tends to begin in the anterior part of the vertebral body adjacent to the intervertebral disk (Figure 3-58, *A*). Irregular, poorly marginated bone destruction within the vertebral body is often associated with a characteristic paravertebral abscess, an accumulation of purulent material that produces a fusiform soft-tissue mass about the vertebra. The spread of tuberculous osteomyelitis causes narrowing of the adjacent intervertebral disk and the extension of infection and bone destruction across the disk to involve the adjacent vertebral body. Unlike bacterial infection, tuberculous osteomyelitis is rarely associated with periosteal reaction or bone sclerosis. In the untreated patient progressive vertebral collapse and anterior wedging lead to a characteristic sharp kyphotic angulation (gibbus deformity) (Figure 3-58, *B*).

Tuberculosis can produce a low-grade chronic infection of the long bones that appears radiographically as a generally destructive lytic process with minimal or no periosteal reaction. The spectrum of radiographic appearances is wide, varying from localized, well-circumscribed, expansile lesions to diffuse uniform, honeycomb-like areas of destruction that are often associated with pathologic fractures. Chronic draining sinuses may develop, especially in children.

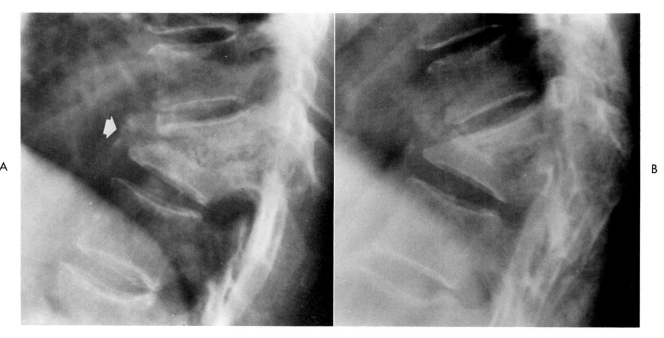

Figure 3-58 A, Initial film demonstrates vertebral collapse and anterior wedging of adjacent midthoracic vertebrae (*arrow*). Residual intervertebral disk space can barely be seen. **B**, Several months later there is virtual fusion of collapsed vertebral bodies, producing characteristic sharp kyphotic angulation (gibbus deformity).

FRACTURES

Fractures are the most common skeletal abnormality seen in a general radiology practice. A fracture is defined as a disruption of bone caused by mechanical forces applied either directly to the bone or transmitted along the shaft of a bone. Although often obvious, some fractures are subtle and difficult to detect. A fracture typically appears as a radiolucent line crossing the bone and disrupting the cortical margins. However, the fracture line may be thin and easily overlooked, whereas overlap of fragments may produce a radiopaque line. Secondary signs of underlying fracture include joint effusion, soft-tissue swelling, and interruption of the normal pattern of bony trabeculae.

Fractures are described and classified by the extent, direction, position, and number of fracture lines and the integrity of the overlying skin (Figure 3-59). A fracture that results in discontinuity between two or more fragments is **complete**; an **incomplete** fracture causes only partial discontinuity, with a portion of the cortex remaining intact. In **closed** fractures, the overlying skin is intact; if the overlying skin is disrupted, the fracture is **open**, or **compound**. Although this is a clinical distinction, the radiographic demonstration of bone clearly protruding through the skin and the presence of air and soft tissues about the fracture site on immediate postinjury radiographs are findings that are highly suggestive of an open fracture.

The direction of a fracture is determined by its relation to the long axis of long and short bones and to the longest axis of irregular bones (e.g., the talus or carpal navicular). A **transverse** fracture runs at a right angle to the long axis of a bone and is most commonly the result of a direct blow or a fracture within pathologic bone. An **oblique** fracture runs a course of approximately 45 degrees to the long axis of the bone and is the result of angulation or angulation and compression forces. A **spiral** fracture encircles the shaft, is generally longer than an oblique fracture, and is caused by torsional forces. **Avulsion** fractures are generally small fragments torn off from bony prominences; they are usually the result of indirectly applied tension forces within attached ligaments and tendons rather than direct blows.

A **comminuted** fracture is composed of more than two fragments. A **butterfly** fragment is an elongated triangular fragment of cortical bone generally detached from two other larger fragments of bone; a **segmental** fracture consists of a segment of the shaft isolated by proximal and distal lines of fracture.

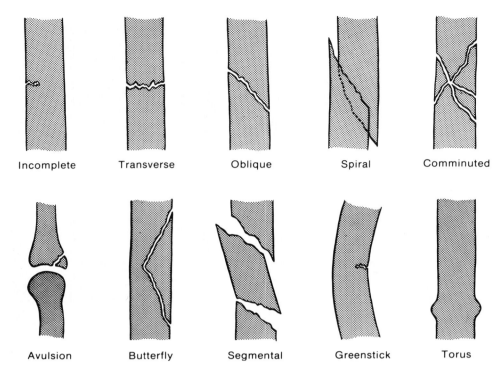

Figure 3-59   Classification of fractures. *(From Eisenberg R: Diagnostic imaging in surgery, New York, McGraw-Hill Book Co, 1987.)*

A **compression** fracture results from a compression force that causes compaction of bone trabeculae and results in decreased length or width of a portion of a bone. Compression fractures most commonly occur in the vertebral body as a result of flexion of the spine; they may also be seen as impacted fractures of the humeral or femoral heads. A **depressed** fracture occurs in the skull or tibial plateau. In the skull a small object with great force can produce a comminuted fracture with portions of the fracture fragment driven inward. In the knee the relatively hard lateral femoral condyle may impact on the relatively soft lateral tibial plateau with sufficient force to push the cortical surface of the tibia into the underlying cancellous bone.

A **stress**, or **fatigue**, fracture is the response of bone to repeated stresses, no one of which is sufficient to cause a fracture. The earliest pathologic process in a stress fracture is osteoclastic resorption, followed by the development of periosteal callus in an attempt to repair and strengthen the bone. A **pathologic** fracture occurs in bone at an area of weakness, caused by such processes as tumor, infection, or metabolic bone disease.

A **greenstick** fracture is an incomplete fracture with the opposite cortex intact. Greenstick fractures are found almost exclusively in infants and children because of the softness of their cancellous bone. A

torus (buckle) fracture is one in which one cortex is intact with buckling or compaction of the opposite cortex. A **bowing** fracture is a plastic deformation caused by a stress that is too great to permit a complete recovery of normal shape but is less than the stress required to produce a fracture.

A fracture is **undisplaced** when a plane of cleavage exists in the bone without angulation or separation. **Displacement** refers to separation of bone fragments; the direction of displacement is described by the relation of the distal fragment with respect to the proximal fragment and is usually measured in terms of the thickness of the shaft. **Angulation** indicates an angular deformity between the axes of the major fragments and is also described by the position of the distal fragment with respect to the proximal one. **Dislocation** refers to displacement of a bone so that it is not in contact with its normal articulation. If there is only partial loss of continuity of the joint surfaces, the displacement is called a **subluxation.**

Radiographs are essential in the diagnosis and management of fractures. Initially, a radiograph documents the clinically suspected fracture and determines whether the underlying bone is normal or whether the fracture is pathologic and has occurred in abnormal bone. After the orthopedic reduction of a fracture, repeat radiographs are required to determine whether the fracture fragments are in good position. Over the next several weeks or months, additional radiographs are obtained to assess fracture healing and to exclude possible complications.

In all cases of trauma, it is essential to have at least two projections of the injured part, preferably taken at 90 degrees to each other. It is also important to demonstrate the joint above and below the fracture to search for a dislocation or second fracture that may have resulted from transmission of the mechanical force. An example of this mechanism is the fracture or dislocation of the head of the fibula that frequently occurs with a fracture of the distal tibia at the ankle.

Fracture treatment

The overall goal of fracture treatment is to restore function and stability with an acceptable cosmetic result and a minimum of residual deformity. In **external**, or **closed**, reduction the fracture is treated by manipulation of the affected body part without surgical incision. **Open reduction** is a surgical procedure in which there is direct or indirect manipulation of the fracture fragments and usually the application or insertion of some type of appliance or device to achieve and maintain the reduction (Figure 3-60). **External fixation** is accomplished by the use of splints or casts; **internal fixation** uses metal plates and screws, wires, rods, or nails, either alone or in combination, to maintain the reduction.

Most reduced fractures are immobilized or protected by an overlying plaster of Paris cast. The radiopaque cast causes some obscuration of fine bony detail and, in severely osteoporotic bone, may make it difficult to visualize the fracture site. Therefore if there is a question of healing that requires the demonstration of early callus formation or if there is a possibility of osteomyelitis, it is essential that the cast be removed by the physician before obtaining radiographs so that there is sufficient visibility of bone detail to resolve these questions.

Fracture healing

The radiographic evidence of fracture healing is a continuous external bridge of callus (calcium deposition) that extends across the line of fracture and unites the fracture fragments (Figure 3-61). The callus is uniformly ossified and approaches the density

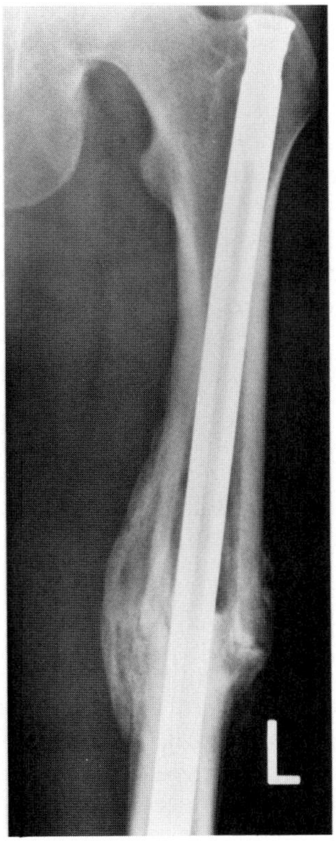

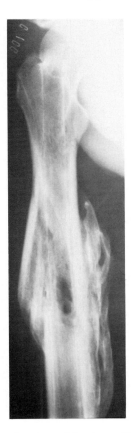

Figure 3-60 Open reduction with internal fixation. Intramedullary rod has been placed across fracture of femoral shaft. Note extensive callus formation about fracture site.

Figure 3-61 Normal union of fracture. There is dense callus formation bridging previous fracture of midshaft of femur. Original fracture line is completely obliterated.

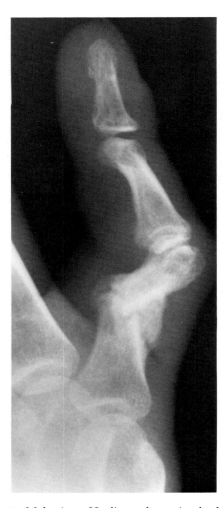

Figure 3-62 Malunion. Healing of proximal phalangeal fracture in poor position led to impairment of normal function.

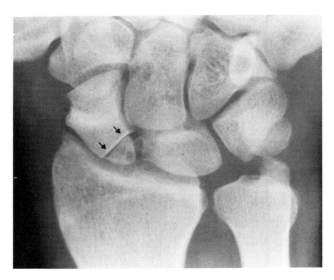

Figure 3-63 Nonunion of fracture of carpal navicular. Twenty years after initial injury, there is smooth, well-defined line of sclerosis (*arrows*) about fracture margin.

of normal bone. It is essential that at least two views be taken (preferably 90 degrees to each other) to be certain that there is callus about the fracture line in all directions. Proper exposure of the radiograph is required because underexposed films may produce the illusion of obliteration of the fracture line by bony trabeculae, whereas a properly exposed film would demonstrate the continued presence of the fracture line and the lack of healing. If the findings are equivocal, conventional tomography or CT may be required to determine the degree of union. "Stress" films, a series of radiographs obtained with the injured part in the neutral position and during the application of stress by a physician or designated assistant on the distal fragment or part in the plane of suspected motion, may demonstrate a change in the alignment of the fragment that indicates a lack of union.

Malunion is the healing of fragments of a fracture in a faulty position. This leads to impairment of normal function or cosmetic appearance that may require surgical correction (Figure 3-62).

Delayed union is an ill-defined term that is arbitrarily applied to any fracture that takes longer to heal than the average fracture at that anatomic location. Delayed union may result from infection or inadequate immobilization or from limited blood supply or loss of bone at the fracture site.

Nonunion refers to a condition in which the fracture healing process has completely stopped and the fragments will remain united even with prolonged immobilization. Radiographically, nonunion characteristically appears as smooth, well-defined sclerosis about the fracture margins with occlusion of the medullary canal by sclerotic bone (Figure 3-63). There is a persistent defect between the fragments, consisting of fibrous tissue and cartilage. Nonunion predominantly occurs in adults, is rare in children, and requires operative intervention to reinitiate the healing process.

Pathologic fractures

Pathologic fractures are those occurring in bone that has been weakened by a pre-existing condition. The most common underlying process is metastatic malignancy or multiple myeloma. In children developmental diseases such as osteogenesis imperfecta, osteopetrosis, or nutritional deficiencies (rickets, scurvy) may result in pathologic fractures. Pathologic fractures also may occur in benign causes of weakened bone, such as simple bone cyst, enchon-

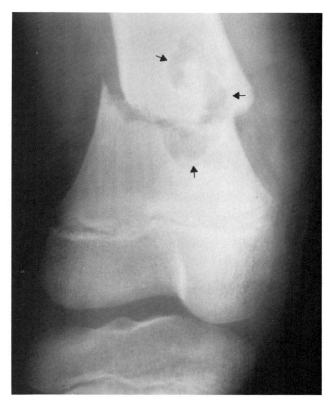

Figure 3-64 Pathologic fracture. There is transverse fracture crossing large benign tumor (*arrows*) of distal femur.

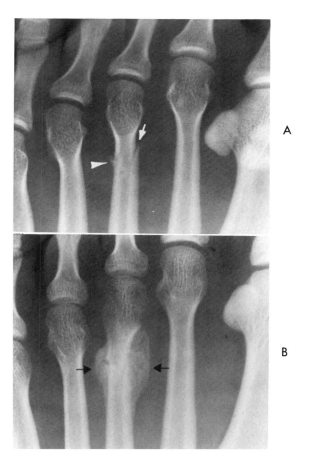

Figure 3-65 Stress fracture of third metacarpal. Initial radiograph was within normal limits. **A,** Radiograph obtained 14 days after onset of symptoms demonstrates thin oblique lucency (*arrow*) interrupting one cortex and small amount of fluffy periosteal callus formation (*arrowhead*) along opposite cortex. There is no evidence of complete fracture line. **B,** Three weeks later, repeat radiograph shows dense callus formation (*arrows*) about fracture site.

droma, aneurysmal bone cysts, and fibrous dysplasia. Metabolic disorders causing a diffuse loss of bone substance (osteoporosis, osteomalacia, hyperparathyroidism) also make the skeleton more susceptible to injury.

Clinically, pathologic fractures arise from minor trauma that would not affect normal bone. Radiographically, the fracture crosses an area of abnormal thinning, expansion, or bone destruction (Figure 3-64). The most frequent sites of pathologic fractures are the spine, femur, and humerus, areas in which metastatic disease is most common. In the spine a pathologic fracture results in collapse of the vertebral body; indeed, a compressed vertebra in a patient older than 40 years of age should suggest underlying myeloma or metastatic disease.

Remember that patients with suspected pathologic fractures must be handled with extreme care lest the radiographer cause either further injury to the bone in question or an additional pathologic fracture in another area.

Stress fractures

Stress (fatigue) fractures are the end result of repeated stresses to a bone that would not be injured by isolated forces of the same magnitude. The type of stress fracture and the site where it occurs vary with the activity. Regardless of location, the activities resulting in stress fractures are usually strenuous, often new or different, and repeated with frequency before producing pain. Stress fractures frequently occur in soldiers during basic training ("march" fracture). The most common sites are the shafts of the second and third metatarsals, the calcaneus, the proximal and distal shafts of the tibia and fibula, the shaft and neck of the femur, and the ischial and pubic rami.

Initially, plain radiographs of the symptomatic area are within normal limits (Figure 3-65, *A*). The stress fracture is first visualized 10 to 20 days after

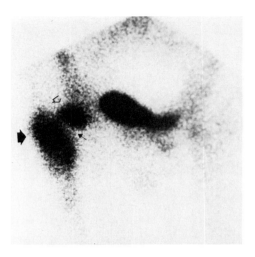

Figure 3-66 Radionuclide bone scan of stress fracture. Markedly increased radionuclide uptake in femoral neck (*open arrow*) and intertrochanteric region (*solid arrow*), with lack of uptake at actual fracture site (*thin arrow*). Plain radiograph and tomograms showed only minimal trabecular disruption and slight callus formation. (*From Dorn HL and Lander PH: AJR 144:343-347, 1985.*)

the onset of symptoms as either a thin line of transverse or occasionally oblique radiolucency or as fluffy periosteal callus formation without evidence of a fracture line. When this radiographic appearance is detected at a site where stress fractures are common, it is important to elicit a history of athletic or other unusual activity as the underlying cause.

Radionuclide bone scans can demonstrate a stress fracture before it can be detected on plain radiographs (Figure 3-66).

Battered-child syndrome

The battered-child syndrome refers to multiple, repeated traumatic injuries in young children caused by parents or guardians. The radiographic findings in this syndrome include multiple fractures of varying age in various stages of healing, fractures of the corners of metaphyses with or without associated epiphyseal displacement, and exuberant subperiosteal new bone formation along the shafts of long bones (Figure 3-67). Skull fractures or widening of the cranial sutures are commonly associated. Another highly suggestive finding is one or more frac-

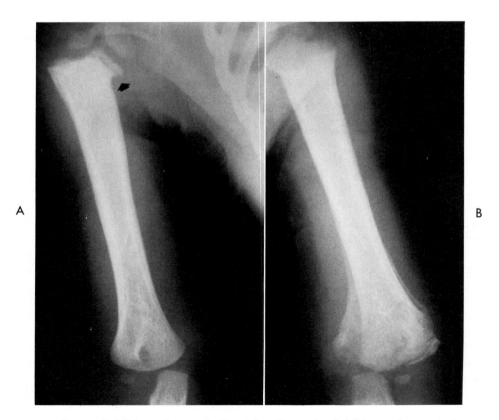

Figure 3-67 Battered-child syndrome. **A,** Frontal radiograph of right arm demonstrates corner fracture (*arrow*) of proximal humerus. **B,** Frontal radiograph of left arm shows healing displaced fracture of distal humerus. (*From Sty JR and Starshak RJ: The role of bone scintigraphy in evaluation of the suspected abused child, Radiology 146:369-375, 1983.*)

tures at otherwise unusual sites (only fractured by direct blows), such as the ribs, scapula, sternum, spine, or lateral ends of the clavicles. Prompt and accurate diagnosis of the battered-child syndrome is essential to minimize the extent of physical and psychologic damage and, in some cases, to prevent a fatal injury.

Common fractures and dislocations

Colles' fracture is a transverse fracture through the distal radius with dorsal (posterior) angulation and often overriding of the distal fracture fragment (Figure 3-68). In more than half the cases there is an associated avulsion fracture of the ulnar styloid process. Colles' fracture is usually caused by a fall on the outstretched hand and is the most common fracture about the wrist.

Navicular fractures are the most common fractures involving the carpal bones. They are usually transverse and occur through the central part (waist) of the bone. Although most navicular fractures can be identified on routine frontal projections of the wrist, subtle fractures may only be identified on specific oblique and angulated projections or on films made using magnification techniques. In some cases

a navicular fracture cannot be detected on the initial examination despite strong clinical suspicion (Figure 3-69, A). In this situation the wrist should be placed in a cast or plaster splint and re-examined (out of plaster) in 7 to 10 days. At this time, resorption of bone at the margins of the fracture widens the fracture line and makes it more apparent radiographically (Figure 3-69, B).

Nonunion is a serious complication of navicular fractures (see Figure 3-63). Its incidence is increased by motion or displacement of the fracture fragments caused either by poor immobilization or by neglected, untreated fractures. Because the blood supply to the navicular is derived primarily from the distal portion, the proximal fragment may become avascular and undergo ischemic necrosis. This appears as an increase in bone density associated with collapse of bone or loss of volume in the affected fragment (Figure 3-70).

A boxer's fracture refers to a transverse fracture of the neck of the fifth metacarpal with volar (palmar) angulation of the distal fragment (Figure 3-71). This injury typically is the result of a blow struck with the fist.

In the detection of fractures about the elbow, a

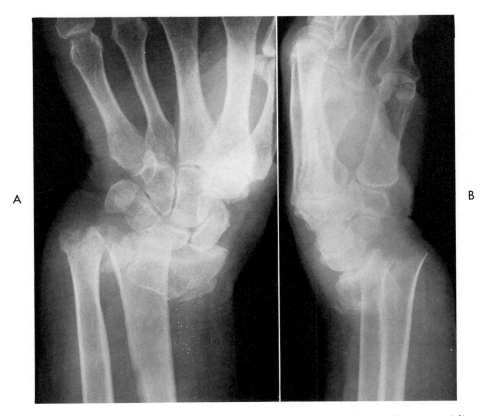

Figure 3-68 Colles' fracture. **A** Frontal and, **B**, lateral projections of wrist show overriding and dorsal displacement of distal fragment. There is also displaced fracture of distal ulna.

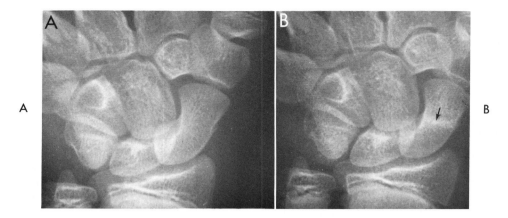

Figure 3-69 Fracture of navicular. **A,** On radiograph obtained immediately after injury, fracture cannot be detected. **B,** On repeat radiograph obtained 3 weeks later, fracture is clearly identified by sclerotic band (*arrow*) of opaque internal callus. (*From Silverman FN: Caffey's pediatric x-ray imaging, Chicago, Year Book Medical Publishers, 1985.*)

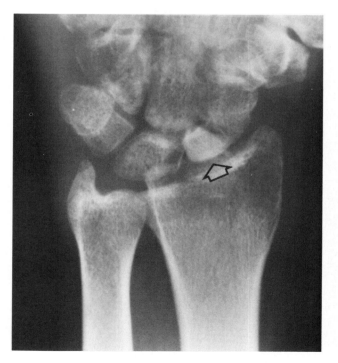

Figure 3-70 Avascular necrosis of navicular fracture. There is increased bone density in avascular proximal fragment (*arrow*).

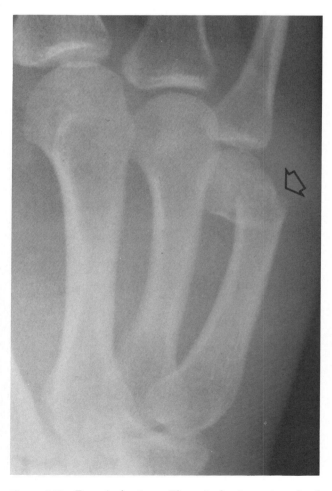

Figure 3-71 Boxer's fracture. There is fracture at neck of fifth metacarpal (*arrow*) with volar angulation of distal fragment.

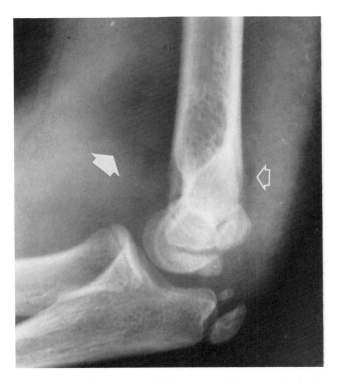

Figure 3-72 Elbow fat pad sign. Anterior fat pad (*solid arrow*) is clearly lifted from its fossa as result of large joint effusion in this child with supracondylar fracture of distal humerus. Normally hidden posterior fat pad is posteriorly displaced by effusion (*open arrow*).

valuable clue is displacement of the normal elbow fat pads (fat pad sign). On lateral projections of the elbow, the anterior fat pad normally appears as a radiolucency closely applied to the anterior surface of the distal end of the humerus. The posterior fat pad is normally hidden in the depths of the olecranon fossa and should not be visible on standard lateral projections of the elbow. Any process producing synovial or hemorrhagic effusion within the elbow joint displaces the fat pads. The normally hidden posterior fat pad is posteriorly displaced and becomes visible as a crescentic lucency behind the lower end of the humerus (Figure 3-72). The anterior fat pad becomes more rounded and further separated from the underlying bone. The posterior fat pad is by far the more sensitive indicator of an elbow joint effusion. Its presence on the lateral projection of the patient with elbow trauma is strongly suggestive of an underlying fracture, especially of the radial head, and indicates the need for oblique projections if no fracture is seen on standard projections. If no fracture is identified, a repeat radiograph obtained 2 weeks or more after appropriate immobilization will often show a fracture by demonstrating a fracture line or callus formation indicating healing.

Most fractures of the forearm involve both the radius and ulna. If only one bone is fractured, it is essential to examine both the elbow and the wrist to exclude the possibility of proximal or distal joint dislocation. A Monteggia fracture (Figure 3-73) refers to an isolated fracture of the shaft of the ulna associated with anterior dislocation of the radius at

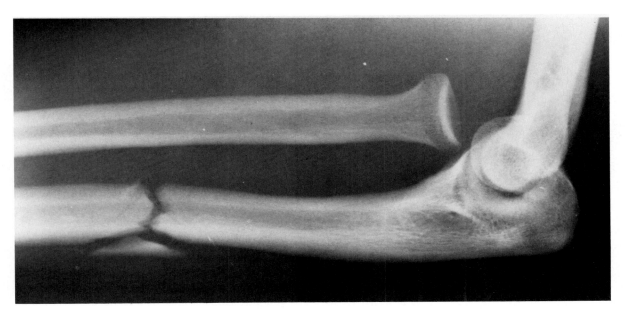

Figure 3-73 Monteggia fracture. Displaced fracture of ulnar shaft is associated with anterior dislocation of radial head.

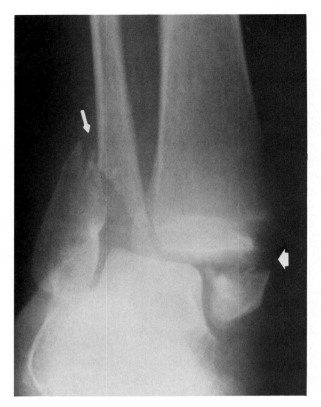

Figure 3-74 Bimalleolar fracture of ankle. There is transverse fracture of medial malleolus (*broad arrow*) associated with low oblique fracture of distal fibula (*thin arrow*).

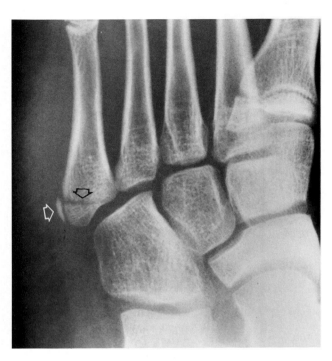

Figure 3-75 Fracture of base of fifth metatarsal. Note that fracture line is transverse (*black arrow*), whereas normal apophysis in this child has vertical orientation (*white arrow*).

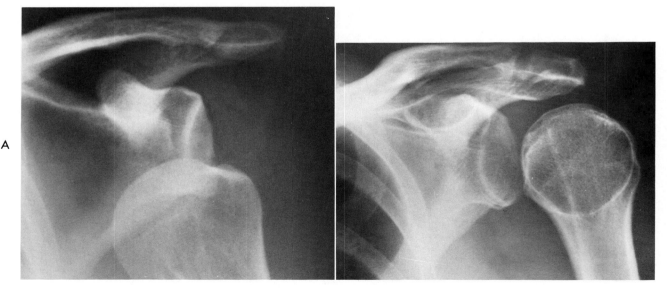

Figure 3-76 Dislocation of shoulder. **A,** Anterior. **B,** Posterior.

the elbow. A Galeazzi fracture refers to the combination of a fracture of the shaft of the radius and dorsal (posterior) dislocation of the ulna at the wrist.

Pott's fracture involves both malleoli (of tibia and fibula) with dislocation of the ankle joint. A bimalleolar fracture refers to one involving both the medial and the lateral malleoli (Figure 3-74). Because of the mechanism of injury, the fracture on one side is transverse, whereas the opposite fracture is oblique or spiral. Trimalleolar fractures involve the posterior lip of the tibia in addition to the medial and lateral malleoli and usually represent fracture dislocations.

One of the most frequent injuries of the foot is a transverse fracture at the base of the fifth metatarsal (Jones' fracture) (Figure 3-75). This fracture represents an avulsion injury that results from plantar flexion and inversion of the foot as in stepping off a curb or falling while walking on stairs. It is important to distinguish this fracture from the longitudinally oriented apophysis that is normally found in children at the lateral margin of the base of the fifth metatarsal.

The shoulder is by far the most commonly dislocated joint in the body (Figure 3-76). About 95% of shoulder dislocations are anterior and the result of external rotation and abduction of the arm. As the anterior displacement occurs, the posterolateral surface of the humeral head impacts against the anterior or anteroinferior surface of the glenoid fossa and may result in a compression fracture of the humeral head, a fracture of the glenoid rim, or both. In most cases, the humeral head is displaced medially and anteriorly and comes to rest beneath the coracoid process.

Dislocations of the hip, with or without associated fracture of the acetabulum, are caused by severe injuries such as automobile collisions, pedestrian accidents, or falls from a great height. Unlike the shoulder, posterior dislocations of the hip are far more common than anterior dislocations and account for 85% to 90% of the cases (Figure 3-77).

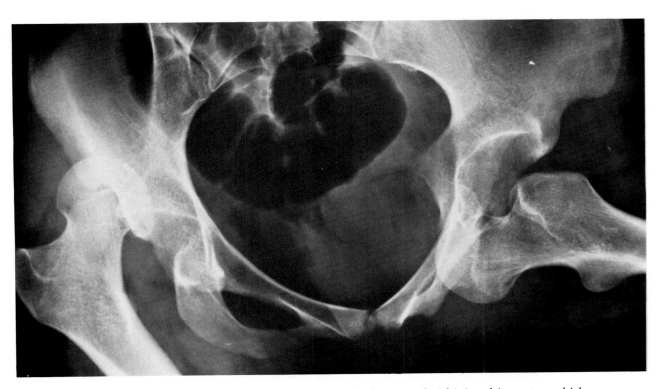

Figure 3-77 Dislocations of hip. Frontal radiograph of teenaged girl injured in motor vehicle collision demonstrates right posterior dislocation and left anterior dislocation of hip. Right posterior dislocation is characterized by typical superolateral displacement of femoral head, fixed adduction, and internal rotation (lesser trochanter superimposed on femoral shaft). Left anterior dislocation is manifested by characteristic inferomedial displacement of femoral head, which has come to overlie obturator foramen; fixed abduction; and external rotation (lesser trochanter depicted in profile). *(From Bassett, LW, Gold, RH, and Epstein HC: AJR 141:385-386, 1983.)*

FRACTURES AND DISLOCATIONS OF THE SPINE

Fractures and dislocations of the spine may be the result of direct trauma, hyperextension-flexion injuries (whiplash), or normal stresses in abnormal bone (osteoporosis, metastatic destruction). In the patient with spinal injury the major goal of the radiographic evaluation is to determine whether a fracture or dislocation is present and whether the injury is stable or unstable. The spine can be considered as consisting of two major columns. The anterior column is composed of the vertebral bodies, intervertebral disks, and anterior and posterior longitudinal ligaments. The posterior column is formed by the facets, apophyseal joints, pedicles, laminae, spinous processes, and all the intervening ligaments. If one of the two columns remains intact, the injury is considered **stable**. If both columns are disrupted, the injury is considered **unstable**.

If there is a strong suspicion of injury to the cervical spine, the initial radiograph should be a horizontal-beam lateral projection with the patient supine. This cross-table lateral radiograph *must* be checked by the physician before any other projections are obtained. It is essential to include all seven cervical vertebrae on the film lest the relatively common injuries of C6 and C7 be overlooked (Figure 3-78). This may require supine oblique projections or films made in the swimmer's projection, in which one arm of the patient is extended over the head while the other arm remains by the side so as to slightly oblique the upper torso and permit visualization of the cervicothoracic junction. A frontal projection of the spine and an open-mouth projection of the atlas and axis (C1 and C2) should be obtained next. In an acutely injured patient, oblique or flexion and extension projections should be performed *only* under the direct supervision of the attending physician. Conventional tomography may be used to

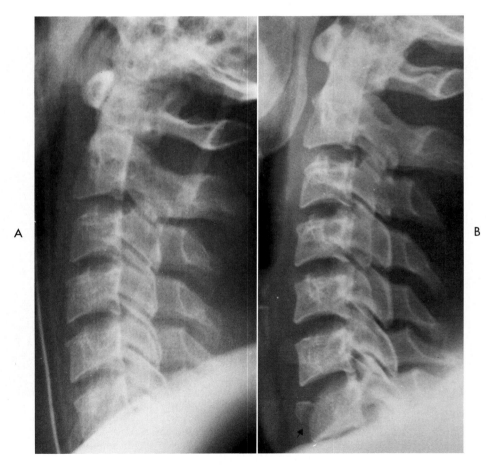

Figure 3-78 Fracture of C7 vertebral body. **A,** On initial lateral radiograph, only upper six cervical vertebrae can be seen. Patient's shoulders overlie seventh cervical vertebra. **B,** With shoulders pulled down to expose seventh cervical vertebra, anterosuperior fracture (*arrow*) is clearly identified.

confirm the presence or absence of a fracture (especially of the posterior elements) and to visualize otherwise obscured areas of the spine such as the craniovertebral and cervicothoracic junctions. CT can precisely localize fracture fragments in relation to the spinal canal and detect otherwise obscure fractures of the posterior elements. Myelography may be performed in patients with a spinal cord injury in the absence of an obvious fracture or dislocation to identify a condition amenable to surgical removal or repair (herniated disk fragment, epidural hematoma of the spinal cord).

There are several types of fractures peculiar to the cervical spine. A **Jefferson fracture** is a comminuted fracture of the ring of the atlas that involves both the anterior and posterior arches and causes displacement of the fragments. The characteristic appearance on frontal radiographs or tomograms is a bilateral offset or spreading of the lateral articular masses of C1 in relation to the apposing articular surfaces of C2 (Figure 3-79).

Fractures of the odontoid process are usually transverse and located at the base of the dens at its junction with the body (Figure 3-80). On an open-mouth view, a lucency between the upper central incisor teeth often overlaps the dens; this must be differentiated from a rare vertical fracture of the dens.

The **hangman's fracture** is the result of acute hyperextension of the head on the neck. This appears as a fracture of the arch of C2 anterior to the inferior facet and is usually associated with anterior subluxation of C2 on C3 (Figure 3-81). Although originally described in patients who had been hanged, this injury is now far more commonly the result of motor vehicle accidents.

Clay shoveler's fracture refers to an avulsion fracture of a spinous process in the lower cervical or upper thoracic spine. The fracture is difficult to dem-

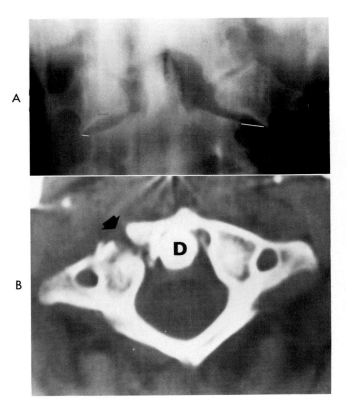

Figure 3-79 Jefferson fracture. **A,** On frontal projection, there is lateral displacement of lateral masses of C1 bilaterally (*white lines*). **B,** CT scan in another patient shows unilateral break in arch of C1 (*arrow*). *D,* Dens.

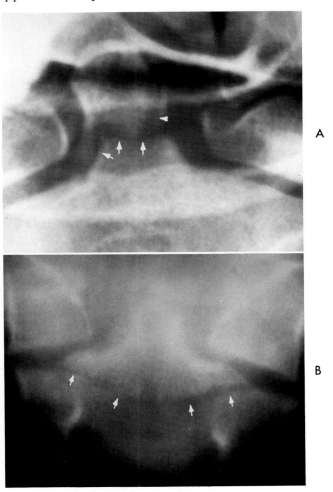

Figure 3-80 Fracture of odontoid process. **A,** Open-mouth frontal projection shows combined oblique and transverse fracture at base of dens (*arrows*). There is also separate cortical fragment on left (*arrowhead*), which most likely remains attached to alar ligament. **B,** In another patient, frontal tomogram shows low fracture (*arrows*) through body of C2.

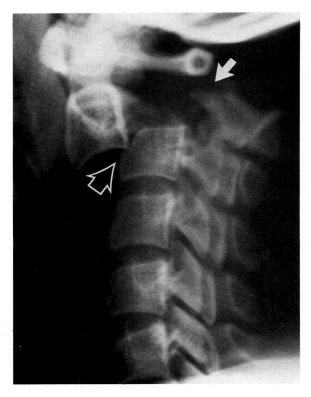

Figure 3-81 Hangman's fracture. Neural arch fracture (*solid arrow*) associated with complete C2-3 subluxation (*open arrow*). (*From Osborn, AG: Head trauma. In Eisenberg RL and Amberg JR, editors: Critical diagnostic pathways in radiology, Philadelphia, JB Lippincott, 1981.*)

onstrate on emergency cross-table lateral radiographs because the shoulders frequently obscure the lower cervical region. The diagnosis can be made on the frontal view by noting the double shadow of the spinous processes caused by the caudad displacement of the avulsed fragment (Figure 3-82). This double–spinous-process sign must be differentiated from a bifid spinous process, which usually lies at a higher level and on a more horizontal plane.

Most fractures of the thoracolumbar spine are due to compressive forces that cause anterior wedging or depression of the superior end plate of a vertebral body (Figure 3-83). The **"seat belt fracture"** refers to a transverse fracture of a lumbar vertebra that is often associated with significant visceral injuries (Figure 3-84). In this condition, a horizontal fracture of the vertebral body extends to involve some or all of the posterior elements.

HERNIATION OF INTERVERTEBRAL DISKS

The intervertebral disks act as shock absorbers between the vertebrae, cushioning the movements of the spine. They consist of a fibrous outer cartilage (annulus) surrounding a central nucleus pulposus, which is the essential part of the disk. The nucleus pulposus is a highly elastic, semifluid mass compressed like a spring between the vertebral surfaces. In youth, it contains a large amount of fluid to cushion the motion of the spine. With increasing age,

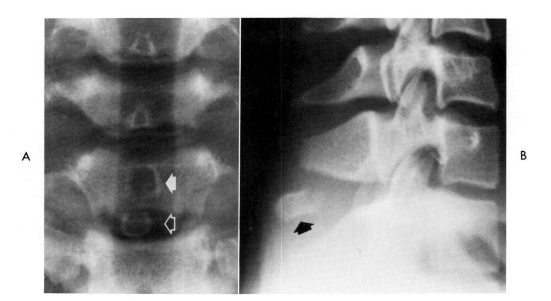

Figure 3-82 Clay shoveler's fracture. **A,** Frontal projection of cervical spine shows characteristic double-spinous-process sign resulting from caudad displacement of avulsed fragment (*open arrow*) with respect to normal position of major portion of spinous process (*solid arrow*). **B,** Lateral projection clearly shows avulsed fragment (*arrow*).

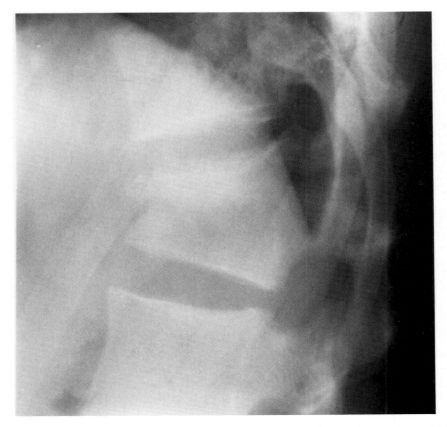

Figure 3-83 Vertebral body fracture. Characteristic anterior wedging of superior end plate of L1 vertebral body.

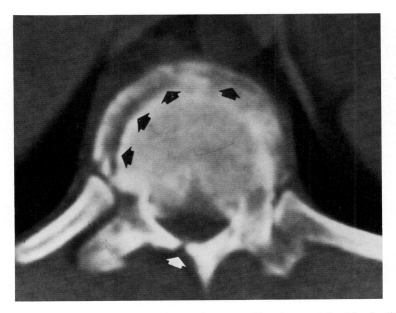

Figure 3-84 Seat belt fracture. CT scan shows fracture of lumbar vertebral body (*black arrows*) associated with lamina fracture at same level (*white arrow*).

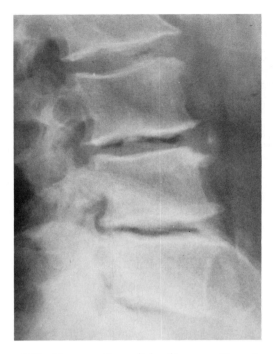

Figure 3-85 Degenerative disk disease. Hypertrophic spurring, intervertebral disk space narrowing, and reactive sclerosis. Note linear lucent collections (*vacuum phenomenon*) overlying several of intervertebral disks.

the fluid and elasticity gradually diminish, leading to degenerative changes and back pain. Protrusion or herniation of a lumbar intervertebral disk is the major cause of severe acute, chronic, or recurring low back and leg pain. It most frequently involves the L4-5 and L5-S1 levels in the lumbar region where it often causes sciatica, pain that radiates down the sciatic nerve to the back of the thigh and lower leg. Other major sites are the C5-6 and C6-7 levels in the neck and the T9 through T12 levels in the thoracic region.

Patients with symptoms suggestive of disk herniation are initially treated conservatively with bed rest, muscle relaxants, and analgesics before being subjected to radiographic studies. Although plain radiographs show characteristic narrowing of the intervertebral disk spaces with hypertrophic spur formation, bony sclerosis, spurs impinging on the neural foramina, and the vacuum phenomenon (lucent collections overlying the intervertebral disks), these findings are nonspecific and frequently occur in patients with minimal symptoms (Figure 3-85). The diagnosis of herniation of an intervertebral disk requires CT, MRI, or myelography to demonstrate impression of the disk on the spinal cord or individual nerve roots (Figures 3-86 to 3-90).

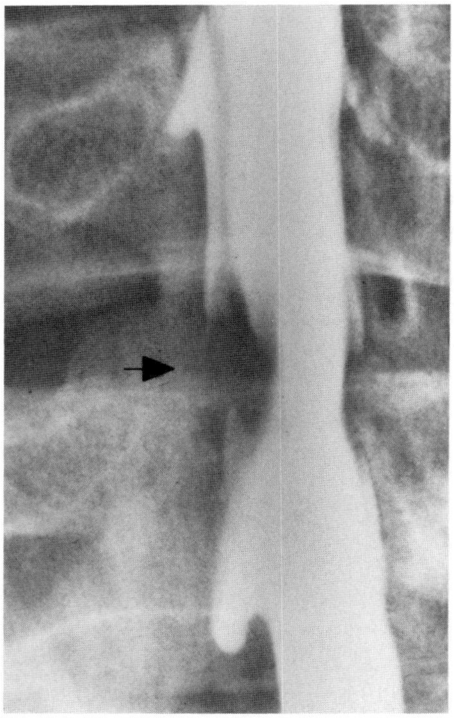

Figure 3-86 Lumbar disk herniation. Myelogram shows extradural lesion (*arrow*) at level of intervertebral disk space. Note amputation of nerve root by disk compression.

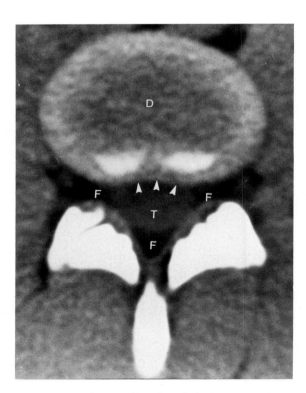

Figure 3-87 CT of normal lumbar disk (*D*) (*arrow*). Normal lumbar intervertebral disk has concave posterior border (*arrowheads*). Note normal epidural fat (*F*) surrounding thecal sac (*T*).

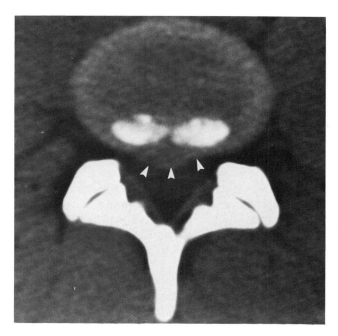

Figure 3-88   Central bulging of intervertebral disk. CT scan shows convex posterior border of disk (*arrowheads*). Note preservation of epidural fat.

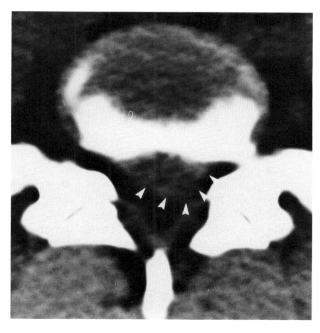

Figure 3-89   Disk herniation at L5-S1 level. CT shows herniation of disk (*arrowheads*) to left with obliteration of epidural fat. (*From Eisenberg RL: Diagnostic imaging in surgery, New York, McGraw-Hill Book Co, 1987.*)

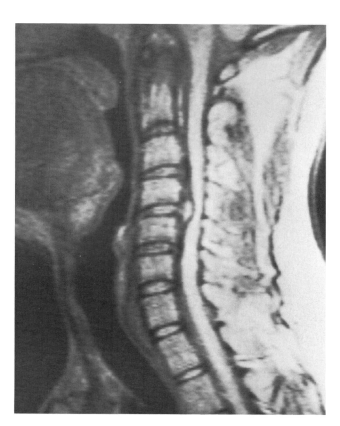

Figure 3-90   MRI of intervertebral disk herniation in cervical region. Note extradural impression on spinal cord (*arrowhead*).

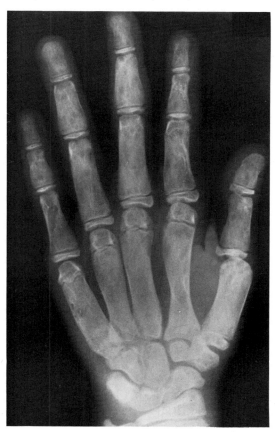

Figure 3-91   Fibrous dysplasia. Smudgy, ground-glass appearance of medullary cavities with failure of normal modeling.

FIBROUS DYSPLASIA

Fibrous dysplasia is a disorder that usually begins during childhood and is characterized by the proliferation of fibrous tissue within the medullary cavity. The disease may be confined to a single bone (monostotic) or the bones of one extremity, or it may be widely distributed throughout the skeleton (polyostotic).

Fibrous dysplasia primarily involves the long bones (especially the femur and tibia), ribs, and facial bones. Fibrous replacement of the medullary cavity typically produces a well-defined radiolucent area, which may vary from completely radiolucent to a homogeneous ground-glass density, depending on the amount of fibrous or osseous tissue deposited in the medullary cavity (Figure 3-91). Irregular bands of sclerosis may cross the cystlike lesion, giving it a multilocular appearance (Figure 3-92). The bone is often locally expanded, and the cortex may be eroded from within, predisposing to pathologic fractures. In severe and long-standing disease, affected bones may be bowed or deformed.

Fibrous dysplasia is the most common cause of an expansile focal rib lesion, which usually has a ground-glass or soap-bubble appearance.

SPONDYLOLYSIS AND SPONDYLOLISTHESIS

Spondylolysis refers to a cleft in the pars interarticularis that is situated between the superior and inferior articular processes of a vertebra. Occurring in about 5% of the population, these clefts are usually bilateral, most commonly involve the fifth lumbar vertebra, and predispose to the forward displacement of one vertebra on the other. Spondylolysis is the term for a defect in the pars interarticularis without displacement; if displacement occurs, the condition is called **spondylolisthesis**.

A plain lateral radiograph of the lower lumbar spine clearly shows any spondylolisthesis and may demonstrate the lucent cleft in the pars interarticularis even if no displacement has occurred (Figure 3-93). In grading spondylolisthesis of the lumbosacral junction on the lateral projection, the superior surface of the sacrum is divided into four equal parts. A forward displacement of the fifth lumbar vertebra up to one fourth the thickness of the sacrum is called a first-degree spondylolisthesis; half the thickness, a second-degree spondylolisthesis, and so on.

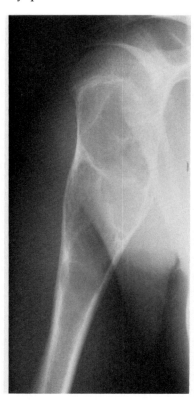

Figure 3-92 Fibrous dysplasia. Expansile lesion of humerus containing irregular bands of sclerosis giving it multilocular appearance.

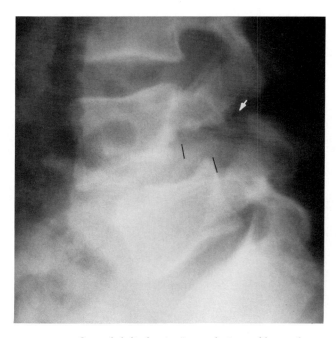

Figure 3-93 Spondylolisthesis. Lateral view of lower lumbar spine shows break in pars interarticularis (*arrow*), with resultant anterior slippage of L4 with respect to L5. Vertical black lines indicate posterior margins of vertebral bodies.

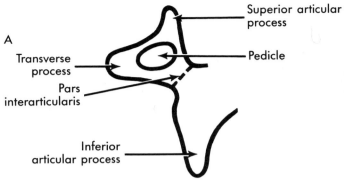

Figure 3-94 Spondylolysis. **A**, Diagram of Scotty dog sign. **B**, Oblique projection of lumbar spine demonstrates defect in pars interarticularis, which appears as fracture through neck of Scotty dog (*arrow*).

The diagnosis of spondylolysis without displacement may require an oblique projection of the lumbar spine, on which the appearance of the posterior elements has been likened to that of a Scotty dog (Figure 3-94). The pedicle and transverse process form the eye and nose; the superior and inferior articular processes form the ear and leg; and the pars interarticularis forms the neck, which is "fractured" in a patient with spondylolysis.

ISCHEMIC NECROSIS OF BONE

Ischemic necrosis of bone results from the loss of blood supply, which in turn can result from such varied conditions as thrombosis, vasculitis, disease of surrounding bone, or single or repeated episodes of trauma disrupting the blood supply. Among the many conditions associated with ischemic necrosis are acute trauma (fracture or dislocation), steroid therapy or Cushing's disease, hemolytic anemia (especially sickle cell disease), chronic alcoholism and chronic pancreatitis, Gaucher's disease, radiation therapy, and caisson disease (a complication of underwater diving, the so-called "bends").

The femoral head is the most frequent site of ischemic necrosis. Initially, the ischemic bone may appear denser than adjacent viable bone. The first sign of structural failure is the development of a radiolucent subcortical band (crescent sign) representing a fracture line (Figure 3-95, *A*). As the disorder pro-

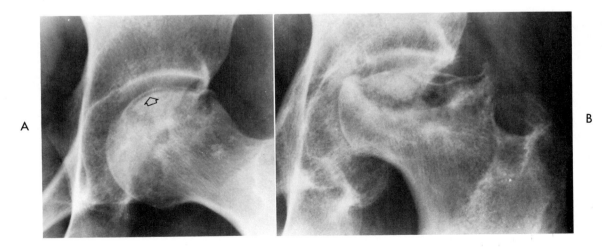

Figure 3-95 Ischemic necrosis of femoral head. **A**, Arclike radiolucent cortical band (crescent sign) (*arrow*) in femoral head represents fracture line. Note lucent cortical band (*arrow*). **B**, Eventually, there is combination of lytic and sclerotic areas with severe flattening of femoral head.

gresses, fragmentation, compression, and resorption of dead bone, along with proliferation of granulation tissue, revascularization, and production of new bone, produce a pattern of lytic and sclerotic areas with flattening of the femoral head and periosteal new bone formation (Figure 3-95, *B*). Mechanical distortion about the hip leads to uneven weight bearing and accelerated secondary osteoarthritis.

It is often necessary to obtain two radiographs in patients with ischemic necrosis. The first is taken with normal density, whereas the second is made with increased kVp to allow for adequate penetration of the more opaque ischemic bone.

Radionuclide bone scanning is more sensitive than plain radiography for detecting changes of ischemic necrosis. In the initial stages of infarction, nuclide activity is absent in the area of involvement. As the disease progresses, this area of decreased activity may become rimmed by a zone of increased activity as a result of the reparative process.

MRI may be even more sensitive than radionuclide bone scanning for detecting ischemic necrosis. Infarction at the end of a bone causes changes in the fatty marrow, sharply reducing the normal intense T1 signal from the marrow so that the infarcted area becomes gray or black (Figure 3-96).

In addition to ischemic changes in the subchondral areas of bone, infarction may involve the shaft of a long bone. In many cases this type of bone infarction is asymptomatic and is detected only on radiographs obtained for another purpose. A mature infarct in the shaft of a bone appears as a densely calcified area in the medullary cavity (Figure 3-97). It may be sharply limited by a dense sclerotic zone or associated with dense streaks extending from the central region. Bone infarction must be differentiated from a calcified enchondroma, which contains amorphous, spotty calcific densities, is not surrounded by a sclerotic rim, and may expand the bone.

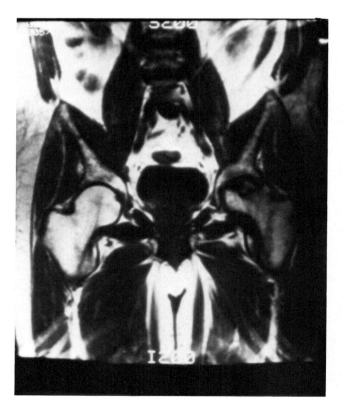

Figure 3-96 Ischemic necrosis. On this T-1 weighted image, ischemic left femoral head has lost normal bright signal intensity and appears dark.

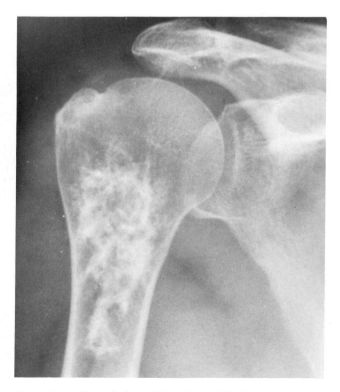

Figure 3-97 Bone infarct. Densely calcified area in medullary cavity of humerus with dense streaks extending from central region.

QUESTIONS

1. The shaft of any long bone is termed the
   A. Epiphysis   C. Metaphysis
   B. Diaphysis   D. Periosteum

2. The end of a long bone is referred to as the
   A. Epiphysis   C. Metaphysis
   B. Diaphysis   D. Periosteum

3. The special types of cells responsible for the diameter growth of bones are
   A. Osteoblasts   C. Chondroblasts
   B. Osteoclasts   D. Both A and B

4. The common area(s) of the body radiographed for bone age determination is/are
   A. Skull   C. Hand
   B. Wrist   D. Both B and C

5. What pathologic condition is present if the posterior elements of one or more vertebrae fail to unite?
   A. Meningocele   C. Myelomeningocele
   B. Spina bifida   D. Spondylolisthesis

6. In patients with advanced osteoporosis, what type of radiographic technique is preferred?
   A. Low kVp; short scale contrast   C. Low kVp; long scale contrast
   B. High kVp; short scale contrast   D. High kVp; long scale contrast

7. The major causes of generalized _____ are aging and postmenopausal hormonal changes.
   A. Osteogenesis imperfecta   C. Osteopetrosis
   B. Osteoporosis   D. Osteomalacia

8. An inherited generalized disorder of connective tissue characterized by multiple fractures and a bluish color of the sclera of the eye is
   A. Osteogenesis imperfecta   C. Osteopetrosis
   B. Osteoporosis   D. Osteomalacia

9. Lack of vitamin D in the diet of infants and children can cause a systemic disease called
   A. Achondroplasia   C. Osteomalacia
   B. Rickets   D. Osteopetrosis

10. A disorder of metabolism causing an increased blood level of uric acid is called
    A. Achondroplasia   C. Gout
    B. Rickets   D. Urasia

11. A benign projection of bone with a cartilage-like cap occurring around the knee in children or adolescents is
    A. Osteochondroma   C. Achondroplasia
    B. Enchondroma   D. Osteoma

12. An example of a malignant bone tumor is
    A. Osteogenic sarcoma   C. Ewing's sarcoma
    B. Chondrosarcoma   D. All of the above

13. The form of noninfectious arthritis characterized by osteoporosis, soft-tissue swelling, and erosions of the metacarpophalangeal joints and ulnar styloid processes is
    A. Reiter's   C. Psoriatic
    B. Rheumatoid   D. Osteoarthritis

14. The extremely common form of arthritis that is characterized by loss of joint cartilage and reactive new bone growth and is part of the normal wear of aging is
    A. Reiter's   C. Psoriatic
    B. Rheumatoid   D. Osteoarthritis

15. Inflammation of the small fluid-filled sacs located around joints that reduce friction is termed
    A. Tendinitis   C. Bursitis
    B. Arthritis   D. Both A and C

16. In what type of fracture is the skin broken?
    A. Open   C. Comminuted
    B. Compound   D. Both A and C

17. What type of fracture consists of more than two fragments?
    A. Open   C. Comminuted
    B. Compound   D. Both A and C

18. What term applies to the new calcium deposits that unite fracture sites?
    A. Bone   C. Periosteum
    B. Callus   D. Both A and C

19. What type of fracture occurs in bone weakened by some pre-existing condition such as a metastatic lesion or multiple myeloma?
    A. Stress   C. Pott's
    B. Colles'   D. Pathologic

20. What is the name for the type of fracture that can occur from falling on the outstretched hand and involves the distal portion of the radius?
    A. Stress   C. Pott's
    B. Colles'   D. Pathologic

21. What name is applied to a fracture involving both malleoli?
    A. Stress   C. Pott's
    B. Colles'   D. Pathologic

22. What is the name applied to the fracture resulting from acute hyperextension of the head on the neck that usually effects C2 and C3?
    A. Hangman's   C. Boxer's
    B. Jefferson   D. Monteggia

23. What area of the spine does a clay shoveler's fracture involve?
A. Lower thoracic and upper lumbar
B. Lumbar only
C. Lower cervical and upper thoracic
D. Cervical only

24. Diagnosis of an intervertebral disk herniation requires which radiographic procedure(s)?
A. Myelography
B. CT
C. MRI
D. A or B or C

25. What medical term refers to a cleft in the pars interarticularis commonly involving the fifth lumbar vertebra?
A. Spondylolisthesis
B. Spondylolysis
C. Spondylitis
D. A or B or C

26. What pathologic condition sometimes occurs after trauma, causing an interrupted blood supply to a bone?
A. Vasculitis
B. Ischemic necrosis
C. Cushing's
D. Stress fracture

27. Place an "H" by those pathologic conditions that are harder to penetrate and an "E" by those that are easier to penetrate:
_____ Callus
_____ Ischemic necrosis
_____ Atrophy
_____ Osteolytic lesions
_____ Acromegaly
_____ Multiple myeloma
_____ Osteoporosis
_____ Osteosclerotic lesions

BIBLIOGRAPHY

Brower AC: Arthritis in black and white, Philadelphia, WB Saunders Co, 1988.

Greenfield GB: Radiology of bone diseases, ed 4, Philadelphia, JB Lippincott Co, 1986.

Resnick D and Niwayama G: Diagnosis of bone and joint disorders, Philadelphia, WB Saunders Co, 1987.

Rogers LF: Radiology of skeletal trauma, New York, Churchill-Livingstone, 1982.

CHAPTER 4

Gastrointestinal System

PREREQUISITE KNOWLEDGE

The student should have a basic knowledge of the anatomy and physiology of the gastrointestinal system. In addition, proper learning and understanding of the material will be facilitated if the student has some clinical experience in gastrointestinal radiography and film evaluation, including a concept of the changes in technique required to compensate for density differences produced by a few of the underlying pathologic conditions.

GOALS

To acquaint the student radiographer with the pathophysiology and radiographic manifestations of all of the common and some of the unusual disorders of the gastrointestinal system

OBJECTIVES

1. Describe the physiology of the gastrointestinal system
2. Identify anatomic structures on both diagrams and radiographs of the gastrointestinal system
3. Be able to define terminology relating to the gastrointestinal system
4. Be able to describe the various pathologic conditions affecting the gastrointestinal system, as well as their radiographic manifestations
5. Be familiar with the changes in technical factors required for obtaining optimal quality radiographs in patients with certain underlying pathologic conditions and contrast studies

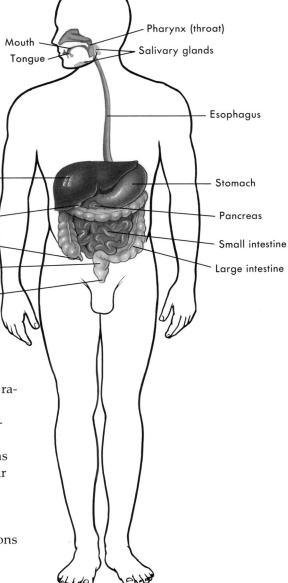

Mouth
Tongue
Pharynx (throat)
Salivary glands
Esophagus
Liver
Stomach
Gallbladder
Pancreas
Appendix
Small intestine
Rectum
Large intestine
Anal canal

RADIOGRAPHER NOTES

Plain abdominal radiographs and contrast studies of the digestive tract remain the most common imaging examinations of the gastrointestinal system. Ultrasound and CT are the major imaging modalities for the pancreas and biliary tract, and MRI is being used in some institutions to screen for hepatic metastases.

Plain abdominal radiographs must show an appropriately wide scale of contrast to demonstrate the many different densities in the abdominal cavity. Depending on the screen-film combination, this requires the use of a kVp in the middle to high range. Bony structures, such as the lumbar spine and its transverse processes, must be well demonstrated, as well as soft-tissue shadows of the liver, kidney, and psoas muscle. For barium studies of the gastrointestinal tract, adequate penetration of the dense barium solution requires a high kVp (about 120 kVp). For double-contrast (air-barium) studies, a kVp in the range of 90 kVp is needed to allow for penetration of the barium combined with excellent visualization of mucosal detail. Gallbladder studies require a shorter scale of contrast than other abdominal examinations and therefore are usually performed using a low to middle range of kVp (about 70 kVp).

As with other body systems, certain pathologic conditions require alterations in technical factors. In patients with ascites, a common complication of advanced cirrhosis, an increased kVp is required to penetrate the additional fluid content of the abdomen. Conversely, a decreased kVp is needed in patients with suspected large or small bowel obstruction because of the excessive amount of gas in the abdominal cavity.

The radiographer usually is called on to assist the radiologist during fluoroscopic examinations of the gastrointestinal tract. Indeed, it is generally the radiographer's task to coerce the patient into drinking and not vomiting the rather unpleasant-tasting contrast material and to urge the patient to turn around several times to provide adequate mucosal coating for the double-contrast upper gastrointestinal series. Similarly, the radiographer may have to convince the patient to retain barium and air during the often uncomfortable barium enema examinations. It is frequently time well spent for the radiographer to fully explain to the patient both the mechanics of the procedure and the extreme importance of patient cooperation.

PHYSIOLOGY OF THE DIGESTIVE SYSTEM

The basic function of the digestive system is to alter the chemical and physical composition of food so that it can be absorbed and used by body cells. This process depends on secretions of the endocrine and exocrine glands and the controlled movement of ingested food through the tract so that absorption can occur.

Digestion begins in the mouth with chewing (**mastication**), the mechanical breakdown of food. The secretion of saliva moistens the food in preparation for swallowing. Swallowing (**deglutition**) is a complex process that requires coordination of many muscles in the head and neck and the precise opening and closing of esophageal sphincters. Digestion continues in the stomach with the churning movement of gastric contents that have been mixed with hydrochloric acid and the proteolytic enzyme pepsin. The resulting milky white **chyme** is propelled through the pyloric sphincter into the duodenum by

rhythmic smooth muscle contractions called **peristalsis**. The greatest amount of digestion occurs in the duodenum, the first part of the small bowel. In addition to intestinal secretions containing mucus and enzymes, digestion in this region is enhanced by secretions of the pancreas and liver. The pancreas secretes enzymes for the digestion of protein (trypsin and chymotrypsin), fat (lipase), and carbohydrate (amylase). It also secretes an alkaline solution to neutralize the acid carried into the small intestine from the stomach. Bile is secreted by the liver, stored in the gallbladder, and enters the duodenum through the common bile duct. Bile is an **emulsifier**, a substance that acts like soap by dispersing the fat into very small droplets that permit it to mix with water.

When digestion is complete, the nutrients are absorbed through the intestinal mucosa into blood capillaries and lymph vessels of the wall of the small bowel. The inner surface area of the small bowel is increased by the formation of numerous fingerlike projections **(villi),** which provide the largest amount of surface area possible for digestion and absorption.

Material that has not been digested passes into the colon, where water and minerals are absorbed and the remaining matter is excreted as feces. If the contents of the lower colon and rectum move at a rate that is slower than normal, extra water is absorbed from the fecal mass to produce a hardened stool and **constipation. Diarrhea** results from increased motility of the small bowel, which floods the colon with an excessive amount of water that cannot be completely absorbed.

The vermiform (worm-shaped) appendix arises from the inferomedial aspect of the cecum about 3 cm below the ileocecal valve. Although the appendix has no functional importance in digestion, it is often classified as an accessory digestive organ merely because of its location.

The liver is the largest gland in the body and is responsible for several vital functions. Liver cells detoxify (make harmless) a variety of poisonous substances that enter the blood from the intestines. Toxic chemicals that are changed to nontoxic compounds in the liver include ammonia (converted to urea and excreted by the kidneys), alcohol, and barbiturates. Liver cells secrete about 1 pint of bile each day. As mentioned, bile is an emulsifier that is essential for the digestion and absorption of dietary fat and the fat-soluble vitamins A, D, E, and K. Bile is a greenish liquid consisting of water, bile salts, cholesterol, and bilirubin (breakdown product of hemoglobin).

Liver cells play a vital role in the metabolism of proteins, fats, and carbohydrates. The liver is the major site of synthesis of the enzymes necessary for various cellular activities throughout the body. Liver cells also synthesize blood proteins, such as albumin, which maintains the correct amount of fluid within blood vessels, and the essential proteins required for blood clotting (fibrinogen and prothrombin). Therefore liver damage may result in edema (excess water in the soft tissues) and a serious bleeding tendency. The liver plays an important role in maintaining the proper level of glucose in the blood by taking up excess glucose absorbed by the small intestine and storing it as **glycogen.** When the level of circulating glucose falls below normal, the liver breaks down glycogen and releases glucose into the bloodstream. Liver cells also store iron and vitamins A, B_{12}, and D.

The gallbladder is a pear-shaped sac that lies on the undersurface of the liver. Its function is to store bile that enters it by way of the hepatic and cystic ducts and to concentrate the bile by absorbing water.

In response to the presence of dietary fat in the small bowel, the gallbladder contracts and ejects the concentrated bile into the duodenum.

The pancreas controls the level of circulating blood glucose by secreting insulin and glucagon in the islands of Langerhans. An increased concentration of glucose in the blood stimulates the beta cells to increase insulin secretion, which decreases the blood glucose level probably by accelerating the transport of glucose into cells. A blood glucose concentration less than normal triggers the alpha cells to secrete glucagon, which accelerates the breakdown of glycogen into glucose by the liver.

As discussed, pancreatic secretions are vital for digestion. Pancreatic enzymes that pass through the pancreatic duct into the duodenum are necessary for the breakdown of protein, carbohydrate, and fat.

ESOPHAGUS

Esophagitis

Reflux

Although the reflux of gastric acid contents is the most common cause of acute esophagitis, infectious and granulomatous disorders, physical injury (caustic agents, radiation injury), and medication may produce a similar inflammatory response. Regardless of the cause, acute esophagitis produces burning chest pain that may simulate the pain of heart disease. The esophagus is often dilated with a loss of effective peristalsis. Nonpropulsive peristaltic waves, ranging from mild tertiary contractions to severe segmental spasms, are an early finding.

Reflux esophagitis develops when the lower esophageal sphincter fails to act as an effective barrier to the entry of gastric acid contents into the distal esophagus. Although there is a higher-than-normal likelihood of gastroesophageal reflux in patients with sliding hiatal hernias, reflux esophagitis can be endoscopically demonstrated in only about one fourth of patients with them. Conversely, esophagitis is often encountered in patients in whom no hiatal hernia can be demonstrated.

A number of radiographic approaches have been suggested for the demonstration of gastroesophageal reflux. One procedure is to increase intraabdominal pressure by straight-leg raising or manual pressure on the abdomen, often with Valsalva's maneuver (forced expiration with the glottis closed). Turning the patient from prone to supine or vice versa may demonstrate reflux of barium from the stomach into the esophagus. A new technique for demonstrating and measuring gastroesophageal reflux is to scan the lower esophagus and stomach after the oral administration of a radioactive sub-

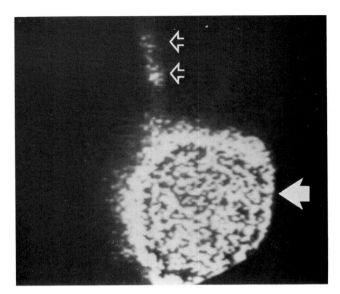

Figure 4-1 Gastroesophageal reflux. Note reflux of orally administered radionuclide into esophagus *(open arrows)* from stomach *(solid arrow).*

stance (Figure 4-1). It must be remembered, however, that the failure to demonstrate reflux radiographically does not exclude the possibility that a patient's esophagitis is related to reflux. As long as typical radiographic findings of reflux esophagitis are noted, there is little reason to persist in strenuous efforts to actually demonstrate retrograde flow of barium from the stomach into the esophagus.

The earliest radiographic findings in reflux esophagitis are detectable on double-contrast studies. They consist of superficial ulcerations or erosions that appear as streaks or dots of barium superimposed on the flat mucosa of the distal esophagus. In single-contrast studies of patients with esophagitis the outer borders of the barium-filled esophagus are not sharply seen, but rather have a hazy, serrated appearance with shallow, irregular protrusions that are indicative of erosions of varying length and depth. Widening and coarsening of edematous longitudinal folds can simulate filling defects. In addition to diffuse erosion, reflux esophagitis can result in large, discrete penetrating ulcers in the distal esophagus (Figure 4-2) or in a hiatal hernia sac (Figure 4-3). Fibrotic healing of diffuse reflux esophagitis or a localized penetrating ulcer may cause narrowing of the distal esophagus. Strictures resulting from reflux esophagitis tend to be smooth and tapering with no demonstrable mucosal pattern (Figure 4-4).

Barrett's esophagus

Barrett's esophagus is a condition related to severe reflux esophagitis in which the normal squa-

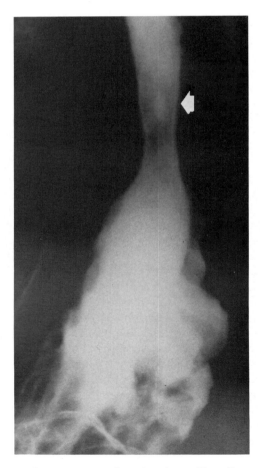

Figure 4-2 Large, penetrating ulcer *(arrow)* in reflux esophagitis.

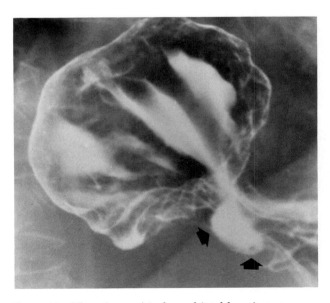

Figure 4-3 Ulcer *(arrows)* in large hiatal hernia sac.

mous lining of the lower esophagus is destroyed and replaced by columnar epithelium similar to that of the stomach. Ulceration in Barrett's esophagus typically occurs at the squamocolumnar junction. Although a hiatal hernia with gastroesophageal reflux is commonly demonstrated, the Barrett's ulcer is usually separated from the hiatal hernia by a variable length of normal-appearing esophagus (Figure 4-5), in contrast to reflux esophagitis, in which the distal esophagus is abnormal down to the level of the hernia. As with reflux esophagitis, fibrotic healing of the ulceration in a Barrett's esophagus often leads to a smooth, tapered stricture (Figure 4-6). In addition to postinflammatory stricture, Barrett's esophagus has an unusually high propensity for developing malignancy in the columnar-lined portion.

These tumors are almost always adenocarcinoma, which is otherwise very rare in the esophagus.

Because the distal esophagus consists of a gastric type of mucosa in Barrett's esophagus, it actively takes up the intravenously injected radionuclide pertechnetate. The demonstration of a continuous concentration of the isotope from the stomach into the distal esophagus to a level that corresponds approximately to that of the ulcer or stricture is indicative of Barrett's esophagus.

Candida and herpes

Candida and herpes are the organisms most often responsible for infectious esophagitis, which usually occurs in patients with widespread malignancy who are receiving radiation therapy, chemotherapy, cor-

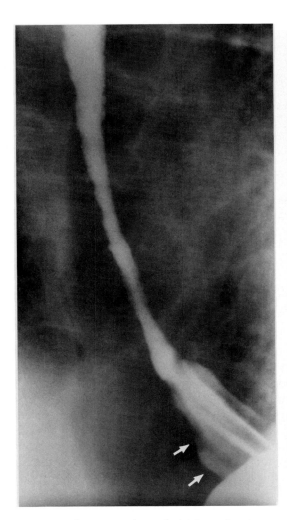

Figure 4-4 Long esophageal stricture due to reflux esophagitis. Note the associated hiatal hernia *(arrows)*.

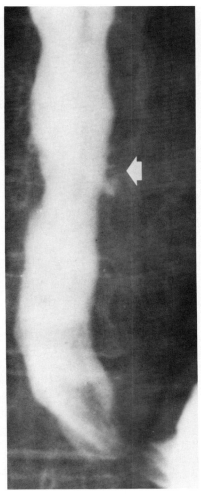

Figure 4-5 Barrett's esophagus. Ulcerations *(arrow)* have developed at a distance from esophagogastric junction.

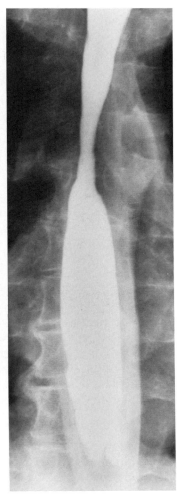

Figure 4-6 Barrett's esophagus. Note smooth, tapered stricture in upper thoracic esophagus.

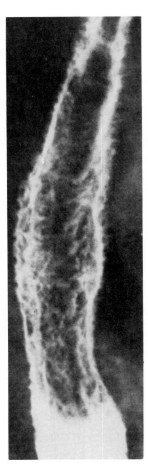

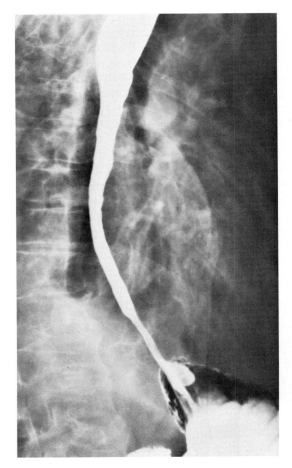

Figure 4-7 *Candida* esophagitis. Multiple ulcers and nodular plaques produce grossly irregular contour of shaggy esophagus. This manifestation of far-advanced candidiasis has become infrequent because of earlier and better treatment of the disease.

Figure 4-8 Corrosive stricture resulting from ingestion of lye.

ticosteroids, or other immunosuppresive agents. It also can develop in patients with AIDS and even in otherwise healthy adults who have received antibiotics (especially tetracycline) for upper respiratory infection. The classic radiographic appearance is an irregular cobblestone pattern with a shaggy marginal contour of the esophagus caused by deep ulcerations and sloughing of the mucosa (Figure 4-7).

Ingestion of corrosive agents

The ingestion of alkaline corrosive agents produces acute inflammatory changes in the esophagus. Superficial penetration of the toxic agent results in only minimal ulceration. Deeper penetration of the submucosa and muscular layers causes sloughing of destroyed tissue and deep ulceration. Drug-induced esophagitis may occur in patients who have delayed esophageal transit time, which permits prolonged

mucosal contact with the ingested substance. The most common drug causing esophageal ulceration is potassium chloride in tablet form. Other medications that can cause esophagitis are weak caustic agents that are harmless when they pass rapidly through the esophagus.

Healing of the intense mucosal and intramural inflammation of acute esophagitis may lead to marked fibrosis and stricture formation. These benign strictures tend to be long lesions with tapered margins and relatively smooth mucosal surfaces (Figure 4-8), in contrast to the irregular narrowing, mucosal destruction and overhanging margins that are generally associated with malignant processes.

Hiatal hernia

Hiatal hernia is the most frequent abnormality detected on upper gastrointestinal examination. Its broad radiographic spectrum ranges from large esophagogastric hernias, in which much of the stomach lies within the thoracic cavity and there is a

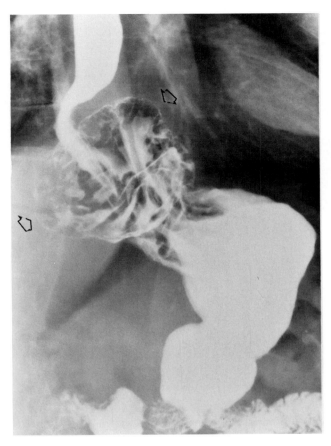

Figure 4-9   Large hiatal hernia *(arrows).*

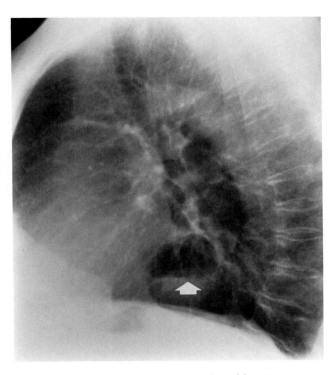

Figure 4-10   Air-fluid level *(arrow)* in hiatal hernia seen on lateral chest radiograph.

predisposition to volvulus (twisting), to small hernias that emerge above the diaphragm only under certain circumstances (related to changes in intra-abdominal or intrathoracic pressure) and easily slide back into the abdomen through the hiatus. The symptoms associated with hiatal hernia, as well as its complications (esophagitis, esophageal ulcer, esophageal stenosis), are related to the presence of esophageal reflux rather than the hiatal hernia itself. Most hiatal hernias do not produce symptoms and are clinically of no importance.

Although the diagnosis of hiatal hernia generally requires a barium study (Figure 4-9), at times a large hiatal hernia may appear on plain chest radiographs as a soft-tissue mass in the posterior mediastinum, often containing a prominent air-fluid level (Figure 4-10).

Cancer of the esophagus

Progressive difficulty in swallowing (dysphagia) in a person older than 40 years of age must be assumed to be due to cancer until proven otherwise. Because the symptoms of esophageal carcinoma tend to ap-

pear late in the course of the disease and since the lack of a limiting outer layer (serosa) commonly permits direct extension of the tumor by the time of initial diagnosis, carcinoma of the esophagus has a dismal prognosis. Most carcinomas of the esophagus are of the squamous cell type. The incidence of carcinoma of the esophagus is far higher in men than in women. There is a strong correlation between excessive alcohol intake, smoking, and esophageal carcinoma.

The earliest radiographic appearance of infiltrating carcinoma of the esophagus is a flat, plaquelike lesion, occasionally with central ulceration, that involves one wall of the esophagus (Figure 4-11). At this stage there may be minimal reduction in the caliber of the lumen. Unless the patient is carefully examined in various positions, this earliest form of esophageal carcinoma can be missed. As the infiltrating cancer progresses, irregularity of the wall is seen, indicating mucosal destruction. Advanced lesions encircle the lumen completely, causing annular constrictions with overhanging margins and often some degree of obstruction. The lumen through the stenotic area is irregular, and mucosal folds are absent or severely ulcerated (Figure 4-12). Less commonly, carcinoma of the esophagus can appear as a localized polypoid mass, often with deep ulceration and a fungating appearance.

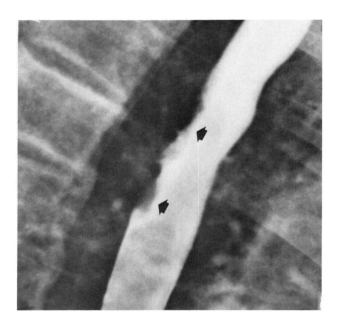

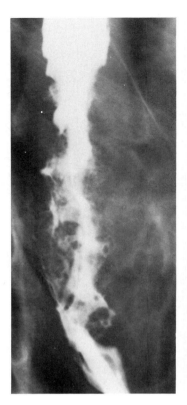

Figure 4-11   Early carcinoma of esophagus. Flat, plaquelike lesion *(arrows)* involves posterior wall of esophagus.

Figure 4-12   Carcinoma of esophagus. Irregular narrowing with ulceration involves extensive segment of thoracic portion of esophagus.

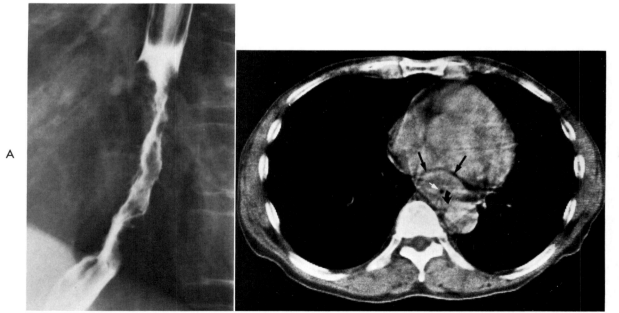

Figure 4-13   CT staging of esophageal carcinoma. **A,** Esophagram demonstrates infiltrating lesion causing irregular narrowing of distal esophagus. **B,** CT scan shows mass of bulky carcinoma *(black arrows)* filling most of lumen *(white arrow)*. Obliteration of fat plane adjacent to aorta *(curved arrow)* indicates mediastinal invasion.

Luminal obstruction as a result of carcinoma causes proximal dilation of the esophagus and may result in aspiration pneumonia. Extension of the tumor to adjacent mediastinal structures may lead to fistula formation, especially between the esophagus and the respiratory tract (see Figure 4-19).

CT has become a major method for staging patients with esophageal carcinoma. It can provide information on tumor size, extension, and resectability that was previously only available at thoracotomy (Figure 4-13). Evidence of spread of tumor includes the obliteration of fat planes between the esophagus and adjacent structures (left atrium, aorta), the formation of a fistula to the tracheobronchial tree, and evidence of metastatic disease (low-density masses in the liver; enlargement of draining lymph nodes).

Esophageal varices

Esophageal varices are dilated veins in the wall of the esophagus that are most commonly the result of increased pressure in the portal venous system (portal hypertension), which is usually a result of cirrhosis of the liver. In patients with portal hypertension, much of the portal blood cannot flow along its normal pathway through the liver to the inferior vena cava and then on to the heart. Instead, it must go by a circuitous collateral route, and increased blood flow through these dilated veins causes the development of esophageal (and gastric) varices. Esophageal varices are infrequently demonstrated in the absence of portal hypertension. "Downhill" varices are produced when venous blood from the head and neck cannot reach the heart because of an obstruction of the superior vena cava caused by tumors or inflammatory disease in the mediastinum. In this situation blood flows "downhill" through the esophageal veins before eventually entering the portal vein, through which it flows to the inferior vena cava and the right atrium.

The characteristic radiographic appearance of esophageal varices is serpiginous thickening of folds, which appear as round or oval filling defects resembling the beads of a rosary (Figure 4-14). Precise technique is required to demonstrate esophageal varices. Complete filling of the esophagus with barium may obscure varices, whereas powerful contractions of the esophagus may squeeze blood out of the varices and make them impossible to detect.

The major complication of esophageal varices is bleeding. Their appearance in patients with cirrhotic liver disease implies significant portal venous hypertension and is an ominous sign, since up to 90% of the deaths from liver disease in patients with cirrhosis occur within 2 years of the diagnosis of varices.

Foreign bodies

A wide spectrum of foreign bodies can become impacted in the esophagus, usually in the cervical esophagus at or just above the level of the thoracic inlet (Figure 4-15). Most metallic objects, such as

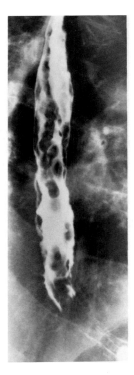

Figure 4-14 Esophageal varices. Note diffuse round and oval filling defects, which resemble rosary beads.

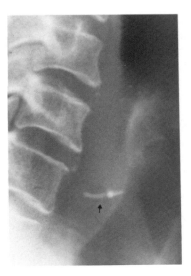

Figure 4-15 Fish bone (arrow) impacted in lower cervical esophagus.

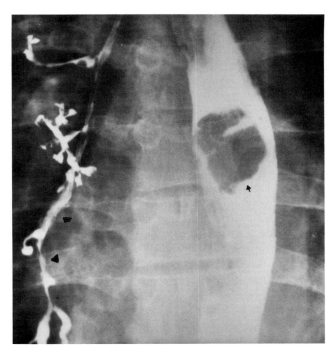

Figure 4-16 Meat impaction in esophagus. Large bolus of hot dog *(arrow)* is trapped in midesophagus of patient with quadriplegia. Note barium in bronchial tree *(arrowheads)* caused by aspiration.

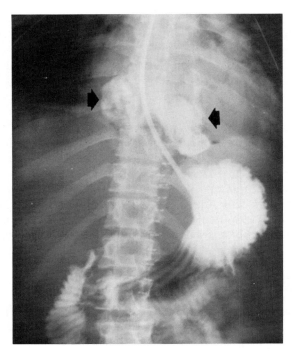

Figure 4-17 Esophageal perforation. Extravasation of contrast material *(arrows)* is seen in previously healthy patient who experienced severe vomiting following excessive ingestion of alcohol.

pins, coins, and small toys, are very radiopaque and are easily visualized on radiographs or during fluoroscopy. Objects made of aluminum and some light alloys may be impossible to detect radiographically because the density of these metals is almost equal to that of soft tissue. It is essential that any suspected foreign body be evaluated on two projections to be certain that the object projected over the esophagus truly lies within it.

Nonopaque foreign bodies in the esophagus, especially pieces of poorly chewed meat, can be demonstrated only after the ingestion of barium (Figure 4-16). Such foreign bodies usually become impacted in the distal esophagus just above the level of the diaphragm and are often associated with a distal stricture. These intraluminal filling defects usually have an irregular surface and may resemble a completely obstructing carcinoma.

Perforation of the esophagus

Perforation of the esophagus may be a complication of esophagitis, peptic ulcer, neoplasm, external trauma, or instrumentation. At times, perforation of a previously healthy esophagus can result from severe vomiting or coughing, often from dietary or alcoholic indiscretion. Complete rupture of the wall of the esophagus may cause the sudden development of severe upper gastric pain simulating myo-

cardial infarction. In the Mallory-Weiss syndrome an increase in intraluminal and intramural pressure associated with vomiting after an alcoholic bout causes superficial mucosal laceration or fissures near the esophagogastric junction that produce severe hemorrhage.

A perforation that extends throughout the entire esophageal wall can lead to free air in the mediastinum or periesophageal soft tissues. The administration of radiopaque contrast material may demonstrate extravasation through the perforation (Figure 4-17) or an intramural dissection channel separated by an intervening lucent line from the normal esophageal lumen.

Tracheoesophageal fistula

Congenital type

Congenital tracheoesophageal (TE) fistulas result from failure of a satisfactory esophageal lumen to develop completely separate from the trachea. Esophageal atresia and TE fistulas are often associated with other congenital malformations involving the skeleton, cardiovascular system, and gastrointestinal tract.

The most common type of TE fistula, type III (85% to 90%), consists of an upper segment ending in a blind pouch at the level of the bifurcation of the

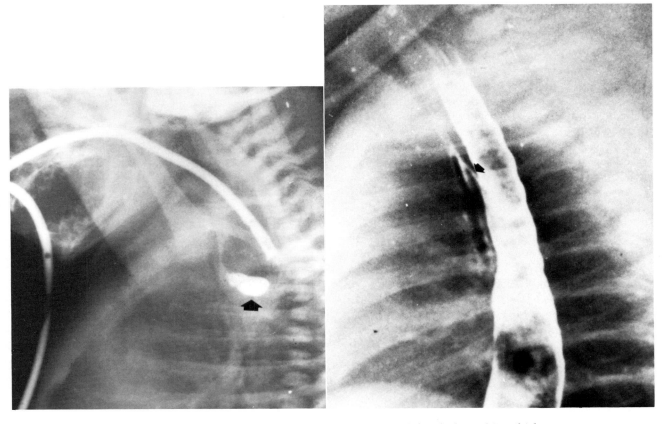

Figure 4-18 Congenital tracheoesophageal fistula. **A,** Type III fistula *(arrow),* in which contrast material injected through feeding tube demonstrates occlusion of proximal esophageal pouch. **B,** Type IV, or H, fistula *(arrow).*

trachea or slightly above it and a lower segment attached to the trachea by a short fistulous tract. Radiographic demonstration of looping of a small esophageal feeding tube indicates that the proximal esophagus ends in a blind pouch (Figure 4-18, *A*). Plain radiographs of the abdomen demonstrate the presence of air in the bowel that has freely entered the stomach through the fistulous connection between the trachea and distal esophagus.

In the next most common type of esophageal anomaly, type I, both the upper and lower segments of the esophagus are blind pouches. This anomaly can be differentiated from the type III lesion only by plain abdominal radiographs, which demonstrate the absence of air below the diaphragm in the type I lesion and air below the stomach in the type III lesion.

In the type II form of TE fistula, the upper esophageal segment communicates with the trachea, whereas the lower segment ends in a blind pouch. Because there is no connection between the trachea and the stomach, there is no radiographic evidence of gas within the abdomen. The oral administration

of contrast material in this condition immediately outlines the tracheobronchial tree.

There are two forms of type IV TE fistula. In one, the upper and lower esophageal segments end in blind pouches, both of which are connected to the tracheobronchial tree. In this case gas is seen in the stomach, and oral contrast material outlines both fistulas and the bronchial tree. In the other form of type IV fistula (H fistula) both the trachea and the esophagus are intact. These two structures are connected by a single fistulous tract that can be found at any level from the cricoid cartilage of the trachea to the tracheal bifurcation (Figure 4-18, *B*). Unlike the other forms of TE fistula, the H fistula may not be identified in infancy and, if it is small and only occasionally causes emptying of material into the lungs, can permit survival into adulthood.

Acquired type

About 50% of acquired fistulas between the trachea and esophagus are due to malignancy in the mediastinum. Almost all the rest result from infectious processes or trauma.

Fistulization between the esophagus and the respiratory tract is a major late complication of esophageal carcinoma and is often a terminal event (Figure 4-19). A fistula can also be a complication of erosion into the esophagus by carcinoma of the lung arising near or metastasizing to the middle mediastinum or by mediastinal metastases from other primary sites. Regardless of therapy, the overall prognosis of malignant TE fistulas is dismal, and more than 80% of patients with this complication die within 3 months from uncontrollable hemorrhage or from pulmonary infection caused by repeated episodes of aspiration pneumonia.

Fistulous communications between the esophagus and the tracheobronchial tree can be the result of esophageal instrumentation and perforation. This is most common after esophagoscopy but may also occur after instrumental dilation of strictures by bouginage, pneumatic dilation of the esophagus for the treatment of achalasia, or even the insertion of a nasogastric tube. Blunt or penetrating trauma to the chest, especially after crush injury, can result in

esophageal perforation and fistulization. After traumatic perforation of the thoracic esophagus, chest radiographs may demonstrate air dissecting within the mediastinum and soft tissues, often with pleural effusion or hydropneumothorax. The introduction of an oral contrast agent may demonstrate the site of perforation and the extent of fistulization.

STOMACH

Gastritis

Inflammation of the stomach can be the result of a variety of irritants including alcohol, corrosive agents, and infection. Alcoholic gastritis may produce thickening of gastric folds (Figure 4-20), multiple superficial gastric erosions, or both. In corrosive gastritis the acute inflammatory reaction heals by fibrosis and scarring, which results in severe narrowing of the antrum and may cause gastric outlet obstruction. In bacterial (phlegmonous) gastritis, inflammatory thickening of the gastric wall causes narrowing of the stomach that may mimic gastric cancer. The diagnosis of infectious gastritis can be made if there is evidence of bubbles of gas (produced by the bacteria) in the stomach wall (Figure 4-21).

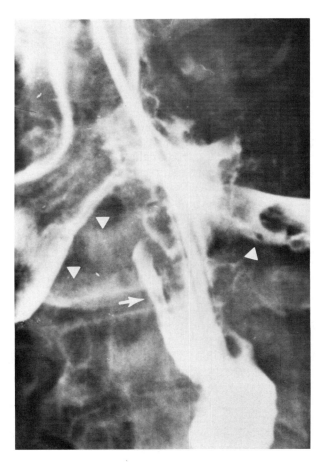

Figure 4-19 Esophagorespiratory fistula between esophagus *(arrow)* and bronchial tree *(arrowheads)*, seen as complication of esophageal carcinoma.

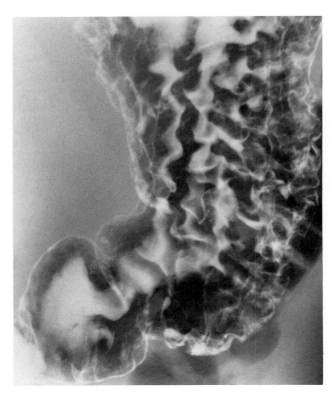

Figure 4-20 Gastritis. Note marked thickening of rugal folds throughout stomach.

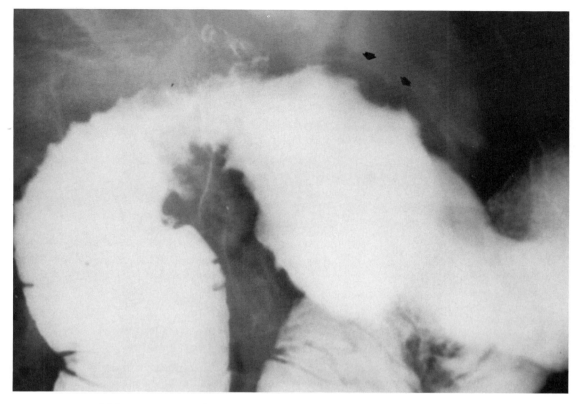

Figure 4-21 Phlegmonous emphysematous gastritis. Note severe, irregular ulceration of distal stomach, with air in wall *(arrows)*.

Chronic atrophic gastritis refers to severe mucosal atrophy (wasting) that causes thinning and a relative absence of mucosal folds, with the fundus or entire stomach having a bald appearance. This is a nonspecific radiographic pattern that can be related to such factors as age, malnutrition, medication, and complications of alcoholism. Chronic atrophic gastritis also occurs in patients with pernicious anemia, who cannot absorb vitamin B_{12} because of an inability of the stomach to secrete intrinsic factor (or hydrochloric acid).

Peptic ulcer disease

Peptic ulcer disease is an inflammatory process involving the stomach and duodenum caused by the action of acid and the enzyme pepsin secreted by the stomach. The spectrum of peptic ulcer disease varies from small and shallow superficial erosions to huge ulcers that may perforate through the bowel wall.

The major complications of peptic ulcer disease are hemorrhage, perforation, and gastric outlet obstruction. Peptic ulcer disease is the most common cause of acute upper gastrointestinal bleeding. Free perforation of a peptic ulcer is the most frequent cause of pneumoperitoneum with peritonitis (see page 162). Narrowing of the lumen of the distal stomach or duodenal bulb caused by peptic ulcer disease is by far the most common cause of gastric outlet obstruction.

Duodenal ulcer

Duodenal ulcer is the most common manifestation of peptic ulcer disease. More than 95% of duodenal ulcers occur in the first portion of the duodenum (duodenal bulb). An unequivocal diagnosis of active duodenal ulcer requires the demonstration of the ulcer crater, which appears in profile as a small collection of barium projecting from the lumen. When seen en face, the ulcer niche appears as a rounded or linear collection of contrast material surrounded by lucent folds that often radiate toward the crater (Figure 4-22). Secondary signs of duodenal ulcer disease are thickening of mucosal folds and deformity of the duodenal bulb. Acute ulcers incite muscular spasm leading to deformity of the margins of the duodenal bulb that may be inconstant and varied during the examination. With chronic ulceration, fibrosis and scarring cause a fixed deformity that persists even though the ulcer heals. Symmetric

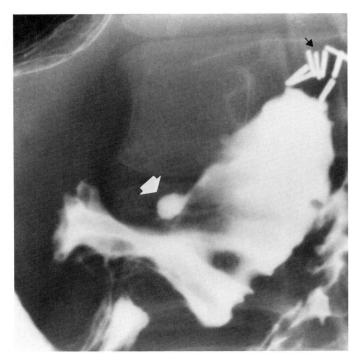

Figure 4-22 Duodenal ulcer. Ulcer niche appears as rounded collection of barium *(white arrow)* surrounded by lucent edema. Of incidental note are multiple surgical clips *(black arrow)*.

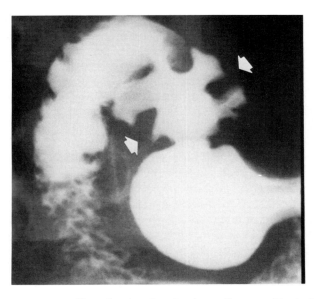

Figure 4-23 Chronic duodenal ulcer disease. Typical clover-leaf deformity is visible *(arrows.)*

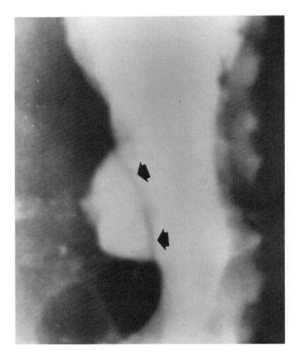

Figure 4-24 Benign gastric ulcer. Penetration of contrast material outside normal barium-filled gastric lumen associated with thin, sharply demarcated, lucent line with parallel straight margins *(arrows)* representing edema at base of ulcer crater.

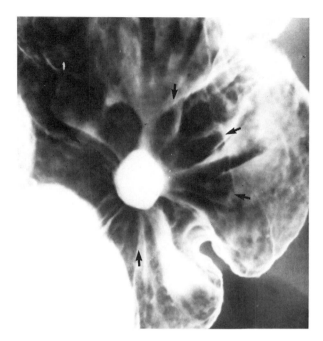

Figure 4-25 Benign gastric ulcer. On *en face* projection, prominent radiating folds extend directly to ulcer. Lucency around ulcer *(arrows)* represents inflammatory mass effect. *(Margulis AR and Burhenne JH, editors: Alimentary tract radiology, ed. 4, St. Louis, The CV Mosby Co, 1989.)*

narrowing of the duodenal bulb in its midportion may produce the typical cloverleaf deformity of chronic duodenal ulcer disease (Figure 4-23).

Gastric ulcer

Unlike duodenal ulcers, which are virtually always benign, up to 5% of gastric ulcers are malignant. Radiographic signs have been described that indicate whether a gastric ulcer is more likely to be benign or malignant. The classic sign of a benign gastric ulcer on profile views is penetration, the clear projection of the ulcer outside the normal barium-filled gastric lumen because the ulcer represents an excavation in the wall of the stomach (Figure 4-24). A thin lucency at the base of the ulcer reflecting mucosal edema caused by inflammatory exudate is another sign of benignancy. When viewed en face, a gastric ulcer appears as a persistent collection of barium surrounded by a halo of edema (Figure 4-25). A hallmark of benign gastric ulcer is radiation of mucosal folds to the edge of the crater. However, since radiating folds can be identified in both malignant and benign ulcers, the character of the folds must be carefully assessed. If the folds are smooth and slender and appear to extend into the edge of the crater, the ulcer is most likely benign (Figure 4-26, *A*). In contrast, irregular folds that merge into

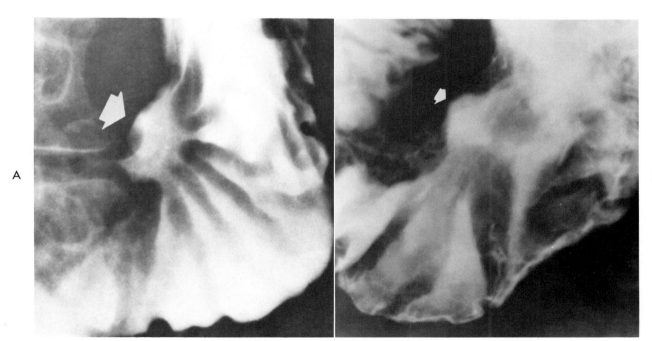

Figure 4-26 Radiating folds in gastric ulcers. **A,** Small, slender folds extending to edge of crater *(arrow)* indicate benign nature of ulcer. **B,** In this malignant gastric ulcer, thick folds radiate to irregular mound of tissue around ulcer *(arrow).*

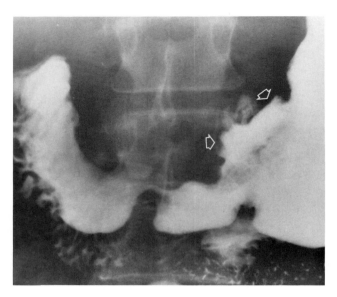

Figure 4-27 Malignant gastric ulcer. There is abrupt transition between normal mucosa and abnormal tissue surrounding irregular gastric ulcer *(arrows).*

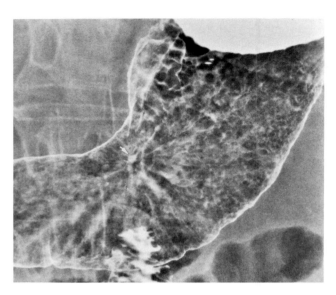

Figure 4-28 Healing of gastric ulcer. Folds converge to residual central depression *(arrow).*

a mound of polypoid tissue around the crater suggest malignancy (Figure 4-26, *B*). Although the size, shape, number, and location of gastric ulcers were formerly suggested as criteria for distinguishing between benign and malignant lesions, these findings are of little practical value. One exception is ulcers in the gastric fundus above the level of the esophagogastric junction, essentially all of which are malignant.

An abrupt transition between the normal mucosa and the abnormal tissues surrounding a gastric ulcer is characteristic of a malignant lesion (Figure 4-27), in contrast to the diffuse and almost imperceptible transition between the normal gastric mucosa and the mound of edema surrounding a benign ulcer. Neoplastic tissue surrounding a malignant ulcer is usually nodular, unlike the smooth contour of the edematous mound around a benign ulcer. A malignant ulcer does not penetrate beyond the normal gastric lumen but remains within it because the ulcer merely represents a necrotic area within an intramural or intraluminal mass.

Most benign gastric ulcers heal completely with medical therapy (Figure 4-28). Complete healing does not necessarily mean that the stomach returns to an absolutely normal radiographic appearance; bizarre deformities can result because of fibrotic retraction and stiffening of the wall of the stomach. Although many malignant ulcers show significant healing, there is almost never complete disappearance of the ulcer crater.

The role of endoscopy in evaluating patients with gastric ulcers is controversial. At present, endoscopy is indicated whenever the radiographic findings are not typical of a benign ulcer, if healing of the ulcer does not progress at the expected rate, or if the mucosa surrounding a healed ulcer crater has a nodular surface or any other feature suggestive of an underlying early gastric cancer.

Superficial gastric erosions

Superficial gastric erosions are ulcerations that are so small and shallow that they are rarely demonstrated on conventional single-contrast upper gastrointestinal examinations. With the increasing use

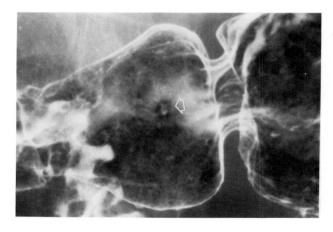

Figure 4-29 Superficial gastric erosions in patient with gastritis. Collection of barium represents shallow erosion surrounded by radiolucent halo *(arrow).*

of double-contrast techniques, a superficial gastric erosion typically appears radiographically as a tiny fleck of barium, which represents the erosion, surrounded by a radiolucent halo, which represents a mound of edematous mucosa (Figure 4-29). Possible factors implicated in the production of superficial gastric erosions include alcohol, anti-inflammatory drugs (aspirin, steroids), Crohn's disease (see page 135), and candidiasis (see page 119).

Cancer of the stomach

Because pain is infrequently an early symptom, carcinoma of the stomach is rarely noted until the disease is far advanced and thus has a dismal prognosis. The incidence of gastric cancer varies widely throughout the world. It is very high in Japan, Chile, and parts of Eastern Europe. It is low in the United States, where for an unknown reason the incidence of the disease has been decreasing. Several conditions appear to predispose persons to the development of carcinoma of the stomach. There is an increased risk of gastric cancer in patients with atrophic gastric mucosa, as a pernicious anemia, and in persons 10 to 20 years after a partial gastrectomy for peptic ulcer disease. A suggestive laboratory sign is achlorhydria, the absence of hydrochloric acid in gastric secretions obtained by means of a stomach tube.

Gastric carcinoma can present a broad spectrum of radiographic appearances. Tumor infiltration of the gastric wall may stimulate intense fibrosis, which produces diffuse thickening, narrowing, and fixa-

tion of the stomach wall (linitis plastica pattern) (Figure 4-30). The stomach is contracted into a tubular structure without normal pliability. This fibrotic process usually begins near the pylorus and progresses slowly upward with the fundus being the area least involved. Another major form of gastric carcinoma is a large polypoid mass. Irregularity and ulceration within the mass suggests malignancy, whereas the presence of a stalk or normal-appearing gastric folds extending to the tumor are signs of benignancy. Ulceration can develop in any gastric carcinoma. This varies from shallow erosions in relatively superficial mucosal lesions to huge excavations within fungating polypoid masses (Figure 4-31).

CT is of major value in the staging and treatment planning of gastric carcinoma, in assessing the response to therapy, and in detecting tumor recurrence (Figure 4-32). Carcinoma of the stomach may appear as thickening of the gastric wall or as an intraluminal mass. Obliteration of the fat planes (covering layers of fat) around the stomach is a reliable indicator of the extragastric spread of tumor. CT can demonstrate direct tumor extension to intra-abdominal organs and distant metastases, especially to the liver.

Lymphoma of the stomach
See later chapter.

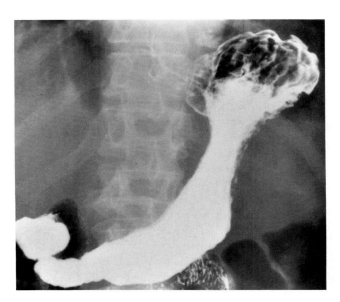

Figure 4-30 Gastric carcinoma producing linitis plastica pattern.

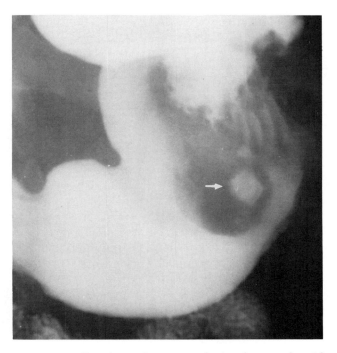

Figure 4-31 Gastric carcinoma producing large polypoid mass with associated ulceration (arrow).

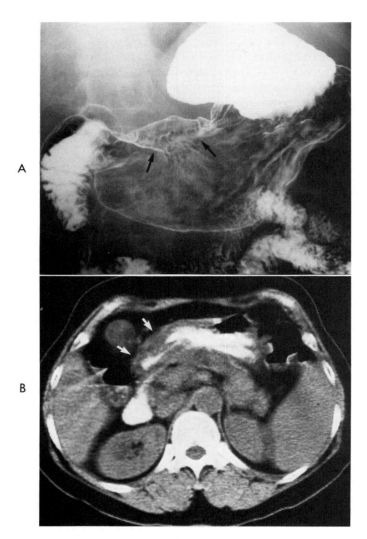

Figure 4-32 CT staging of gastric carcinoma. **A,** Double-contrast study demonstrates large lesser-curvature mass *(arrows)*. **B,** CT scan shows narrowing of antrum by gastric carcinoma *(white arrows),* and adjacent lymph node metastases *(curved arrow).*

SMALL BOWEL

Small bowel obstruction

Fibrous adhesions caused by previous surgery or peritonitis account for almost 75% of all small bowel obstructions. External hernias (inguinal, femoral, umbilical, incisional) are the second most frequent cause. Other general causes of mechanical small bowel obstruction include luminal occlusion (gallstone, intussusception) and intrinsic lesions of the bowel wall (neoplastic or inflammatory strictures, vascular insufficiency).

Distended loops of small bowel containing gas and fluid can usually be recognized within 3 to 5 hours of the onset of complete obstruction. Almost all gas proximal to a small bowel obstruction represents swallowed air. On upright or lateral decubitus projections, the interface between gas and fluid forms a straight horizontal margin. Gas-fluid levels are occasionally present normally, but more than two gas-fluid levels in small bowel distal to the duodenum are generally considered to be abnormal (Figure 4-33). Although the presence of gas-fluid levels at different heights in the same loop has traditionally been considered evidence for mechanical obstruction, an identical pattern can also be demonstrated in some patients with adynamic ileus.

As time passes, the small bowel may become so distended as to be almost indistinguishable from the colon. To make the critical differentiation between small and large bowel obstruction, it is essential to determine which loops of bowel contain abnormally large amounts of air. Small bowel loops generally occupy the more central portion of the abdomen, whereas colonic loops are positioned laterally around the periphery of the abdomen or inferiorly in the pelvis (Figure 4-34). Gas within the lumen of the small bowel outlines the thin valvulae conniventes, which completely encircle the bowel. In contrast, colonic haustral markings are thicker and farther apart and occupy only a portion of the transverse diameter of the bowel.

The site of obstruction can usually be predicted with considerable accuracy if the number and position of dilated bowel loops are analyzed. The presence of a few dilated loops of small bowel located high in the abdomen (in the center or slightly to the left) indicates an obstruction in the distal duodenum or jejunum. The involvement of more small bowel loops suggests a lower obstruction. As additional loops are affected, they appear to be placed one above the other upward and to the left, producing a characteristic stepladder appearance (Figure 4-35). The point of obstruction is always distal to the lowest loop of dilated bowel.

In patients with complete mechanical small bowel obstruction, little or no gas is found in the colon. This is a valuable point in the differentiation between mechanical obstruction and adynamic ileus, in which gas is seen within distended loops throughout the bowel. Although a small amount of gas or fecal accumulations may be present at an early stage of a small bowel obstruction (Figure 4-34), the detection of a large amount of gas in the colon effectively eliminates this diagnosis.

The bowel proximal to an obstruction can contain no gas but be completely filled with fluid. This may produce a confusing picture of a normal-appearing abdomen or a large soft-tissue abdominal mass.

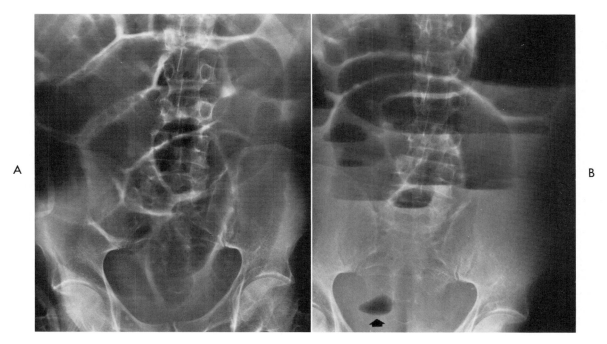

Figure 4-33 Small bowel obstruction. **A,** Supine and, **B,** upright projections demonstrate large amounts of gas in dilated loops of small bowel with multiple prominent air-fluid levels. Single, small collection of gas *(arrow)* remains in colon.

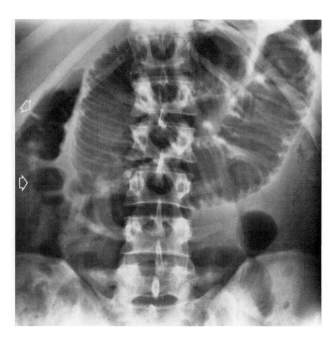

Figure 4-34 Small bowel obstruction. Dilated loops of small bowel occupy central portion of abdomen, with non-dilated cecum and ascending colon positioned laterally around periphery of abdomen *(arrows)*.

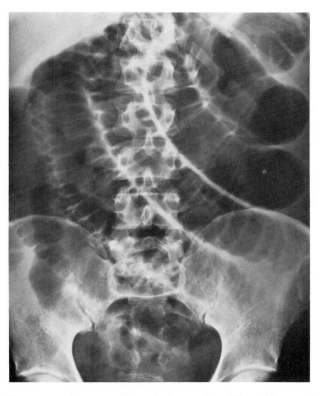

Figure 4-35 Low small bowel obstruction. Dilated loops of gas-filled bowel appear to be placed one above other, upward and to left, producing characteristic stepladder appearance.

Plain abdominal radiographs are occasionally not sufficient for a distinction to be made between small and large bowel obstruction. In these instances a carefully performed barium enema examination will document or eliminate the possibility of large bowel obstruction. If it is necessary to determine the precise site of small bowel obstruction, barium can be administered in either a retrograde (by means of an enema) or an antegrade (by way of the mouth) manner. Oral barium (*not* water-soluble agents) is the most effective contrast material for demonstrating the site of small bowel obstruction (Figure 4-36). The large amount of fluid proximal to a small bowel obstruction prevents any trapped barium from hardening or increasing the degree of obstruction. The density of barium permits excellent visualization far into the intestine, unlike water-soluble agents, which are lost to sight because of dilution and absorption. It must be emphasized that if plain radiographs clearly demonstrate a mechanical small bowel obstruction, *any* contrast examination is unnecessary.

Strangulation of bowel caused by interference with the blood supply is a serious complication of small bowel obstruction. In a closed-loop obstruction (volvulus, incarcerated hernia), both the loops going toward (afferent) and away from (efferent) the area of narrowing become obstructed. The involved segments are usually filled with fluid and appear radiographically as a tumorlike soft-tissue mass. A closed loop is a clinically dangerous form of obstruction, since the continuing outpouring of fluid into the enclosed space can raise intraluminal pressure and rapidly lead to occlusion of the blood supply to that segment of bowel. Because venous pressure is normally lower than arterial pressure, blockage of venous outflow from the strangulated segment occurs before obstruction of the mesenteric arterial supply. Ischemia can rapidly cause necrosis of the bowel with sepsis, peritonitis, and a potentially fatal outcome.

Adynamic ileus

Adynamic ileus is a common disorder of intestinal motor activity in which fluid and gas do not progress normally through a nonobstructed small and large bowel. A variety of neural, hormonal, and metabolic

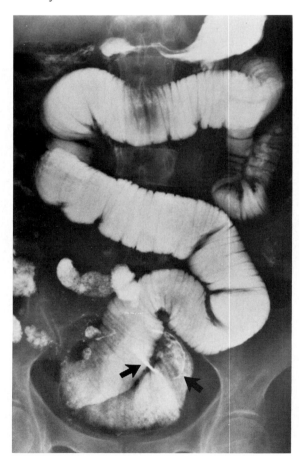

Figure 4-36 Barium upper gastrointestinal series demonstrates impacted bezoar *(arrows)* to be cause of small bowel obstruction.

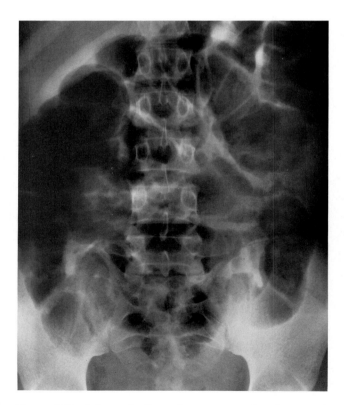

Figure 4-37 Adynamic ileus. Large amounts of gas and fluid are retained in loops of dilated small and large bowel. Entire small and large bowel appear almost uniformly dilated with no demonstrable point of obstruction.

factors can precipitate reflexes that inhibit intestinal motility. Adynamic ileus occurs to some extent in almost every patient who undergoes abdominal surgery. Other causes of adynamic ileus include peritonitis, medication that decreases intestinal peristalsis (atropine-like effect), electrolyte and metabolic disorders, and trauma. The clinical appearance of patients with adynamic ileus varies from minimal symptoms to generalized abdominal distention with a marked decrease in the frequency and intensity of bowel sounds.

The radiographic hallmark of adynamic ileus is the retention of large amounts of gas and fluid in dilated small and large bowel. Unlike the appearance in mechanical small bowel obstruction, the entire small and large bowel in adynamic ileus appears almost uniformly dilated with no demonstrable point of obstruction (Figure 4-37).

There are two major variants of adynamic ileus. **Localized ileus** refers to an isolated distended loop of small or large bowel (sentinel loop) that is often associated with an adjacent acute inflammatory process. The portion of the bowel involved can offer a clue to the underlying disease. Localized segments of the jejunum or transverse colon are frequently dilated in patients with acute pancreatitis. Similarly, the hepatic flexure of the colon can be distended in acute cholecystitis, the terminal ileum can be dilated in acute appendicitis, the descending colon can be distended in acute diverticulitis, and dilated loops can be seen along the course of the ureter in acute ureteral colic (Figure 4-38). Unfortunately, isolated segments of distended small bowel are commonly seen in patients with abdominal pain and thus the "sentinel loop" may be found guarding the wrong area.

Colonic ileus refers to selective or disproportionate gaseous distention of the large bowel without an obstruction (Figure 4-39). Massive distention of the cecum, which is often horizontally oriented, characteristically dominates the radiographic appearance. Colonic ileus usually accompanies or follows an acute abdominal inflammatory process or abdominal surgery. The clinical presentation and the findings on plain abdominal radiographs simulate those of mechanical obstruction of the colon. A barium enema examination is usually necessary to exclude an obstructing lesion.

Crohn's disease (regional enteritis)

Crohn's disease is a chronic inflammatory disorder of unknown cause that most often involves the terminal ileum but can affect any part of the gastrointestinal tract. Although it can occur at any age, Crohn's disease is most common in young adults. The underlying cause is unknown, although there appears to be some psychogenic element; stress or emotional upsets are frequently related to the onset or relapse of the disease.

The granulomatous inflammatory process in Crohn's disease is frequently discontinuous, with diseased segments of bowel separated by apparently

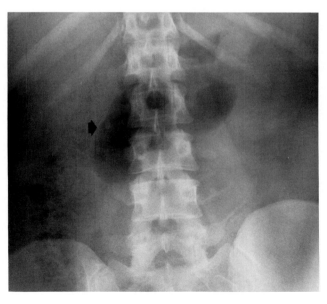

Figure 4-38 Localized ileus in patient with acute ureteral colic. Arrow points to impacted ureteral stone.

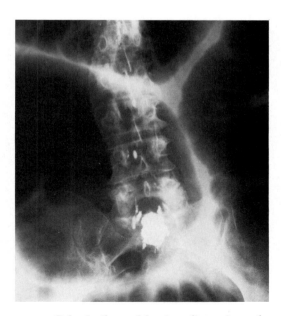

Figure 4-39 Colonic ileus. Massive distension of small bowel without obstruction in pateint with severe diabetes and electrolyte abnormalities.

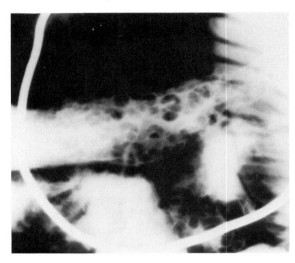

Figure 4-40 Crohn's disease. Cobblestone appearance is produced by transverse and longitudinal ulcerations separating islands of thickened mucosa and submucosa.

healthy portions ("skip areas"). Diffuse inflammation with edema involves all layers of the intestinal wall. Ulceration is common, and fistulas running in the bowel wall or extending to other organs are not infrequent.

The clinical spectrum of Crohn's disease is broad,

ranging from a relatively benign course with unpredictable acute attacks and remissions to severe diarrhea and an acute abdomen. Although acute Crohn's disease may produce right lower quadrant pain simulating appendicitis, there is often blood in the stools in Crohn's disease as a result of bleeding from the intensely congested mucous membranes. Small bowel obstruction and fistula formation occur in up to half of patients. Rectal fissures and perirectal abscesses occur in about one third.

In the small bowel the earliest radiographic changes of Crohn's disease include irregular thickening and distortion of mucosal folds caused by submucosal inflammation and edema. Transverse and longitudinal ulcerations can separate islands of thickened mucosa and submucosa, leading to a characteristic rough cobblestone appearance (Figure 4-40). Rigid thickening of the entire bowel wall produces pipelike narrowing. Continued inflammation and fibrosis can result in a severely narrowed, rigid segment of small bowel in which the mucosal pattern is lost (string sign) (Figure 4-41). When several areas of small bowel are diseased, involved seg-

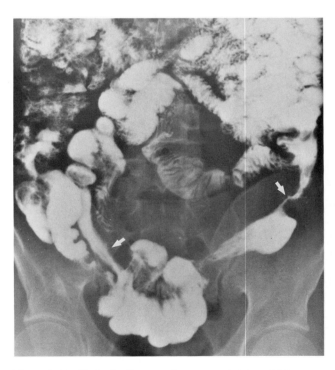

Figure 4-41 Crohn's disease. Arrows point to widely separated areas of disease (skip lesions), which appear as markedly narrowed segments of small bowel (string sign).

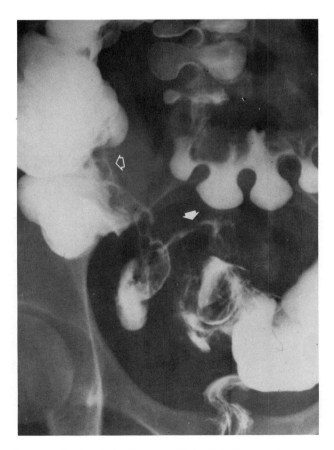

Figure 4-42 Crohn's disease. Note fistulization between terminal ileum and sigmoid colon *(solid arrow)* as well as along cecum *(open arrow)*.

ments of varying length are often sharply separated from radiographically normal segments (skip lesions).

Fistula formation is a hallmark of chronic Crohn's disease found in at least half of all patients with this condition (Figure 4-42). The diffuse inflammation of the serosa and mesentery in Crohn's disease causes involved loops of bowel to be firmly matted together by fibrous peritoneal and mesenteric bands. Fistulas apparently begin as ulcerations that burrow through the bowel wall into adjacent loops of small bowel and colon. In addition to fistulas between loops of bowel, a characteristic finding in Crohn's disease is the appearance of fistulous tracts ending blindly in abscess cavities surrounded by dense inflammatory tissue. These abscess cavities can produce palpable masses, persistent fever, or pain. Although less common than bowel-bowel fistulas, internal fistulas extending from the bowel to the bladder or vagina can occur. A common complication is the development of external gastrointestinal fistulas, which usually extend to the perianal area and may be associated with fissures and perirectal abscesses.

Whenever possible, Crohn's disease is treated with medications, and surgery is only performed if complications require it. Surgical resection of an involved segment of small bowel is associated with a high incidence of Crohn's disease recurring adjacent to the anastomosis.

Malabsorption disorders

The term **malabsorption disorders** refers to a multitude of conditions in which there is defective absorption of carbohydrates, proteins, and fats from the small bowel. Regardless of the cause, malabsorption results in steatorrhea—the passage of bulky, foul-smelling, high-fat-content stools that float.

Many of the diseases causing malabsorption produce radiographic abnormalities in the small bowel, although malabsorption can exist without any detectable small bowel changes. The two major radiographic appearances are (1) small bowel dilation with normal folds (Figure 4-43) and (2) a pattern of generalized, irregular, distorted small bowel folds (Figure 4-44).

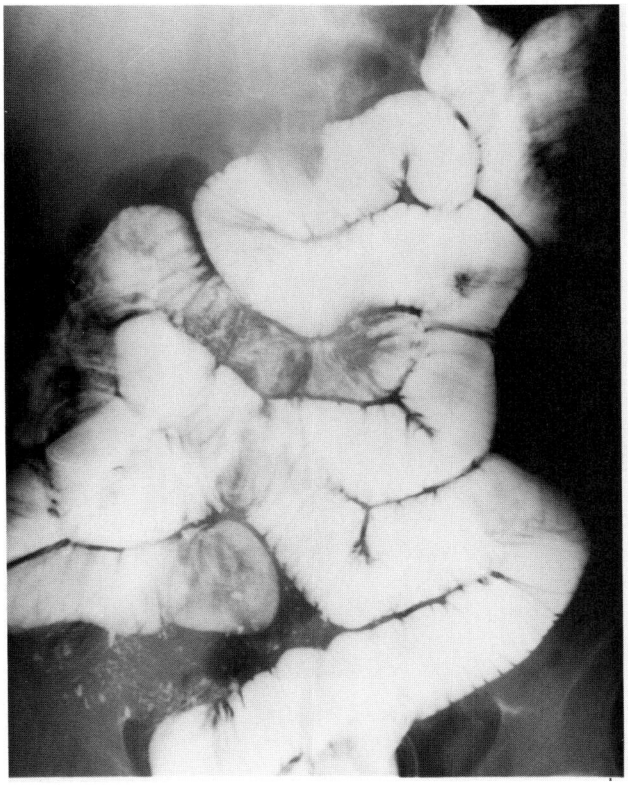

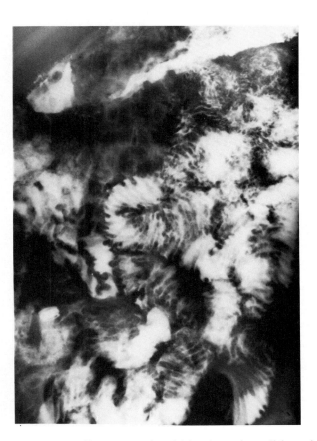

Figure 4-43 Diffuse dilation of entire small bowel with excessive intraluminal fluid in patient with malabsorption caused by sprue.

Figure 4-44 Diffuse, irregular thickening of small bowel folds in patient with malabsorption secondary to Whipple's disease.

Intussusception

Intussusception is a major cause of bowel obstruction in children; it is much less common in adults. Intussusception is the telescoping of one part of the intestinal tract into another because of peristalsis, which forces the proximal segment of bowel to move distally within the ensheathing outer portion. Once such a lead point has been established, it gradually progresses forward and causes increased obstruction. This can compromise the vascular supply and produce ischemic necrosis of the intussuscepted bowel.

In children, intussusception is most common in the region of the ileocecal valve. The clinical onset tends to be abrupt, with severe abdominal pain, blood in the stool ("currant jelly"), and often a palpable right-sided mass. If the diagnosis is made early and therapy instituted promptly, the mortality rate of intussusception in children is less than 1%. However, it treatment is delayed more than 48 hours after the onset of symptoms, the mortality rate increases dramatically. In adults, intussusception is often chronic or subacute and is characterized by irregular recurrent episodes of colicky pain, nausea, and vomiting. A specific cause of intussusception often cannot be detected in children. In adults, however, the leading edge is frequently a polypoid tumor with a stalk (pedunculated) or an inflammatory mass.

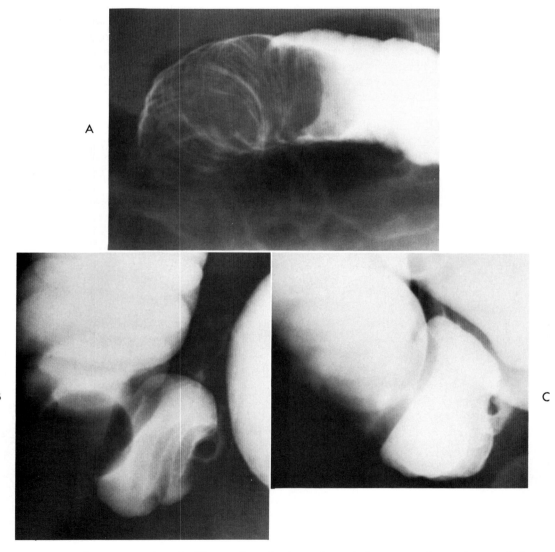

Figure 4-45 Intussusception. **A,** Obstruction of colon at hepatic flexure produces characteristic coiled-spring appearance of intussuscepted bowel. **B,** Partial and, **C,** complete reduction of intussusception by careful barium enema examination.

Radiographically, an intussusception produces the classic coiled-spring appearance of barium trapped between the intussusceptum and the surrounding portions of bowel (Figure 4-45, *A*). Reduction of a colonic intussusception can sometimes be accomplished by a barium enema examination (Figure 4-45, *B,* and *C*), although great care must be exercised to prevent excessive intraluminal pressure that may lead to perforation of the colon. If a colonic intussusception is reduced in an adult, a repeat barium enema examination is necessary to determine whether an underlying polyp or tumor is present.

APPENDICITIS

Acute appendicitis develops when the neck of the appendix is blocked by a fecalith or by postinflammatory scarring that creates a closed-loop obstruction within the organ. Because of inadequate drainage, fluid accumulates in the obstructed portion and serves as a breeding ground for bacteria. High intraluminal pressure causes distention and thinning of the appendix distal to the obstruction that interferes with the circulation and may lead to gangrene and perforation. If the process evolves slowly, adjacent organs (terminal ileum, cecum, omentum) may wall off the appendiceal area so that a localized abscess develops; rapid vascular compromise may permit free perforation with the spilling of fecal material into the peritoneal cavity and the development of generalized peritonitis.

The clinical symptoms of acute appendicitis are usually so characteristic that there is no need for routine radiographs to make the correct diagnosis. The presence of severe right lower quadrant pain, low-grade fever, and slight leukocytosis, especially in younger adults, is presumed to be evidence of appendicitis. However, in some patients, especially the elderly, the clinical findings may be obscure or minimal. In addition, because the appendix is mobile and may be in unusual locations, the pain of acute appendicitis may mimic cholecystitis, diverticulitis, or pelvic inflammatory disease. When the symptoms are confusing, radiographic examination may be necessary for prompt diagnosis and surgical intervention before perforation occurs.

Plain abdominal radiographs may demonstrate a round or oval, laminated calcified fecalith in the appendix (appendicolith) (Figure 4-46). Surgical experience suggests that the presence of an appendicolith in combination with symptoms of acute appendicitis usually implies that the appendix is gangrenous (necrotic) and likely to perforate. Most appendicoliths are located in the right lower quadrant overlying the iliac fossa. Depending on the

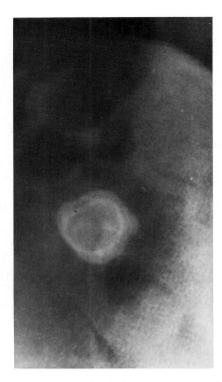

Figure 4-46 Laminated calcification in appendicolith.

length and position of the appendix, however, an appendicolith can also be seen in the pelvis or in the right upper quadrant (retrocecal appendix), where it can simulate a gallstone.

Because of the danger of perforation, barium enema examination is usually avoided in acute appendicitis. If it is performed, an irregular impression of the base of the cecum (caused by inflammatory edema), in association with failure of barium to enter the appendix, is a characteristic finding. Nevertheless, failure of barium to fill the appendix is not a reliable sign of appendicitis, since the appendix does not fill in about 20% of normal patients. Partial filling of the appendix with distortion in its shape or caliber strongly suggests acute appendicitis (Figure 4-47), especially if there is a cecal impression. In contrast, a patent (open) appendiceal lumen effectively excludes the diagnosis of acute appendicitis, especially when barium extends to fill the rounded appendiceal tip.

In the past few years, high-resolution ultrasound with a graded compression technique has proved to be of clinical value in diagnosing questionable cases of acute appendicitis. Initially the sonographic visualization of a noncompressible appendix was considered diagnostic of acute appendicitis. More recent studies show the importance of measuring the width of the appendix's walls. A diagnosis of appendicitis

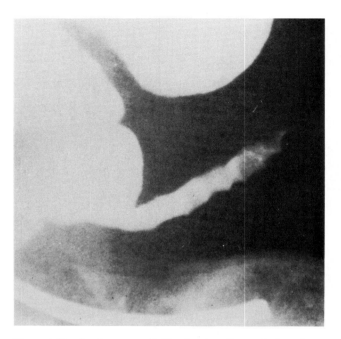

Figure 4-47 Acute appendicitis. Spot radiograph from barium enema examination shows incomplete filling of appendix. *(Rice RP et al: The barium enema in appendicitis: spectrum of appearances and pitfalls, Radiographics 4:393-409, 1984).*

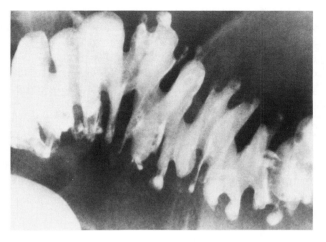

Figure 4-48 Diverticulosis. Typical saw tooth configuration produced by thickened circular muscle associated with multiple diverticula.

could be made in adult patients with persistent right lower quadrant pain and a visualized appendix greater than 6 mm in diameter. If the maximal diameter of the appendix was 6 mm or less, these authors suggested a period of close clinical observation rather than early surgery, as long as no compelling evidence of appendicitis existed or multiple appendicoliths were identified at sonography. Using this approach, they concluded that sonography should significantly reduce the rate of false-negative appendectomies—especially in women, in whom surgery for a noninflamed appendix occurs in up to 40% of cases.

COLON

Diverticulosis

Colonic diverticula are outpouchings that represent acquired herniations of mucosa and submucosa through the muscular layers at points of weakness in the bowel wall. The incidence of colonic diverticulosis increases with age. Rare in persons less than 30 years of age, diverticula can be demonstrated in up to half of persons over 60 years of age. Diverticula occur most commonly in the sigmoid colon and decrease in frequency in the proximal colon. Although most patients with diverticulosis have no symptoms, a substantial number have chronic or intermittent

lower abdominal pain, frequently related to meals or emotional stress, and alternating bouts of diarrhea and constipation. Bleeding may be caused by inflammatory erosion of penetrating blood vessels at the base of the diverticulum.

Colonic diverticula appear radiographically as round or oval outpouchings of barium projecting beyond the confines of the lumen. They vary in size from barely visible dimples to saclike structures 2 cm or more in diameter. Giant sigmoid diverticula of up to 25 cm in diameter, which probably represent slowly progressing chronic diverticular abscesses, may appear as large, well-circumscribed, lucent cystic structures in the lower abdomen.

Diverticula are usually multiple and tend to occur in clusters, although a solitary diverticulum is occasionally found. With multiple diverticula, deep criss-crossing ridges of thickened circular muscle can produce a characteristic series of sacculations (saw-tooth configuration) (Figure 4-48).

Diverticula also commonly occur in the esophagus and duodenum and infrequently may develop in the jejunum and ileum.

Diverticulitis

Diverticulitis is a complication of diverticular disease of the colon, especially in the sigmoid region, in which perforation of a diverticulum leads to the development of a peridiverticular abscess. It is estimated that up to 20% of patients with diverticulosis eventually develop acute diverticulitis. Retained fecal material trapped in a diverticulum by the narrow opening of the diverticular neck causes inflammation of the mucosal lining that leads to perforation of the diverticulum. This usually results in a local-

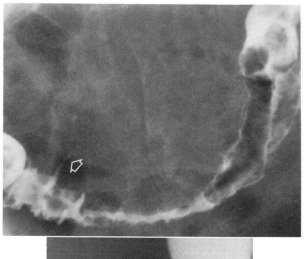

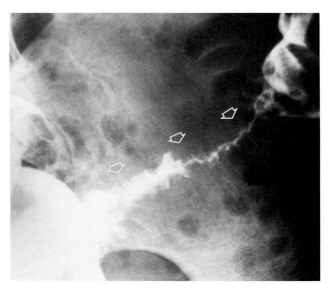

Figure 4-50 Sigmoid diverticulitis. Severe narrowing of long, involved portion of sigmoid colon *(arrows)* in patient with no radiographically detectable diverticula.

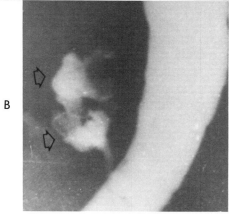

Figure 4-49 Diverticulitis. **A,** Thin projection of contrast *(arrow)* implies extravasation from colonic lumen. Note severe spasm of sigmoid colon caused by intense adjacent inflammation. **B,** Obvious contrast filling of pericolic abscess *(arrows).*

ized peridiverticular abscess that is walled off by fibrous adhesions. The inflammatory process may localize within the wall of the colon and produce an intramural mass, or it may dissect around the colon, causing segmental narrowing of the lumen. Extension of the inflammatory process along the colon wall can involve adjacent diverticula, resulting in a longitudinal sinus tract along the bowel wall. A common complication of diverticulitis is the development of fistulas to adjacent organs (bladder, vagina, ureter, small bowel).

The radiographic diagnosis of diverticulitis requires direct or indirect evidence of diverticular perforation. The most specific sign is extravasation, which can appear either as a tiny projection of contrast material from the tip of a diverticulum (Figure 4-49, *A*) or as obvious filling of a pericolic abscess (Figure 4-49, *B*). A more common, although some-

what less specific, sign of diverticulitis is the demonstration of a pericolic soft-tissue mass that is due to a localized abscess and represents a walled-off perforation. This extraluminal mass appears as a filling defect causing eccentric narrowing of the bowel lumen. The adjacent diverticula are spastic, irritable, and attenuated and frequently seem to drape over the mass. It is important to remember, however, that a peridiverticular abscess caused by diverticulitis can occur without radiographically detectable diverticula (Figure 4-50).

Severe spasm or fibrotic healing of diverticulitis can cause rigidity and progressive narrowing of the colon that simulates annular carcinoma. Although radiographic distinction from carcinoma may be impossible, findings favoring the diagnosis of diverticulitis include the involvement of a relatively long segment, a gradual transition from diseased to normal colon, a relative preservation of mucosal detail, and fistulous tracts and intramural abscesses. At times, colonoscopy or surgery may be required to make a definitive diagnosis.

Ulcerative colitis

Ulcerative colitis is primarily a disease of young adults that is highly variable in severity, clinical course, and ultimate prognosis. The etiology is unknown, although an autoimmune cause has been suggested and a psychogenic factor may be involved because the condition is often aggravated by stress. The onset of the disease, as well as subsequent exacerbations, can be insidious or abrupt. The main symptoms include bloody diarrhea, abdominal pain, fever, and weight loss. A characteristic feature of ulcerative colitis is alternating periods of remission and relapse. Most patients have intermittent episodes of symptoms with complete remission between attacks. In fewer than 15% of patients, ulcerative colitis is an acute severe process with a far higher incidence of serious complications such as toxic megacolon (extreme dilation of a segment of colon with systemic toxicity) and free perforation into the peritoneal cavity.

In the radiographic evaluation of a patient with known or suspected ulcerative colitis, plain abdominal radiographs are essential. Large nodular protrusions of hyperplastic mucosa, deep ulcers outlined by intraluminal gas, or polypoid changes along with a loss of haustral markings (normal indentations in the wall of the colon) suggest the diagnosis. Plain abdominal radiographs can also demonstrate evidence of toxic megacolon, a dramatic and ominous complication of ulcerative colitis that is characterized by extreme dilation of a segment of colon (Figure 4-51), or of an entire diseased colon, combined with systemic toxicity (abdominal pain and tenderness, tachycardia, fever, and leukocytosis). Toxic megacolon can lead to spontaneous perforation of the colon, which can be dramatic and sudden and can cause irreversible shock. Because there is such a high danger of spontaneous perforation, barium enema examination is absolutely contraindicated during a recognized attack of toxic megacolon.

Ulcerative colitis has a strong tendency to begin in the rectosigmoid area. Although by radiographic

criteria alone the rectum appears normal in about 20% of patients with ulcerative colitis, true rectal sparing is infrequent, and there is usually evidence of disease on sigmoidoscopy or rectal biopsy. Although ulcerative colitis may spread to involve the entire colon (pancolitis), isolated right colon disease with a normal left colon does not occur. The disease is almost always continuous, without evidence of the skip areas seen in Crohn's disease. Except for "backwash ileitis" (minimal inflammatory changes involving a short segment of terminal ileum), ulcerative colitis does not involve the small bowel, a feature distinguishing it from Crohn's disease, which may involve both the large and the small intestines.

On double-contrast studies, the earliest detectable radiographic abnormality in ulcerative colitis is fine granularity of the mucosa corresponding to the hyperemia and edema seen endoscopically (Figure 4-52). Once superficial ulcers develop, small flecks of adherent barium produce a stippled mucosal pattern. As the disease progresses, the ulcerations become deeper. Extension into the submucosa may produce broad-based ulcers with a collar-button appearance (Figure 4-53). Perirectal inflammation can cause widening of the soft-tissue space between the anterior sacrum and the posterior rectum (retrorectal space).

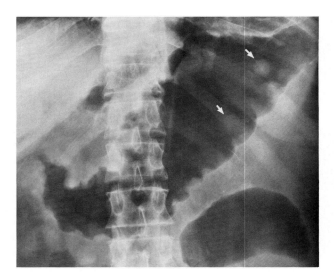

Figure 4-51 Toxic megacolon in ulcerative colitis. Note dilation of transverse colon with multiple pseudopolypoid projections extending into lumen *(arrows)*.

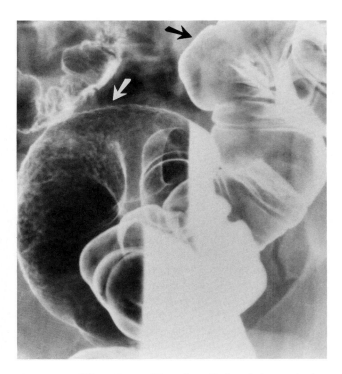

Figure 4-52 Ulcerative colitis primarily involving rectosigmoid. Distal rectosigmoid mucosa *(white arrow)* is finely granular, compared with normal-appearing mucosa *(black arrow)* in the more proximal colon.

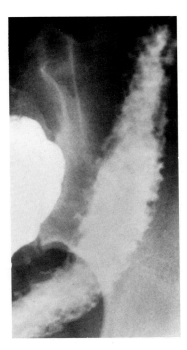

Figure 4-53 Ulcerative colitis. Progression of disease results in deep ulceration (collar-button ulcers) extending into submucosal layer.

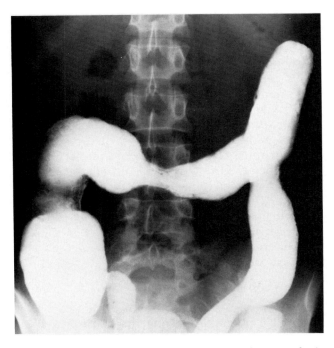

Figure 4-54 Chronic ulcerative colitis (lead-pipe colon). Muscular hypertrophy and spasm cause shortening and rigidity of colon with loss of haustral markings.

With chronic disease, fibrosis and muscular spasm cause progressive shortening and rigidity of the colon (Figure 4-54). The haustral pattern is absent, and the bowel contour is relatively smooth because of ulcer healing and subsequent re-epithelial-ization. Eventually, the colon may appear as a symmetric, rigid tubular structure (lead-pipe colon).

Carcinoma of the colon is about 10 times more frequent in patients with ulcerative colitis than in the general population. During the first 10 years of

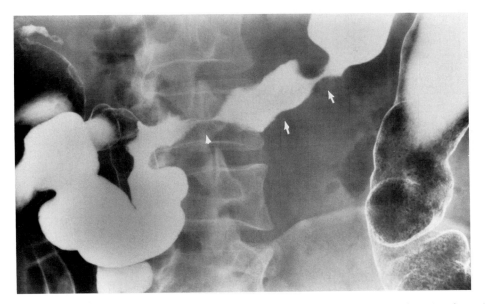

Figure 4-55 Carcinoma of colon developing in patient with long-standing chronic ulcerative colitis. Long, irregular lesion with bizarre pattern is visible in transverse colon *(arrows)*.

disease, there is only a small risk of malignancy. Thereafter, it is estimated that there is a 20% chance per decade that a patient with ulcerative colitis will develop carcinoma. Malignant lesions in ulcerative colitis generally occur at a much younger age than the general population and tend to be extremely virulent. Carcinoma of the colon in patients with chronic ulcerative colitis often appears as a bizarre stricture rather than with the more characteristic polypoid or apple-core appearance of a primary colonic malignancy (Figure 4-55). The tumor typically produces a narrowed segment with an eccentric lumen, irregular contours, and margins that are rigid and tapered. Because it is frequently difficult to distinguish carcinoma from benign stricture in patients with ulcerative colitis, colonscopy or surgery is often required for an unequivocal diagnosis.

Crohn's colitis

Crohn's disease of the colon is identical to the same pathologic process involving the small bowel and must be distinguished from ulcerative colitis. The proximal portion of the colon is most frequently involved in Crohn's disease; associated disease of the terminal ileum is seen in up to 80% of the patients. Unlike ulcerative colitis, in Crohn's colitis the rectum is often spared, and isolated rectal disease very rarely occurs. Crohn's disease usually has a patchy distribution, with involvement of multiple noncontiguous segments of colon (skip lesions), unlike the continuous colonic involvement in ulcerative colitis. Perirectal abnormalities (fissures, abscesses, fistulas)

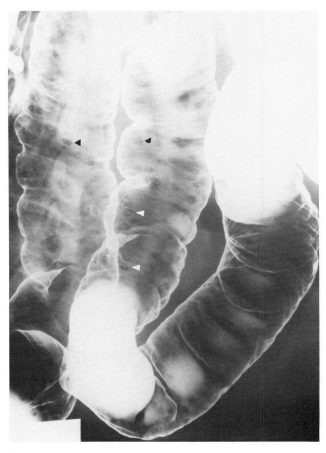

Figure 4-56 Diffuse aphthous ulcers *(arrowheads)* in early Crohn's colitis. *(Caroline DF and Evers K: Colitis, Radiol Clin North Am 25:47-66, 1987.)*

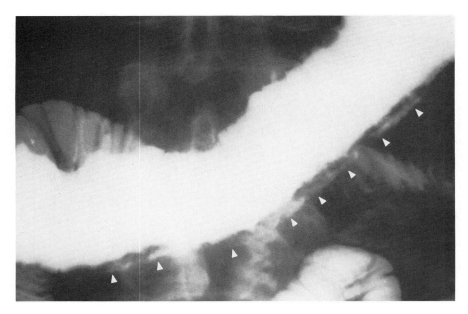

Figure 4-57 Crohn's colitis. Note long intramural fistula *(arrowheads)* in transverse colon. *(Lichtenstein JE: Radiol Clin North Am 25:3-23, 1987.)*

occur at some point during the course of disease in half of patients with Crohn's colitis but are rare in ulcerative colitis.

The earliest radiographic findings of Crohn's disease of the colon are seen on double-contrast examinations. Isolated tiny, discrete erosions (aphthous ulcers) appear as punctate collections of barium with a thin halo of edema around them (Figure 4-56). Aphthous ulcers in Crohn's disease have a patchy distribution against a background of normal mucosa, unlike the blanket of abnormal granular mucosa seen in ulcerative colitis.

As Crohn's colitis progresses, the ulcers become deeper and more irregular, with a great variation in size, shape, and overall appearance. Deep linear, transverse, and longitudinal ulcers often separate intervening mounds of edematous but nonulcerating mucosa, producing a characteristic cobblestone appearance (Figure 4-40). If the penetrating ulcers extend beyond the contour of the bowel, they can coalesce to form long tracts running parallel to the long axis of the colon (Figure 4-57). The penetration of ulcers into adjacent loops of bowel or into the bladder, vagina, or abdominal wall causes fistulas that can often be demonstrated radiographically.

Inflammatory and fibrotic thickening of the bowel wall leads to narrowing of the lumen and stricture formation. Occasionally, an eccentric stricture with a suggestion of overhanging edges can be difficult to distinguish from annular carcinoma (Figure 4-58).

In most instances, however, characteristic features of Crohn's disease elsewhere in the colon (deep ulcerations, pseudopolyps, skip lesions, sinus tracts, fistulas) clearly indicate the correct diagnosis.

Patients with Crohn's colitis appear to have a higher incidence of developing colon cancer than the general population, although this association is less striking than between colon cancer and ulcerative colitis. Carcinoma complicating Crohn's colitis is most common in the proximal portion of the colon and usually appears radiographically as a fungating mass with typical malignant features, unlike the mildly irregular stricture characteristic of colon cancer in patients with ulcerative colitis.

Ischemic colitis

Ischemic colitis is characterized by the abrupt onset of lower abdominal pain and rectal bleeding. Diarrhea is common, as is abdominal tenderness on physical examination. Most patients are older than 50 years of age, and many have a history of prior cardiovascular disease.

The initial radiographic appearance of ischemic colitis is fine superficial ulceration caused by inflammatory edema of the mucosa. As the disease progresses, deep penetrating ulcers, pseudopolyps, and characteristic "thumbprinting" can be demonstrated. Thumbprinting refers to sharply defined, fingerlike indentations along the margins of the colon wall (Figure 4-59). In most cases the radiographic

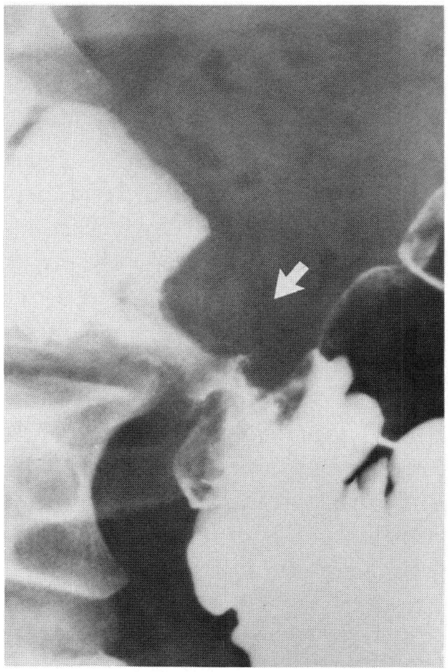

Figure 4-58 Chronic Crohn's colitis. Benign stricture with overhanging edges in transverse colon simulates carcinoma *(arrow)*.

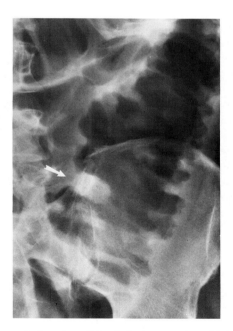

Figure 4-59 Ischemic colitis. Soft-tissue polypoid densities *(arrow)* protrude into lumen of descending colon in patient with acute abdominal pain and rectal bleeding.

appearance of the colon returns to normal within 1 month if good collateral circulation is established. Extensive fibrosis during the healing phase can cause tubular narrowing and a smooth stricture. If blood flow is insufficient, acute bowel necrosis and perforation may result.

Irritable bowel syndrome

The term **irritable bowel syndrome** refers to several conditions that have an alteration in intestinal motility as the underlying pathophysiologic abnormality. Patients with this condition may complain primarily of chronic abdominal pain and constipation (spastic colitis), chronic intermittent watery diarrhea, often without pain, or alternating bouts of constipation and diarrhea. Although there are no specific radiographic findings in the irritable bowel syndrome, patients with this condition usually undergo a barium enema examination to exclude another chronic disorder as the cause of the symptoms. When the patient is symptomatic, the barium enema may demonstrate areas of irritability and spasticity and accentuated haustration, although similar radiographic findings may be observed in normal asymptomatic persons, especially those who have received laxatives and enemas.

Cancer of the colon

Carcinoma of the colon and rectum is the leading cause of death from cancer in the United States, although it can be more easily diagnosed than most other malignant neoplasms. About half of colon carcinomas occur in the rectum and sigmoid, where they can be felt by rectal examination or seen with a sigmoidoscope. Carcinoma of the colon and rectum is primarily a disease of older persons, with a peak incidence in the 50- to 70-year range. Two diseases predispose to development of cancer of the colon: long-standing ulcerative colitis and familial polyposis, a hereditary disease in which innumerable polyps develop in the colon and elsewhere in the intestinal tract.

Because cancer of the colon is curable if discovered early in the course, delay in diagnosis is the most significant factor in the poor prognosis. There is considerable evidence to suggest that many, if not most, carcinomas of the colon arise in pre-existing polyps. Therefore the early diagnosis of colonic cancer is basically an exercise in polyp detection. Malignant polyps (Figure 4-60) tend to be sessile lesions (without stalks) with an irregular or lobulated surface, unlike benign polyps that are usually smooth and often have a stalk (pedunculated). Other radiographic criteria suggesting that a polyp is malignant include large size (especially if greater than 2 cm in

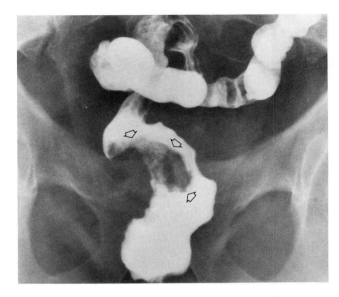

Figure 4-60 Carcinoma of rectum. Bulky lesion *(arrows)* could be felt on rectal examination.

diameter), retraction or indentation (puckering) of the colon wall seen on profile view at the site of origin of a sessile polyp, and evidence of interval growth of a polyp on sequential examinations.

Annular carcinoma (apple-core, napkin-ring) is one of the most typical forms of primary colonic malignancy (Figure 4-61). Annular carcinomas appear to arise from flat plaques of tumor (saddle lesions) that involve only a portion of the circumference of the colon wall. Unless there is meticulous care in searching for an area of minimal straightening or slight contour defects, the small and subtle, but lethal, saddle carcinomas can easily be overlooked. As the tumor grows, it characteristically infiltrates the bowel wall rather than forming a bulky intraluminal mass. This produces a classic bilateral contour defect with ulcerated mucosa, eccentric and irregular lumen, and overhanging margins. Progressive constriction of the bowel can cause complete colonic obstruction, most commonly in the sigmoid region.

Ulceration is common in carcinoma of the colon. It can vary from an excavation within a large fungating mass to mucosal destruction within an annular apple-core tumor.

A patient with carcinoma of the colon has a 1% risk of having multiple synchronous (same time) colon cancers. Therefore it is essential to carefully examine the rest of the colon once an obviously malignant lesion has been detected. In addition, such a patient has a 3% risk of developing additional metachronous cancers at a later date.

CT is a major modality for staging carcinoma of the colon and in assessing tumor recurrence

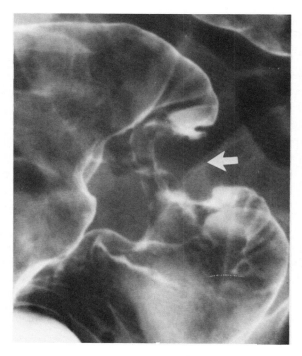

Figure 4-61 Annular carcinoma of sigmoid colon. Note sharply defined proximal and distal margins of this relatively short, apple-core lesion *(arrow).*

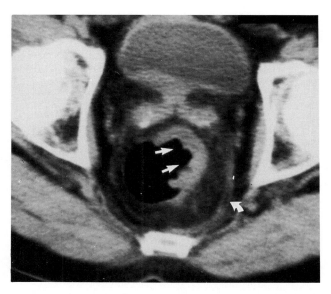

Figure 4-62 CT of rectal carcinoma. Note a soft-tissue mass on lateral wall of rectum containing central ulceration *(straight arrows).* Thickening of perirectal fascia *(curved arrow),* presence of multiple lymph nodes (on more cephalad images), and increased soft-tissue density of perirectal fat suggested tumor extension beyond bowel wall, which was confirmed at surgery. *(Butch RJ: In Taveras JM and Ferrucci JT, editors: Radiology: diagnosis-imaging-intervention, Philadelphia, JB Lippincott, 1987.)*

(Figure 4-62). Carcinoma causes asymmetric or circumferential thickening of the bowel wall with narrowing and deformity of the lumen. CT can demonstrate local extension of tumor to the pelvic organs as well as lymphadenopathy and metastases to the adrenal glands or liver.

Large bowel obstruction

About 70% of large bowel obstructions are a result of primary colonic carcinoma. Diverticulitis and volvulus account for most other cases. Colonic obstructions tend to be less acute than small bowel obstructions; the symptoms develop more slowly, and fewer fluid and electrolyte disturbances are produced.

The radiographic appearance of colonic obstruction depends on the competency of the ileocecal valve. If the ileocecal valve is competent, obstruction causes a large, dilated colon with a markedly distended, thin-walled cecum and little small bowel gas. The colon distal to the obstruction is usually collapsed and free of gas. If the ileocecal valve is incompetent, there is distention of gas-filled loops of both colon and small bowel that may simulate an adynamic ileus.

The major danger in colonic obstruction is perforation. If the ileocecal valve is competent, the colon

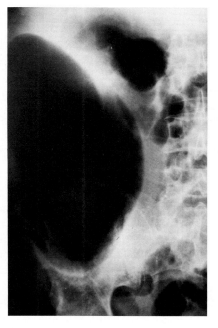

Figure 4-63 Large bowel obstruction. Huge dilation of cecum (to 13 cm in diameter) without perforation.

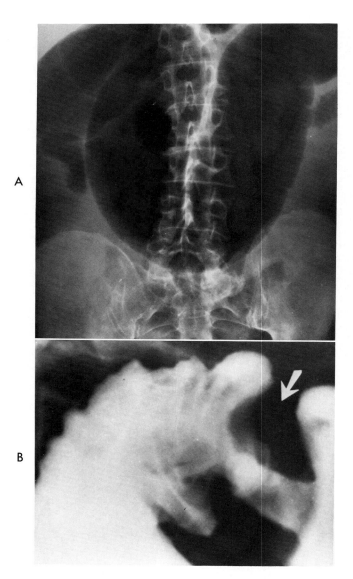

Figure 4-64 Large bowel obstruction caused by annular carcinoma of sigmoid. **A,** Plain abdominal radiograph demonstrates pronounced dilation of gas-filled transverse and ascending colon. **B,** Barium enema demonstrates typical apple-core lesion *(arrow)* producing the colonic obstruction.

behaves like a closed loop, and the increased pressure caused by the obstruction cannot be relieved. Because the cecum is spherical and has a large diameter, it is the most likely site for perforation. In acute colonic obstruction, perforation is very likely if the cecum distends to more than 10 cm; in intermittent or chronic obstruction, however, the cecal wall can become hypertrophied, and the diameter of the cecum can greatly exceed 10 cm without perforation (Figure 4-63). In the patient with suspected large bowel obstruction, a low-pressure barium enema can be safely performed and will demonstrate the site and often the cause of the obstruction (Figure 4-64).

Volvulus of the colon

Volvulus refers to a twisting of the bowel on itself that may lead to intestinal obstruction. Because twisting of the bowel usually requires a long, movable mesentery, volvulus of the large bowel most frequently involves the cecum and sigmoid colon. The transverse colon, which has a short mesentery, is rarely affected by volvulus.

Cecal volvulus

The ascending colon and the cecum may have a long mesentery as a fault of rotation and fixation during the embryonic development of the gut. This situation predisposes to volvulus, with the cecum twisting on its long axis. It should be stressed, however, that only a few patients with an extremely mobile cecum ever develop cecal volvulus.

In cecal volvulus the distended cecum tends to be displaced upward and to the left, although it can be found anywhere within the abdomen. A pathognomonic sign of cecal volvulus is a kidney-shaped mass (representing the twisted cecum) with the twisted and thickened mesentery mimicking the renal pelvis (Figure 4-65, *A*). A barium enema examination is usually required for definite confirmation of the diagnosis. This study demonstrates obstruction of the contrast column at the level of the stenosis, with the tapered edge of the column pointing toward the site of the twist (Figure 4-65, *B*).

Sigmoid volvulus

A long, redundant loop of sigmoid colon can undergo a twist on its mesenteric axis and form a closed-loop obstruction. In sigmoid volvulus the greatly inflated sigmoid loop appears as an inverted U-shaped shadow that rises out of the pelvis in a vertical or oblique direction and can even reach the level of the diaphragm. The affected loop appears devoid of haustral markings and has a sausage or balloon shape. A barium enema examination demonstrates an obstruction to the flow of contrast material at the site of volvulus and marked distention of the rectum. The lumen of the sigmoid tapers toward the site of stenosis, and a pathognomonic bird's beak appearance is produced (Figure 4-66).

Hemorrhoids

Hemorrhoids are varicose veins of the lower end of the rectum that cause pain, itching, and bleeding. As with varicose veins in the leg, hemorrhoids are due to increased venous pressure. The most com-

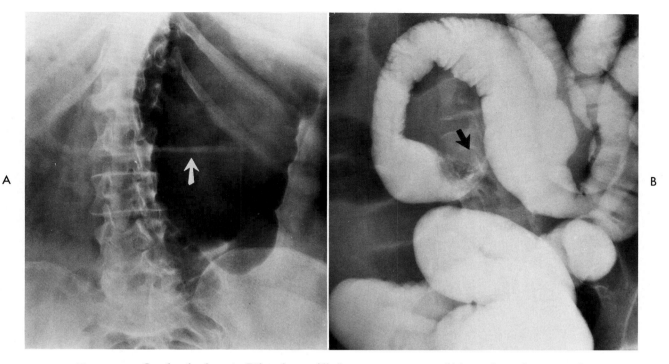

Figure 4-65 Cecal volvulus. **A,** Dilated, gas-filled cecum appears as kidney-shaped mass with torqued and thickening mesentery *(arrow)* mimicking renal pelvis. **B,** Barium enema examination demonstrates obstruction of contrast column at level of stenosis *(arrow)* with tapered edge of column pointing toward torsion site.

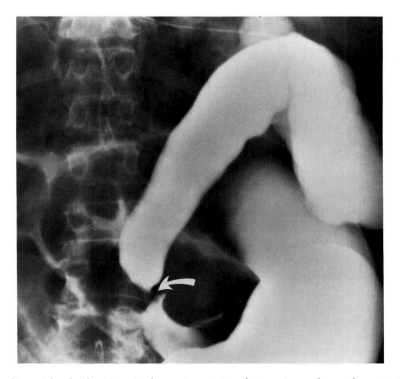

Figure 4-66 Sigmoid volvulus. Luminal tapering at site of stenosis produces characteristic bird's-beak configuration.

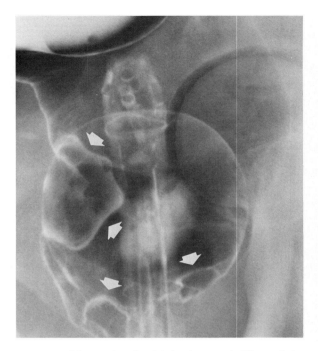

Figure 4-67 Hemorrhoids. Multiple rectal filling defects *(arrows)* simulate polyps.

mon cause of increased pressure is chronic constipation with resulting excessive muscular straining needed to empty the bowel. Increased venous pressure can also be produced by a pelvic tumor or a pregnant uterus.

On barium enema examinations, hemorrhoids occasionally can produce single or multiple rectal filling defects that simulate polyps (Figure 4-67). The proper diagnosis can easily be made by inspection, digital examination, or direct vision through the anoscope.

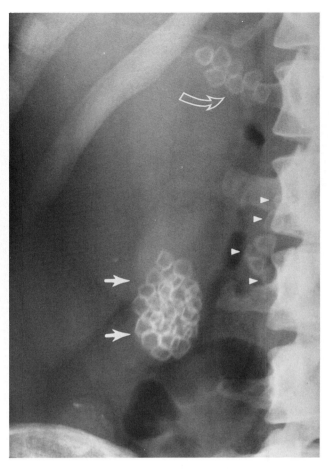

Figure 4-68 Calculi in gallbladder *(solid arrows)* and bile ducts *(open arrow)*. Calculi *(arrowheads)* lie in common bile duct, some of which overlie spine and are difficult to detect. *(Courtesy Stephen R. Baker, New York, N.Y.)*

GALLBLADDER

Gallstones (cholelithiasis)

Gallstones can develop whenever bile contains insufficient bile salts and lecithin in proportion to cholesterol to maintain the cholesterol in solution. This situation can result from a decrease in the amount of bile salts present (because of decreased reabsorption in the terminal ileum as a result of inflammatory disease or surgical resection) or can be caused by increased hepatic synthesis of cholesterol. Because cholesterol is not radiopaque, most gallstones are radiolucent and visible only on contrast examinations or ultrasound. In up to 20% of patients, however, gallstones contain sufficient calcium to be detectable on plain abdominal radiographs (Figure 4-68). Gallstones can have a central nidus (focus) of calcification, be laminated (alternating opaque and

lucent rings), or have calcification around the periphery. Occasionally, a nonopaque stone may contain gas-filled fissures that produce the "Mercedes-Benz" sign, a characteristic triradiate pattern similar to the German automobile trademark (Figure 4-69).

Oral cholecystography (OCG) has been the traditional technique for the diagnosis of gallstones, although it has been replaced in most institutions by ultrasound (see below). Gallstones appear as freely movable filling defects in the opacified gallbladder. They fall by gravity to the dependent portion of the gallbladder and frequently layer out at a level that depends on the relation of the specific gravity of the stone to that of the surrounding bile (Figure 4-70). Solitary gallstones are usually rounded; multiple stones are generally faceted.

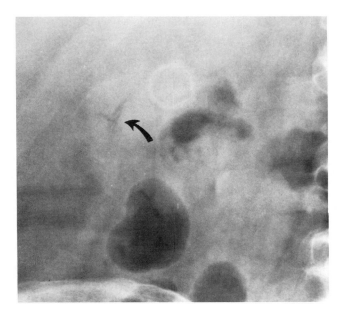

Figure 4-69 Mercedes-Benz sign of fissuring in gallstone *(arrow)*. Note adjacent gallstone with radiopaque rim.

Large numbers of stones can have a sandlike or gravel-like consistency and be visible only when they layer out on radiographs obtained with the patient in an erect or lateral decubitus position using a horizontal beam. Infrequently, a gallstone is coated with tenacious mucus and adheres to the gallbladder wall.

Malabsorption of the radiopaque contrast, hepatocellular dysfunction (serum bilirubin $\geq$ 2 mg/dl), and intrinsic disease of the gallbladder (cystic duct obstruction, chronic cholecystitis) can lead to nonvisualization of the gallbladder on OCG. If these causes can be excluded, failure of the gallbladder to opacify after the administration of two doses of oral cholecystographic contrast material is highly reliable evidence of gallbladder disease.

Ultrasound is now the major imaging modality for demonstrating gallstones. This noninvasive technique is equal in accuracy to OCG, is independent of hepatic function, and does not rely on patient compliance in taking oral contrast agents. In addition to imaging the gallbladder, ultrasound can provide important additional information by effectively demonstrating the biliary tree and hepatic parenchyma. Gallstones appear on ultrasound as foci of high-amplitude echoes associated with posterior acoustic shadowing (Figure 4-71). The mobility of free-floating gallstones may be demonstrated by performing the examination with the patient in various positions.

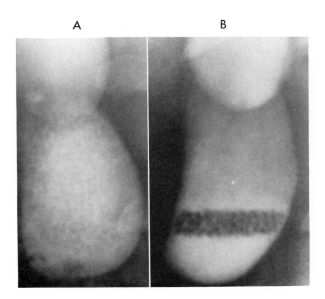

Figure 4-70 Oral cholecystogram showing multiple gallstones. **A,** With the patient supine, the stones are poorly defined and have a gravel-like consistency. **B,** On an erect film taken with a horizontal beam, the innumerable gallstones layer out and are easily seen.

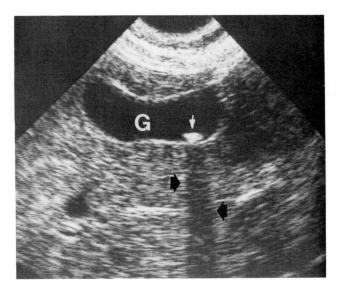

Figure 4-71 Ultrasound of gallstones. Echogenic focus *(white arrow)* in otherwise sonolucent gallbladder *(G)* represents large gallstone. Note acoustic shadowing immediately inferior to stone *(black arrows)*.

Acute cholecystitis

Acute cholecystitis usually follows obstruction of the cystic duct by an impacted gallstone. Either ultrasound or radionuclide scanning can be used. The sonographic diagnosis of acute cholecystitis requires the demonstration of a distended gallbladder containing gallstones. Important additional findings include edema of the gallbladder wall and focal tenderness elicited directly over the gallbladder. A normal gallbladder ultrasound virtually excludes the diagnosis of acute cholecystitis. Because many disorders may mimic acute cholecystitis, ultrasound can also be used to evaluate the remainder of the right upper quadrant to detect any other acute abnormality.

The normal radionuclide cholescintigram demonstrates the bile ducts, the gallbladder, and early excretion of radionuclide into the duodenum and proximal jejunum within 30 minutes of the intravenous injection of isotope (Figure 4-72, *A*). Failure to accumulate radioactivity in the gallbladder is highly sensitive and specific for cystic duct obstruction (Figure 4-72, *B*). If associated with appropriate symptoms, this finding is virtually diagnostic of acute cholecystitis.

Emphysematous cholecystitis

Emphysematous cholecystitis is a rare condition in which the growth of gas-forming organisms in the gallbladder is facilitated by stasis and ischemia caused by cystic duct obstruction (most often by stones). Emphysematous cholecystitis occurs most frequently in elderly men and in patients with poorly controlled diabetes mellitus. Plain abdominal radiographs demonstrate gas in the gallbladder lumen that dissects into the wall or pericholecystic tissues to produce the pathognomonic appearance of a rim of lucent bubbles or streaks of gas outside of and roughly parallel to the gallbladder lumen (Figure 4-73).

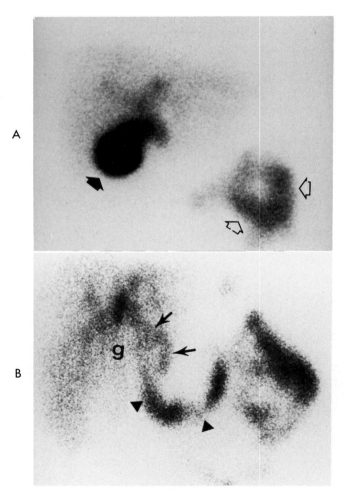

Figure 4-72 Acute cholecystitis. **A,** Normal radionuclide cholescintigram demonstrates bile ducts, gallbladder *(solid arrow)*, and early excretion of radionuclide into duodenum and proximal jejunum *(open arrows)*. **B,** In patient with acute cholecystitis, cholescintigram shows no visualization of gallbladder *(g)* but good visualization of common bile duct *(arrows)* and duodenum *(arrowheads)*, indicating obstruction of cystic duct. *(Harned RE: In Eisenberg RL and Amberg JR, editors: Critical diagnostic pathways in radiology, Philadelphia, JB Lippincott, 1981.)*

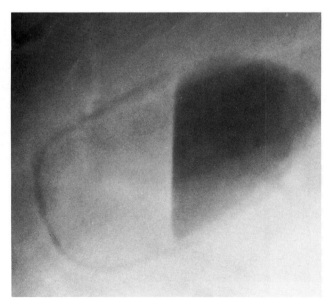

Figure 4-73 Emphysematous cholecystitis. Gas is found in both lumen and wall of gallbladder. *(Eisenberg RL: Gastrointestinal radiology: a pattern approach, ed 2, Philadelphia, 1990, JB Lippincott Co.)*

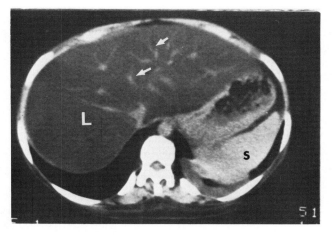

Figure 4-75 Fatty infiltration of liver in cirrhosis. CT scan shows generalized decrease in attenuation value of liver *(L)*, which is far less than that of spleen *(S)*. Portal veins appear as high-density structures *(arrows)* surrounded by background of low-density hepatic fat.

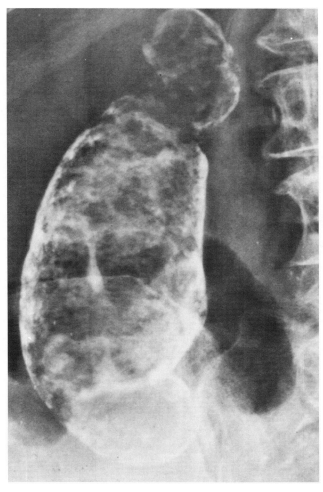

Figure 4-74 Porcelain gallbladder. Note extensive mural calcification around perimeter of gallbladder.

Porcelain gallbladder

Porcelain gallbladder refers to extensive calcification in the wall of the gallbladder, which forms an oval density that corresponds to the size and shape of the organ (Figure 4-74). The term reflects the blue discoloration and brittle consistency of the gallbladder wall. The calcification in a porcelain gallbladder can appear as a broad continuous band in the muscular layers or be multiple and punctate and occur in the glandular spaces of the mucosa. The detection of extensive calcification in the wall of the gallbladder should suggest the possibility of carcinoma. Although a porcelain gallbladder is uncommon in cases of carcinoma of the gallbladder, there is a striking incidence of carcinoma in porcelain gallbladders (up to 60% of the cases). Therefore, even if they are asymptomatic, patients with porcelain gallbladders are usually subjected to prophylactic cholecystectomy.

LIVER

Cirrhosis of the liver

Cirrhosis refers to chronic destruction of liver cells and structure with nodular regeneration of liver parenchyma and fibrosis. The major cause of cirrhosis is chronic alcoholism, in which damage to the liver is related either to the toxic effect of alcohol or the malnutrition that frequently accompanies chronic alcoholism. Other causes of liver destruction leading to cirrhosis include postnecrotic viral hepatitis, hepatotoxic drugs and chemicals that destroy liver cells, disease of the bile ducts (primary and secondary biliary cirrhosis), and excessive deposition of iron pigment within the liver (hemochromatosis). Regardless of the cause, the destroyed liver cells are replaced by fibrous connective tissue that has no liver cell function. Initially the liver is enlarged because of regeneration, but it eventually becomes smaller as the fibrous connective tissue contracts and the surface becomes bumpy and nodular.

Cirrhosis causes many physiologic changes that can be detected clinically and/or radiographically. In alcoholic cirrhosis a large amount of fat accumulates within the liver. This fatty infiltration is beautifully demonstrated on CT. In normal individuals the liver always appears brighter than the spleen, whereas in cirrhosis the liver is much darker because of the large amount of fat (Figure 4-75). The portal veins appear as high-density structures surrounded by a background of low density caused by hepatic fat, the opposite of the normal pattern of portal veins as low-density channels on noncontrast scans.

Nodular regeneration of the liver combined with fibrosis causes obstruction of the portal vein, which drains blood from the gastrointestinal tract through the liver before emptying into the inferior vena cava near the heart. Increased pressure within this vessel causes marked enlargement of the spleen (splenomegaly). Because blood cannot flow through the obstructed portal vein, it must find an alternative route to bypass the liver. This leads to the development

of collateral circulation, with large dilated veins becoming prominent on the abdominal wall in the area of the umbilicus. Another alternative route for blood to return to the heart is the periesophageal veins, which dilate to become esophageal varices that can rupture and lead to fatal hemorrhage (Figure 4-14).

Destruction of liver cells substantially decreases the ability of the organ to synthesize proteins, such as albumin and several of the multiple factors required for blood clotting. A deficiency of albumin (hypoalbuminemia) results in fluid leaking out of the

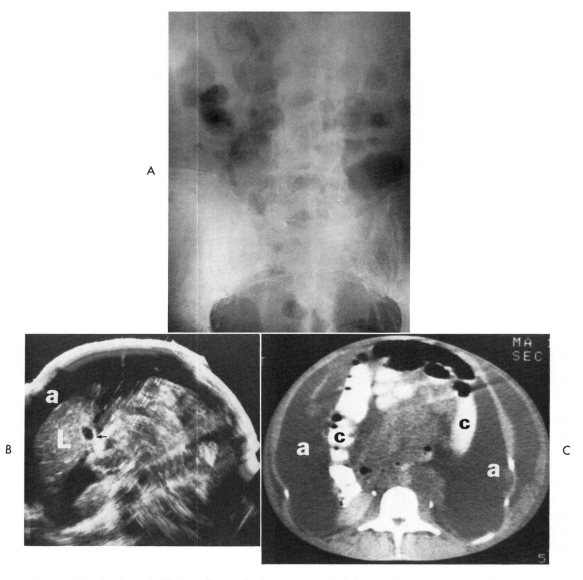

Figure 4-76 Ascites. **A,** Plain radiograph shows general abdominal haziness (ground-glass appearance). **B,** On ultrasound, large amount of sonolucent ascitic fluid *(a)* separates liver *(L)* and other soft-tissue structures from anterior abdominal wall. Note relative thickness of gallbladder wall *(arrow)*. **C,** CT scan through lower abdomen shows huge amount of low-density ascitic fluid *(a)* with medial displacement of ascending and descending colon *(c)*.

circulation and the development of generalized edema. Edema can be seen as swelling of the lower extremity; when it involves the wall of the intestinal tract, edema can produce regular, uniform thickening of small bowel folds.

One of the most characteristic symptoms of cirrhosis is the accumulation of fluid in the peritoneal cavity (ascites), which causes characteristic abdominal distention. Ascites develops because of a combination of albumin deficiency and increased pressure within obstructed veins, which permits fluid to leak into the abdominal cavity. Large amounts of ascitic fluid are easily detectable on plain abdominal radiographs as a general abdominal haziness (ground-glass appearance) (Figure 4-76, *A*). With the patient in a supine position the peritoneal fluid tends to gravitate to dependent portions of the pelvis and accumulate within the pelvic peritoneal reflections, thus filling the recesses on both sides of the bladder and producing a symmetric density resembling dog's ears. Smaller amounts of fluid (300 to 1000 ml) may widen the flank stripe and obliterate the right lateral inferior margin of the liver (hepatic angle). Ascites is exquisitely shown on ultrasound as a mobile, echofree fluid region shaped by adjacent structures (Figure 4-76, *B*) or on CT as an extravisceral collection of fluid with a low attenuation value (Figure 4-76, *C*).

Cirrhosis may lead to the development of jaundice, either from destruction of liver cells or obstruction of bile ducts. Because the liver cannot perform its usual task of inactivating the small amounts of female sex hormones secreted by the adrenal glands in both men and women, men with cirrhosis often develop breast enlargement (gynecomastia). The inability of necrotic liver cells to detoxify harmful substances leads to an accumulation of ammonia and other poisonous material in the circulation. The patient becomes confused and disoriented, develops a typical flapping tremor or shaking, becomes abnormally sleepy (somnolence), and may lapse into potentially fatal hepatic coma.

Hepatocellular carcinoma

In the United States, primary liver cell carcinoma most commonly occurs in patients with underlying diffuse hepatocellular disease, especially alcoholic or postnecrotic cirrhosis. The clinical presentation varies from mild right upper quadrant discomfort and weight loss to hemorrhagic shock from massive intraperitoneal bleeding, which reflects rupture of the tumor into the peritoneal cavity. Invasion of the biliary tree may produce obstructive jaundice.

CT is the modality of choice in diagnosing hepatocellular carcinoma. The tumor appears as a large

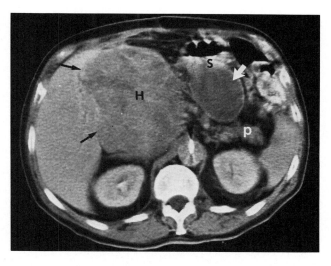

Figure 4-77 Hepatocellular carcinoma. CT scan shows huge mass *(H)* with attenuation value slightly less than that of normal liver. Black arrows point to interface between tumor and normal liver. Of incidental note is pancreatic pseudocyst *(white arrow)* in lesser sac between stomach *(S)* and pancreas *(p)*.

mass, with an attenuation value close to normal parenchyma, that tends to alter the contour of the liver by projecting beyond its outer margin (Figure 4-77). After the rapid administration of intravenous contrast material, there usually is dense, diffuse, and non-uniform enhancement of the tumor. Unlike metastases, hepatocellular carcinoma tends to be solitary or produce a small number of lesions. Hepatocellular carcinoma tends to invade the hepatic and portal venous systems, and tumor thrombi within these veins are well demonstrated on CT.

Although the overall prognosis of hepatocellular carcinoma remains bleak, radiographic studies can determine whether the patient can successfully undergo surgical removal of the tumor. If the tumor is confined to one lobe of the liver and there is no evidence of metastases, arteriography is usually indicated to demonstrate the precise surgical anatomy and to detect small, staining tumor nodules that cannot be identified with noninvasive imaging techniques.

Hepatic metastases

Metastases are by far the most common malignant tumors involving the liver. Although some types of metastases (especially mucinous carcinoma of the colon or rectum) may produce diffuse, finely granular calcifications seen on plain radiographs, the diagnosis of hepatic metastases usually requires CT, ultrasound, MRI, or radionuclide studies. CT and

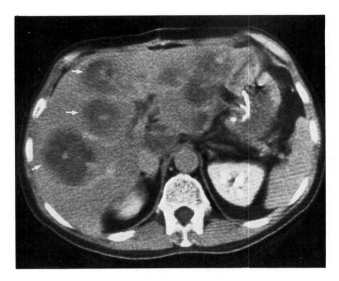

Figure 4-78 Hepatic metastases. CT scan shows multiple low-density metastases with high-density centers *(arrows)*.

MRI are probably the most sensitive techniques for detecting hepatic metastases. On CT, most metastases are relatively well marginated and appear less dense than normal liver parenchyma (Figure 4-78). Although frequently detectable on noncontrast scans, most metastatic lesions are best seen as areas of increased density adjacent to normally enhancing hepatic parenchyma after the administration of intravenous contrast material. MRI demonstrates liver metastases as areas of low signal intensity on T1 sequences and extremely bright lesions on T2 sequences.

Ultrasound and radionuclide scans can demonstrate hepatic metastases, but these modalities are slightly less sensitive than CT. CT has the additional advantage of being able to detect extrahepatic metastases, such as to abdominal lymph nodes.

PANCREAS

Acute pancreatitis

Acute pancreatitis is an inflammatory process in which protein- and lipid-digesting enzymes become activated within the pancreas and begin to digest the organ itself. Occasionally, this necrotic process extends into blood vessels, causing bleeding (acute hemorrhagic pancreatitis) that may be life-threatening.

The most common cause of acute pancreatitis is excessive alcohol consumption. Less frequently, acute pancreatitis is related to gallstones, which may enter the common bile duct and obstruct the ampulla of Vater and force bile to reflux into the pancreas and cause an inflammatory reaction.

Acute pancreatitis usually presents with the sudden onset of severe, steady abdominal pain that radiates to the back and may suggest a perforated ulcer. Nausea and vomiting are common, and jaundice may develop if inflammatory edema of the head of the pancreas is sufficient to obstruct the common bile duct. If a large area of the pancreas is affected, the absence of lipid enzymes from the pancreas prevents the proper absorption of fat, leading to the malabsorption syndrome. On blood tests and urinalysis, there is typically a high level of the pancreatic enzyme amylase, which confirms the diagnosis of acute pancreatitis.

Plain abdominal radiographs are often normal in the patient with acute pancreatitis; even when abnormal, the findings are usually nonspecific and consistent with any intra-abdominal inflammatory disease. The most frequent abnormalities include a localized adynamic ileus, usually involving the jejunum ("sentinel loop"); generalized ileus with diffuse gas-fluid levels; isolated distention of the duodenal sweep; and localized distention of the transverse colon to the level of the splenic flexure (colon cutoff sign). Pancreatic calcifications indicate that the patient has chronic pancreatitis, and moreover they may suggest an exacerbation of the inflammatory disease.

Ultrasound and CT are the imaging modalities that most precisely define the degree of pancreatic inflammation and the pathways of its spread throughout the abdomen. They also are of great clinical importance in the early diagnosis of complications of acute pancreatitis, such as abscess, hemorrhage, and pseudocyst formation.

CT in acute pancreatitis demonstrates diffuse or focal enlargement of the gland. In the normal patient the margins of the pancreas are sharply delineated by surrounding peripancreatic fat. Spread of inflammation and edema beyond the confines of the pancreas obscures the peripancreatic soft tissues and often thickens the surrounding fascial planes (Figure 4-79).

Acute pancreatitis may alter both the size and the parenchymal echogenicity of the gland on ultrasound examination. Although the pancreas usually enlarges symmetrically and retains its initial shape, nonspecific enlargement of the pancreatic head or tail can simulate focal pancreatic carcinoma. The accompanying interstitial inflammatory edema causes the pancreas to appear relatively sonolucent when compared with the adjacent liver (Figure 4-80). One limitation of ultrasound in patients with acute pancreatitis is the frequent occurrence of adynamic ileus with excessive intestinal gas, which may prevent adequate visualization of the gland.

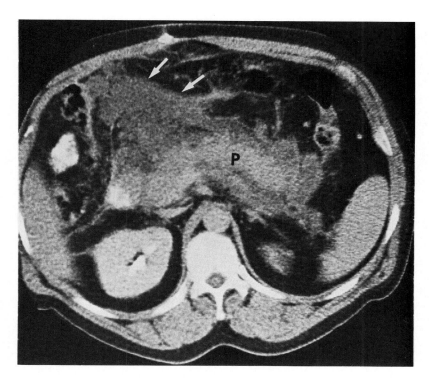

Figure 4-79 Acute pancreatitis. CT scan demonstrates diffuse enlargement of pancreas *(P)* with obliteration of peripancreatic fat planes by inflammatory process. Note extension of inflammatory reaction into transverse mesocolon *(arrows)*. *(From Jeffrey RB, Federle MD, and Laing FC: Computed tomography of mesenteric involvement in fulminant pancreatitis, Radiology 147:185-192, 1983.)*

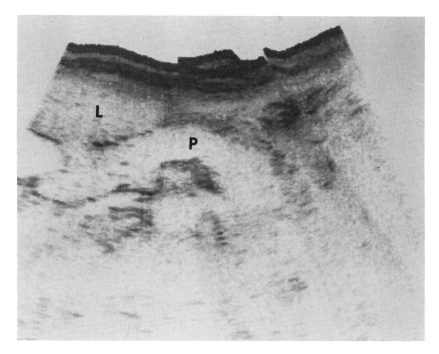

Figure 4-80 Acute pancreatitis. Transverse sonogram demonstrates diffuse enlargement of gland *(P)* with retention of its normal shape. Note relative sonolucency of pancreas when compared with echogenicity of adjacent liver *(L)*.

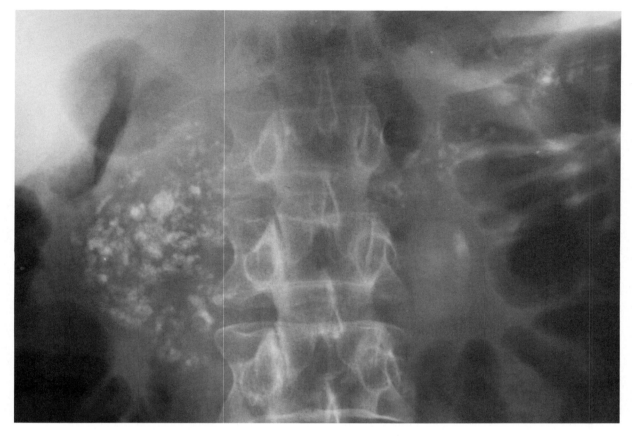

Figure 4-81   Chronic pancreatitis. Diffuse pancreatic calcifications.

Chronic pancreatitis

Pancreatic calcifications are an essentially pathogno-monic finding in chronic pancreatitis, developing in about one third of patients with this disease (Figure 4-81). The small, irregular calcifications are seen most frequently in the head of the pancreas and can extend upward and to the left to involve the body and tail of the organ.

On ultrasound examination, the major feature of chronic pancreatitis is an alteration of the intrinsic echo pattern caused by calcification and fibrosis. The pancreas may be atrophic as a result of fibrous scar-ring or appear significantly enlarged during recur-rences of acute inflammation. Dilation of the pan-creatic duct as a result of gland atrophy and obstruc-tion can be seen, although a similar pattern can be produced by the ductal obstruction in pancreatic cancer. CT can also demonstrate ductal dilation, cal-cification, and atrophy of the gland in patients with chronic pancreatitis. However, since similar infor-mation can be obtained less expensively and without ionizing radiation by ultrasound, CT is usually re-served for patients with chronic pancreatitis in

whom technical factors make ultrasound subopti-mal.

Enlargement of the pancreatic head can cause widening and pressure changes on the inner aspect of the duodenal sweep on barium studies. This pro-duces narrowing of the lumen (double-contour ef-fect) and spiny protrusions of mucosal folds (spic-ulation) that can be indistinguishable from pan-creatic carcinoma.

Pancreatic pseudocyst

Pancreatic pseudocysts are loculated (walled off) fluid collections arising from inflammation, necrosis, or hemorrhage associated with acute pancreatitis or trauma (Figure 4-82). On ultrasound examination, a pseudocyst typically appears as an echo-free cystic structure with a sharp posterior wall (Figure 4-83). Hemorrhage into the pseudocyst produces a com-plex fluid collection containing septations or echo-genic areas. CT demonstrates pseudocysts as sharply marginated, fluid-filled collections that are often best delineated after the administration of in-travenous contrast material (Figure 4-84).

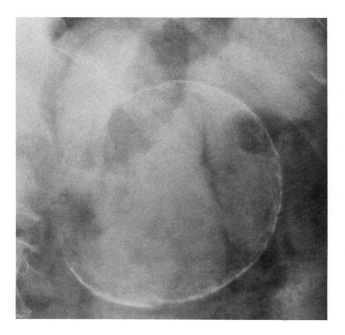

Figure 4-82 Calcified pancreatic pseuodcyst.

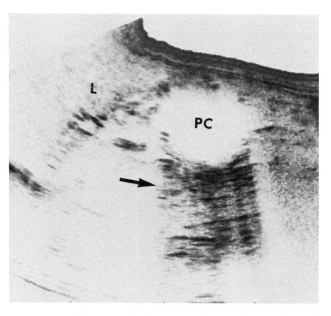

Figure 4-83 Ultrasound of pancreatic pseudocyst. Longitudinal sonogram of right upper quadrant demonstrates irregularly marginated pseudocyst *(PC)* with acoustic shadowing *(arrow). L,* Liver.

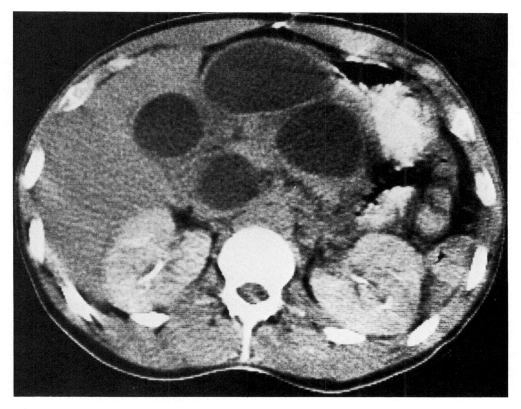

Figure 4-84 Multiple pancreatic pseudocysts. CT scan following intravenous administration of contrast material demonstrates four sharply marginated, fluid-filled collections.

Large pseudocysts are visible on plain radiographs of the abdomen when they displace the gasfilled stomach and bowel. Similarly, pseudocysts in the head of the pancreas can cause pressure defects and widening of the duodenal sweep, whereas those arising from the body or tail of the pancreas can displace and deform the stomach, proximal jejunum, or colon. However, since ultrasound is highly accurate in diagnosing pancreatic pseudocysts, it has completely replaced plain abdominal radiographs and barium studies, which display only indirect signs.

Pseudocysts may undergo spontaneous resolution or persist as chronic collections that may require surgical intervention. Because ultrasound is relatively inexpensive and without ionizing radiation, serial sonograms are usually used to monitor the progression of a pancreatic pseudocyst.

Cancer of the pancreas

The most common pancreatic malignancy is adenocarcinoma, which often is far advanced before it is detected and thus has an extremely poor survival rate. Several less common pancreatic tumors are hormone-secreting neoplasms of the islet cells of the islands of Langerhans. Production of insulin by an insulinoma can lower blood sugar, leading to attacks of weakness, unconsciousness, and insulin shock. Ulcerogenic islet cell tumors (gastrinomas) produce the Zollinger-Ellison syndrome, which is characterized by intractable ulcer symptoms, hypersecretion of gastric acid, and diarrhea. Diarrheagenic islet cell tumors produce the WDHA syndrome; this acronym stands for *w*atery *d*iarrhea, *h*ypokalemia (low serum potassium), and *a*chlorhydria (low serum chloride), which are major features of the clinical picture. ACTH production by pancreatic islet cell tumors causes Cushing's syndrome; the release of serotonin by pancreatic tumors may cause the carcinoid syndrome. Because these functional islet cell tumors usually become apparent by their hormonal effects rather than by the consequences of tumor bulk, they are often small and difficult to detect.

Because it is noninvasive and relatively inexpensive, ultrasound is often the initial screening in a patient suspected of pancreatic carcinoma. Ultrasound can demonstrate most tumors greater than 2 cm in diameter that lie in the head of the pancreas; lesions in the body and tail of the pancreas are more difficult to detect by this modality. Pancreatic carcinoma typically causes the gland to have an irregular contour and a semisolid pattern of intrinsic echoes (Figure 4-85).

CT is the most effective modality for detecting pancreatic cancer in any portion of the gland and

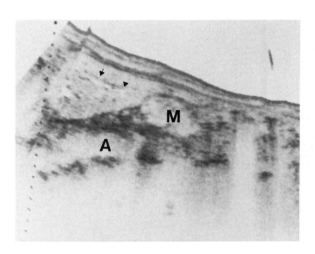

Figure 4-85 Carcinoma of pancreas. Longitudinal sonogram demonstrates irregular mass *(M)* with semisolid pattern of intrinsic echoes. Note associated dilation of intrahepatic bile ducts *(arrows)*. A, Aorta.

for defining its extent. CT can demonstrate the mass of the tumor and ductal dilation and invasion of neighboring structures. After the administration of intravenous contrast material, the relatively avascular tumor appears as an area of decreased attenuation when compared with the normal pancreas. CT is the best procedure for staging pancreatic carcinoma and may prevent needless surgery in patients with nonresectable lesions. This technique may permit detection of hepatic metastases or involvement of regional vessels and adjacent retroperitoneal lymph nodes.

Cytologic examination of tissue obtained by percutaneous fine-needle aspiration under ultrasound or CT guidance can often provide the precise histologic diagnosis of a neoplastic mass, thus making surgical intervention unnecessary.

Carcinoma of the head of the pancreas often causes obstructive jaundice and the appearance of narrowing of the distal common bile duct on transhepatic cholangiography, or ERCP (Figure 4-87). Percutaneous biliary drainage may represent an alternative to surgical intervention for relieving biliary obstruction in patients with pancreatic carcinoma who cannot be cured. Although the transhepatic insertion of biliary drainage tubes does not alter the dismal prognosis, it can reduce patient morbidity and the need for hospitalization.

Barium upper gastrointestinal series demonstrate distortion of the mucosal pattern and configuration of the duodenal sweep in about half of patients with carcinoma of the head of the pancreas. Early or small lesions, however, rarely produce detectable radio-

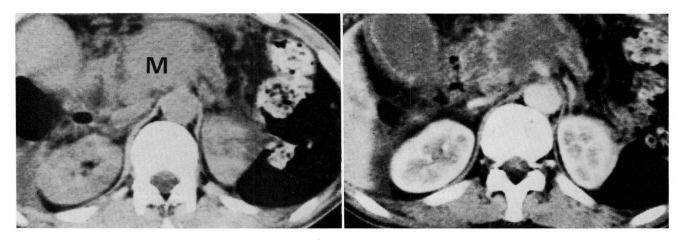

Figure 4-86 Carcinoma of pancreas. *(From Federle MP and Goldberg HL: In Moss AA, Gamsu G, and Genant HG, editors: Computed tomography of the body, Philadelphia, 1983, WB Saunders Co.)*

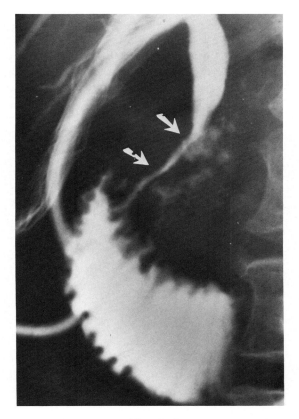

Figure 4-87 Carcinoma of head of pancreas. Transhepatic cholangiogram shows irregular narrowing of common bile duct *(arrows)*. Calcifications reflect underlying chronic pancreatitis.

graphic abnormalities; tumors of the body or tail of the pancreas must be quite large to be visible on barium examinations.

PNEUMOPERITONEUM

Free air in the peritoneal cavity associated with significant abdominal pain and tenderness is often caused by perforation of a gas-containing viscus and indicates a surgical emergency. Less frequently, pneumoperitoneum results from abdominal, gynecologic, intrathoracic, or iatrogenic causes and does not require operative intervention.

The radiographic demonstration of free air in the peritoneal cavity is a valuable sign in the diagnosis of perforation of the gastrointestinal tract. As little as 1 cc (ml) of free intraperitoneal gas can be identified. Free air is best demonstrated by examination of the patient in the upright position with a horizontal beam (Figure 4-88). Because the gas rises to the highest point in the peritoneal cavity, it accumulates beneath the domes of the diaphragm. Free intraperitoneal gas appears as a sickle-shaped lucency that is easiest to recognize on the right side between the diaphragm and the homogeneous density of the liver. On the left, the normal gas and fluid shadows present in the fundus of the stomach can be confusing. The free air is shown to best advantage if the patient remains in an upright (or lateral decubitus) position for 10 minutes before a radiograph is obtained.

If the patient is too ill to sit or stand, a lateral

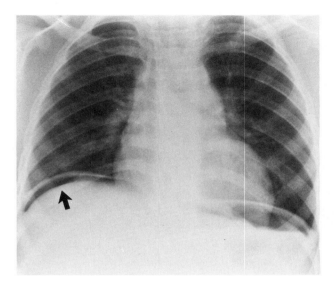

Figure 4-88 Pneumoperitoneum. Gas accumulating beneath dome of right hemidiaphragm *(arrow)* appears as sickle-shaped lucency on this erect chest film, obtained with horizontal beam.

decubitus view (preferably with the patient on the left side) can be used. In this position, free air moves to the right and collects between the lateral margin of the liver and the abdominal wall (Figure 4-89). Some gas also collects in the right iliac fossa and, when large amounts are involved, can be seen along the flank down to the pelvis.

When the patient is in the supine position, free intraperitoneal gas accumulates between the intestinal loops and is much more difficult to demonstrate. However, a large quantity of gas can be diagnosed indirectly because it permits visualization of the outer margins of the intestinal wall (Figure 4-90). The distinct demonstration of the inner and outer contours of the bowel wall is often the only sign of pneumoperitoneum in patients in such poor condition that they cannot be turned on their side or be examined upright.

In children, pneumoperitoneum can be manifest as a generalized greater-than-normal lucency of the entire abdomen. An important sign of pneumoperitoneum on the supine radiograph is demonstration of the falciform ligament. This almost vertical, curvilinear, water-density shadow in the upper abdomen to the right of the spine is outlined only when there is gas on both sides of it, as in a pneumoperitoneum (Figure 4-91).

The most frequent cause of pneumoperitoneum with associated inflammation is perforation of a peptic ulcer, either gastric or duodenal. Colonic perforations, especially those involving the cecum, give the most abundant quantities of free intraperitoneal gas. Septic infection of the peritoneal cavity by gas-forming organisms can result in the production of a substantial amount of gas and the radiographic appearance of pneumoperitoneum. Pneumoperitoneum can also develop after penetrating injuries of

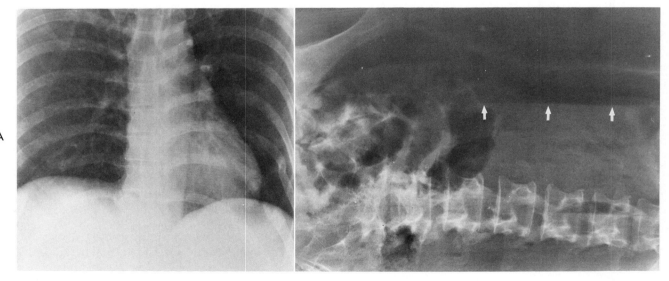

A   B

Figure 4-89 Pneumoperitoneum. **A,** Semi-erect projection obtained without a horizontal beam shows no evidence of free intraperitoneal gas beneath domes of diaphragm. **B,** On lateral decubitus projection obtained with horizontal beam on same patient, free intraperitoneal gas is clearly seen collecting under right side of abdominal wall *(arrows)*. Gas can even be seen extending down flank to region of pelvis.

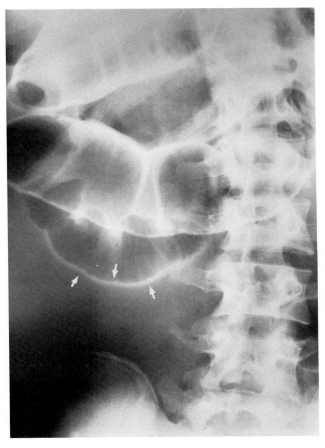

Figure 4-90 Double-wall sign of pneumoperitoneum demonstrated on supine projection. Large quantities of free intraperitoneal gas may be diagnosed indirectly because gas permits visualization of both inner and outer margins of intestinal wall *(arrows)*.

the abdominal wall and after blunt trauma causing rupture of a hollow viscus.

Iatrogenic pneumoperitoneum is generally asymptomatic and usually follows abdominal surgery. Postoperative pneumoperitoneum can be radiographically detectable for up to 3 weeks after surgery, but usually can no longer be demonstrated after the first postoperative week. Rarely, free air in the peritoneal cavity may be the result of perforation during an endoscopic procedure.

SPLEEN

Enlargement

Enlargement of the spleen (splenomegaly) is associated with numerous conditions, including infections (subacute bacterial endocarditis, tuberculosis, infectious mononucleosis, malaria), connective tissue disorders, neoplastic hematologic disorders

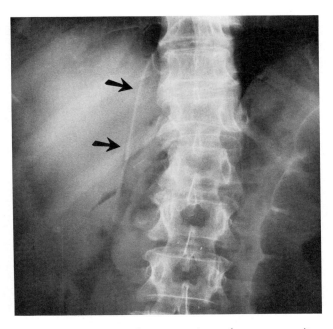

Figure 4-91 Falciform ligament sign of pneumoperitoneum. On supine projection, falciform ligament appears as curvilinear water-density shadow *(arrows)* in upper abdomen to right of spine. This finding implies that there is pneumoperitoneum with gas on both sides of ligament.

(lymphoma, leukemia), hemolytic anemia and hemoglobinopathies, and portal hypertension (cirrhosis).

Plain abdominal radiographs can demonstrate the inferior border of the enlarged spleen well below the costal margin. An enlarged spleen can elevate the left hemidiaphragm, impress the greater curvature of the barium-filled stomach, and displace the entire stomach toward the midline. Splenomegaly can also cause downward displacement of the left kidney and the splenic flexure of the colon.

CT is of value when it is unclear whether a mass felt in the left upper quadrant represents an enlarged spleen or a separate abdominal mass. When splenomegaly is present, CT findings may suggest the cause of the splenic enlargement by demonstrating a tumor (Figure 4-92), abscess, or cyst. Associated abdominal lymph node enlargement suggests lymphoma; characteristic alterations in the size and shape of the liver and prominence of collateral venous structures in the splenic hilum suggest that splenomegaly is a result of cirrhosis and portal hypertension.

Rupture

Rupture of the spleen is usually caused by trauma. Infrequently, it may be a complication of palpation of a spleen enlarged by infection (especially infec-

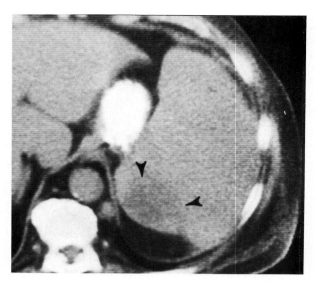

Figure 4-92 Lymphoma of spleen. CT scan shows focal low-attenuation lesion *(arrowheads)* posteriorly in markedly enlarged spleen. *(Koehler RE: Spleen. In Lee JKT, Sagel SS, and Stanley RJ, editors: Computed body tomography, New York, Raven Press, 1983.)*

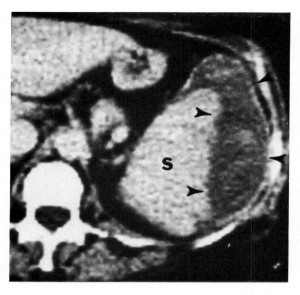

Figure 4-93 Traumatic subcapsular splenic hematoma. Contrast-enhanced CT scan shows hematoma as large zone of decreased attenuation *(arrowheads)* that surrounds and flattens lateral and anteromedial borders of adjacent spleen *(S)*. *(Koehler RE: Spleen. In Lee JKT, Sagel SS, and Stanley RJ, editors: Computed body tomography, New York, Raven Press, 1983.)*

tious mononucleosis) or leukemia. In many patients suffering traumatic rupture of the spleen, the severity of clinical symptoms and the rapid loss of blood into the abdominal cavity require immediate surgery without radiographic investigation. However, in patients in whom bleeding stops temporarily or in whom there is slow bleeding over several days, radiographic studies may be of diagnostic value.

CT is the best imaging procedure for screening patients with blunt abdominal trauma for the presence of splenic injury. Indeed, its almost 100% sensitivity in detecting splenic injury has substantially decreased the need for abdominal arteriography and exploratory surgery. Subcapsular hematomas ap-

pear on CT as crescentic collections of fluid that flatten or indent the lateral margin of the spleen (Figure 4-93). Splenic lacerations, which may occur with or without an accompanying subcapsular hematoma, produce a CT appearance of splenic enlargement, an irregular cleft or defect in the splenic border, and free blood in the peritoneal cavity.

Before the advent of CT, splenic arteriography was the procedure of choice for demonstrating splenic rupture. Major positive findings include extravasation of contrast material into the splenic parenchyma; obstruction of a major splenic artery; and vascular defects in an enlarged spleen, indicating sites of rupture and hematoma.

QUESTIONS

1. Visualization of which of the following structures is an indication of the correct contrast scale of a plain abdominal radiograph?
   I.   Liver, kidneys, and psoas muscle shadows
   II. Lumbar spine and transverse processes
   III. Kidneys and psoas muscle shadows
   IV. Lumbar spine and psoas shadows
   A. Both I and IV   C. I only
   B. Both I and II   D. IV only

2. The rhythmic smooth muscle contractions found in the upper gastrointestinal system are called
   A. Chyme   C. Peristalsis
   B. Digestion   D. Mastication

3. The greatest amount of digestion occurs in which portion of the intestines?
   A. Duodenum   C. Ileum
   B. Jejunum   D. Colon

4. Detoxification of poisonous substances takes place in which organ?
   A. Kidneys   C. Pancreas
   B. Liver   D. Spleen

5. Which organ controls the level of glucose in the circulating blood?
   A. Kidneys   C. Pancreas
   B. Liver   D. Spleen

6. The telescoping of one part of the intestinal tract into another is termed _____.
   A. Intussusception   C. Crohn's disease
   B. Volvulus   D. Ileus

7. Twisting of the bowel upon itself is termed

   _____.
   A. Intussusception   C. Crohn's disease
   B. Volvulus   D. Ileus

8. What is now considered to be the major imaging modality for the demonstration of gallstones?
   A. OCG   C. CT
   B. MRI   D. Ultrasound

9. What is the major cause of cirrhosis in the United States and Europe?
   A. Hepatitis   C. Alcoholism
   B. Elevated choles-   D. Cholecystitis
      terol

10. Rupture of the spleen as a result of blunt abdominal trauma can best be demonstrated by what imaging procedure?
    A. OCG   C. CT
    B. MRI   D. Ultrasound

11. If a patient is too ill to stand, what projection can be used to demonstrate pneumoperitoneum?
    A. Right lateral decubitus, patient on left side
    B. Right lateral decubitus, patient on right side
    C. Left lateral decubitus, patient on left side
    D. Left lateral decubitus, patient on right side

12. Extensive calcification in the wall of the gallbladder is termed _____.
    A. Cholelithiasis   C. Cholecystitis
    B. Porcelain gallblad- D. A or B
       der

13. Varicose veins of the rectum are termed

    _____.
    A. Polyps   C. Ulcerations
    B. Hemorrhoids   D. Carcinomas

14. *Apple-core* and *napkin-ring* are common descriptive terms for annular carcinoma of the

    _____.
    A. Small intestine   C. Jejunum
    B. Stomach   D. Colon

15. Crohn's disease occurs in what organ(s)?
    A. Colon   C. Stomach
    B. Small bowel D. All of the above

16. Large amounts of gas and fluid in uniformly dilated loops of small and large bowel, often seen after abdominal surgery, is termed

    _____.
    A. Adynamic ileus   C. Colonic ileus
    B. Localized ileus   D. Ileus

17. What medical term is used to denote difficulty in swallowing?
    A. Mastication   C. Deglutition
    B. Dysphagia   D. B and C

18. Gastric contents that have mixed with hydrochloric acid and pepsin are called _____.
    A. Chyme   C. Enzyme
    B. Digest   D. Emulsifier

19. To demonstrate esophageal reflux, the patient is often asked to perform the _____.
    A. Trendelenberg's   C. Fowler's maneuver
       maneuver   D. Valsalva maneuver
    B. Sims maneuver

20. An abnormal accumulation of fluid in the peritoneal cavity is termed _____.
    A. Pneumoperito-   C. Volvulus
       neum   D. Hydroperitoneum
    B. Ascites

21. Herniations, or outpouchings, of the walls of a hollow organ are termed _____.
    A. Ulcers   C. Hemorrhoids
    B. Diverticula   D. Polyps

22. A colon intussusception can sometimes be reduced by what radiographic procedure?
    A. Upper GI series   C. Enteroclysis
    B. Small bowel series D. Barium enema

23. Patients over the age of 40 with a history of difficulty in swallowing are usually assumed, until proved otherwise, to have what pathologic condition?
    A. Esophageal varices   C. Esophageal fistula
    B. Esophageal carci-   D. Esophageal hernia
       noma

24. What is the most common manifestation of peptic ulcer disease?
    A. Gastric ulcer   C. Duodenal ulcer
    B. Esophageal ulcer   D. Peritoneal ulcer

25. If loops of bowel are distended by abnormally large amounts of air and are occupying the central portion of the abdomen, the patient most likely has a _____.
    A. Small bowel ob-   C. Gastric obstruction
       struction   D. A and B
    B. Large bowel ob-
       struction

BIBLIOGRAPHY

Eisenberg RL: Gastrointestinal radiology: a pattern approach, Philadelphia, JB Lippincott Co, 1990.

Gedgaudas-McClees RK: Gastrointestinal imaging, New York, Churchill-Livingstone, 1987.

Jones B and Braver JM: Essentials of gastrointestinal radiology, Philadelphia, WB Saunders Co, 1982.

Margulis AR and Burhenne HJ: Alimentary tract radiology, ed 4, St. Louis, The CV Mosby Co, 1989.

Meyers MA: Dynamic radiology of the abdomen, New York, Springer-Verlag, 1988.

CHAPTER 5

Urinary System

PREREQUISITE KNOWLEDGE

The student should have a basic knowledge of the anatomy and physiology of the urinary system. In addition, proper learning and understanding of the material will be facilitated if the student has some clinical experience in urinary radiography and film evaluation.

GOALS

To acquaint the student radiographer with the pathophysiology and radiographic manifestations of all of the common and some of the unusual disorders of the urinary system

OBJECTIVES

1. Describe the physiology of the urinary system
2. Identify anatomic structures on both diagrams and radiographs of the urinary system
3. Be able to define terminology relating to the urinary system
4. Be able to describe the various pathologic conditions affecting the urinary system and their radiographic manifestations
5. Be familiar with the changes in technical factors required for obtaining optimal quality radiographs

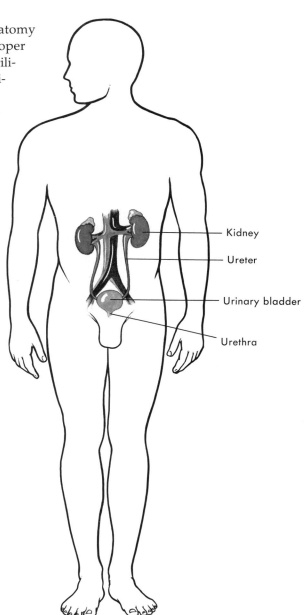

Kidney

Ureter

Urinary bladder

Urethra

RADIOGRAPHER NOTES

Although ultrasound and CT are being used with increasing frequency, plain radiography with contrast material introduced intravenously or by means of a catheter remains a major technique for imaging the urinary system. For excretory urography, the radiographer is responsible for preparing sterile injections of contrast material in addition to proper operation of equipment and positioning of the patient. In some instances the radiographer may have to perform these functions in an operating room using sterile technique.

All radiographic studies begin with a "scout" film that is obtained before the injection of any contrast material. The radiographer should evaluate this film for proper technique and positioning so that any required alterations can be made on subsequent radiographs during the procedure. A film with correct density and contrast should demonstrate the kidney and psoas muscle shadows and the lumbar vertebrae and their transverse processes. A correctly positioned film should show all of both kidneys down to the superior portion of the pubic bones (to ensure that all of the bladder is included). The radiograph must be in a true anteroposterior position with the pelvis appearing symmetric and the spinous processes of the lumbar vertebrae projected over the central portions of the vertebral bodies. The radiologist evaluates the scout radiograph to make certain that the technique and positioning are appropriate for the clinical problem and to evaluate proper patient preparation. The radiograph is also checked for any radiopaque calculi or other abnormality that might be obscured after the injection of contrast material.

The radiographer must be alert to the possibility of an allergic reaction whenever contrast agents are used. It is essential that the radiographer be aware of the proper procedures to follow in the event of an allergic reaction and be able to initiate and maintain basic life support until advanced life support personnel have arrived. Depending on departmental policy, it is usually the radiographer's responsibility to assist during resuscitation procedures. Therefore it is essential that the radiographer be familiar with the contents of the emergency cart and be responsible for ensuring that the cart is completely stocked with appropriate medications.

All radiographs of the urinary system must be made with the patient in full exhalation so that the diaphragm assumes its highest position and does not compress the abdominal contents. Depending on the specific area being evaluated, the radiographer may have to perform oblique or erect projections, coned-down views of the kidneys or bladder, tomograms, or films made with abdominal compression. In certain pathologic conditions radiographs must be obtained at precisely timed intervals, and delayed films may be necessary.

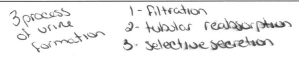

PHYSIOLOGY OF THE URINARY SYSTEM

The urinary system consists of the kidneys, ureters, and bladder. The functional unit of the kidney is the nephron. Each kidney contains more than a million nephrons, which filter waste products from the blood, reabsorb water and nutrients (e.g., glucose, amino acids) from the tubular fluid, and secrete excess substances in the form of urine. In an average person, about 190 L of water is filtered out of glomerular blood each day. This enormous amount is many times the total volume of blood in the body. However, only a small proportion of this water (1 to 2 L) is excreted in the urine. Therefore more than 99% of water is reabsorbed into tubular blood.

The formation of urine begins in the **glomerulus**, a tuft of capillaries with very thin walls and a large surface area. The blood pressure within the glomerulus is higher than that in the surrounding **Bowman's capsule**. This causes the filtration of fluid into Bowman's capsule that is equivalent to plasma containing neither protein nor red blood cells (if the nephron is healthy). The initial urine proceeds into the **proximal convoluted tubule**, where a large amount of water and virtually all nutrients are reabsorbed by means of blood capillaries surrounding the tubules. The amount of sodium and chloride reabsorbed is determined by the concentration of these substances in the body and occurs at a variable rate designed to keep the osmotic pressure of the body constant. This process is greatly influenced by two hormones, antidiuretic hormone (ADH) secreted by the posterior pituitary gland and aldosterone secreted by the adrenal glands.

After passing through the proximal tubule, the fluid flows through the **loop of Henle**, a complex structure consisting of a descending limb, a loop, and an ascending limb. In addition to reabsorption of salt and water, the loop of Henle permits the excretion of a concentrated urine by actively secreting substances such as potassium (K^+) and hydrogen (H^+) ions, and some drugs. In this way the kidney plays an essential role in maintaining **electrolyte** (salt) **balance** and **acid-base balance** of blood and body fluids.

To maintain a healthy metabolism, the pH must be maintained in the very limited range of 7.35 to 7.45. If the pH of blood is lower than this (too acidic), the kidney excretes an acid urine to remove H^+; if the pH of blood is higher than 7.5 (too alkaline), the kidney preserves H^+ and secretes an alkaline urine.

Eventually, urine passes from the **collecting tubules**, whose openings are in the papillae, into the calyces, and on to the funnel-shaped renal pelvis and tubular ureters. Peristaltic waves (about 1 to 5/min) force the urine down the ureters and into the bladder. The ureters enter the bladder through an oblique tunnel that functions as a valve to prevent backflow of urine into the ureters (vesicoureteral reflux) during bladder contraction.

The bladder acts as a reservoir for the urine before it leaves the body. The openings of the two ureters lie at the posterior corners of the triangular-shaped floor (**trigone**), and the urethral opening is situated at the anterior and lower corner. Filling of the bladder (about 250 ml in the average person) stimulates autonomic nerve endings in the wall that are perceived as a distended sensation and the desire to void (**micturate**). A complicated sequence of bladder contractions and relaxation of the sphincter muscles permits the bladder to expel urine from the body through the urethra. Voluntary contraction of the external sphincter to prevent or terminate micturition is learned and is possible only if the motor system is intact. Nervous system injury (cerebral hemorrhage, cord injury) results in involuntary emptying of the bladder at intervals (**incontinence**).

The kidney is also important in the production of red blood cells and the control of blood pressure. **Erythropoietin,** a substance produced by the kidney, stimulates the rate of production of red blood cells. Therefore renal failure is often associated with a severe anemia. The juxtaglomerular apparatus refers to specialized cells within renal arterioles that secrete

renin, an enzyme that acts with one of the plasma proteins to produce **angiotensin.** Decreased blood flow through these arterioles increases the secretion of renin and thus the blood level of angiotensin, which constricts peripheral arterioles throughout the body and elevates the blood pressure.

CONGENITAL/HEREDITARY DISEASES OF THE URINARY TRACT

Anomalies of number and size

Unilateral **renal agenesis** (solitary kidney) is a rare anomaly that may be associated with a variety of other congenital malformations (Figure 5-1). Before the diagnosis can be made, it is essential to exclude a nonfunctioning, diseased kidney or a prior nephrectomy. Ultrasound or CT can demonstrate the absence of renal tissue. A solitary kidney tends to be larger than expected, reflecting compensatory hypertrophy.

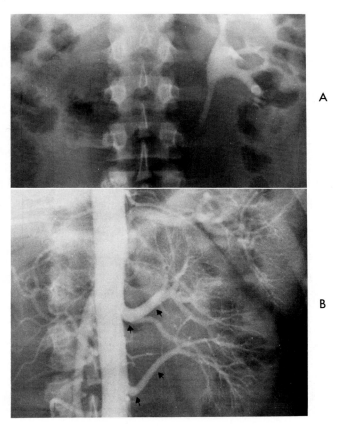

A

B

Figure 5-1 Solitary kidney. **A,** Excretory urogram demonstrates normal left kidney with no evidence of right renal tissue. **B,** Aortogram shows two renal arteries to left kidney *(arrows)* and no evidence of right renal artery, thus confirming diagnosis of unilateral renal agenesis.

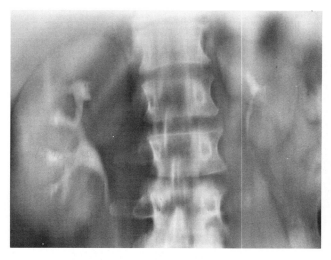

Figure 5-2 Hypoplastic kidney with compensatory hypertrophy. Small left kidney (miniature replica of a normal kidney) has good function and normal relation between amount of parenchyma and size of collecting system. Markedly enlarged right kidney represents compensatory hypertrophy.

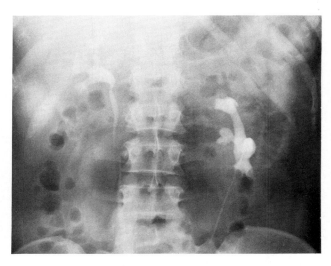

Figure 5-3 Malrotation of left kidney. Note apparent lateral displacement of upper ureter and elongation of pelvis.

A **supernumerary kidney** is also a rare anomaly. The third kidney is usually small and rudimentary and possesses a separate pelvis, ureter, and blood supply.

A small, **hypoplastic** kidney often appears as a miniature replica of a normal kidney, with good function and normal relation between the amount of parenchyma and the size of the collecting system (Figure 5-2). Renal hypoplasia must be differentiated from an acquired atrophic kidney, which is small and contracted because of vascular or inflammatory disease that has reduced the volume of renal parenchyma.

Compensatory hypertrophy is an acquired condition that develops when one kidney is forced to perform the function normally carried out by two kidneys (Figure 5-2). This phenomenon may follow unilateral renal agenesis, atrophy, or nephrectomy. The ability of the kidney to undergo compensatory hypertrophy is greatest in children and diminishes in adulthood.

Anomalies of rotation, position, and fusion

Malrotation of one or both kidneys may produce a bizarre appearance of the renal parenchyma, calyces, and pelvis that suggests a pathologic condition when in reality the kidney is otherwise entirely normal (Figure 5-3). Abnormally positioned kidneys **(ectopic kidney)** may be found in various locations, from the true pelvis **(pelvic kidney)** (Figure 5-4) to

above the diaphragm **(intrathoracic kidney)** (Figure 5-5). Whenever only one kidney is seen on excretory urography, a full view of the abdomen is essential to search for an ectopic kidney. Although the ectopic kidney usually functions, the nephrogram and the pelvocalyceal system may be obscured by overlying bone and fecal contents.

Horseshoe kidney is the most common type of fusion anomaly. In this condition both kidneys are malrotated and their lower poles are joined by a band of normal renal parenchyma (isthmus) or connective tissue (Figure 5-6). The ureters arise from the kidneys anteriorly instead of medially and the lower pole calyces point medially rather than laterally. The pelves are often large and flabby and may simulate obstruction. **Crossed ectopia** refers to a situation in which an ectopic kidney lies on the same side as the normal kidney and is most commonly fused with it. **Complete fusion** of the kidneys is a rare anomaly that produces a single irregular mass that has no resemblance to a renal structure. The resulting bizarre appearance has been given such varied names as disk, cake, lump, and doughnut kidney.

Anomalies of renal pelvis and ureter

Duplication (duplex kidney) is a common anomaly that may vary from a simple bifid pelvis to a completely double pelvis, ureter, and ureterovesical orifice. The ureter draining the upper renal segment

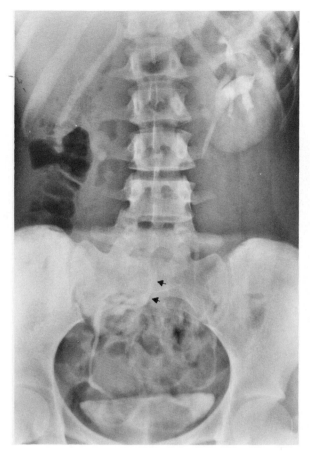

Figure 5-4 Pelvic kidney. Arrows point to collecting system.

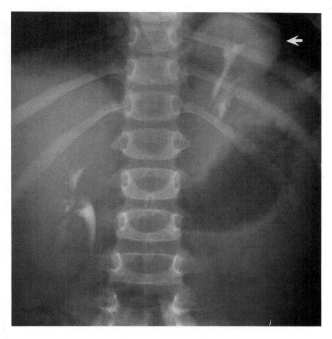

Figure 5-5 Intrathoracic kidney *(arrow)*.

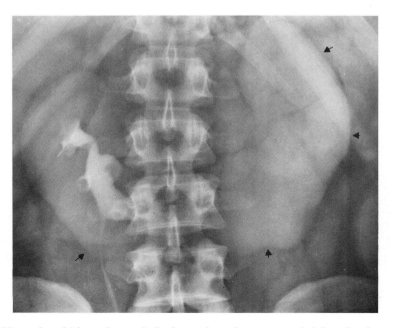

Figure 5-6 Horseshoe kidney *(arrows)*. Prolonged nephrogram and delayed calyceal filling on left are caused by obstructing stone at ureteropelvic junction on that side.

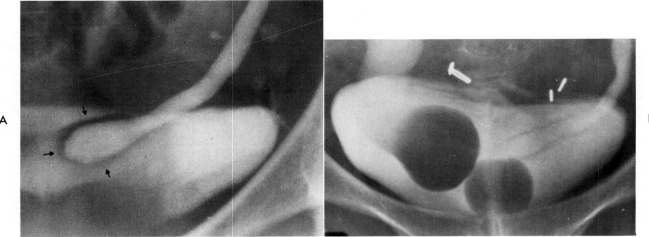

Figure 5-7 Simple ureteroceles. **A,** Unilateral ureterocele *(arrows)* filled with contrast material. **B,** Bilateral ureteroceles without contrast material appear as radiolucent masses in bladder.

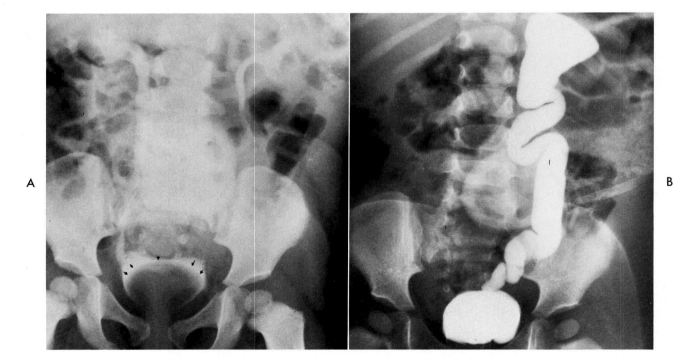

Figure 5-8 Ectopic ureteroceles. **A,** Excretory urogram demonstrates large lucency *(arrows)* filling much of bladder. There is slight downward and lateral displacement of visualized pelvocalyceal system on left. **B,** Cystogram shows contrast material refluxing to fill markedly dilated collecting system draining upper pole of left kidney. Note severe dilation and tortuosity of ureter.

enters the bladder below the ureter draining the lower renal segment. Complete duplication can be complicated by obstruction or by vesicoureteral reflux with infection. Vesicoureteral reflux and infection more commonly involve the ureter draining the lower renal segment; obstruction more frequently affects the upper pole, where it can cause a hydronephrotic mass that displaces and compresses the lower calyces.

Ureterocele

A ureterocele is a cystic dilation of the distal ureter near its insertion into the bladder. In the simple (adult) type the opening in the ureter is situated at or near the normal position in the bladder, usually with stenosis of the ureteral orifice and with varying degrees of dilation of the proximal ureter. The stenosis leads to prolapse of the distal ureter into the bladder and dilation of the lumen of the prolapsed segment. The appearance on excretory urography depends on whether opaque medium fills the ureterocele. If it is filled, the lesion appears as a round or oval density surrounded by a thin radiolucent halo representing the wall of the prolapsed ureter and the mucosa of the bladder (cobra head sign) (Figure 5-7, A). When the ureterocele is not filled with contrast material, it appears as a radiolucent mass within the opacified bladder in the region of the ureteral orifice (Figure 5-7, B).

Ectopic ureteroceles are found almost exclusively in infants and children; most are associated with ureteral duplication. On excretory urography, an ectopic ureterocele typically appears as a large, eccentric filling defect impressing the floor of the bladder (Figure 5-8). The ureterocele arises from the ureter draining the upper segment of the duplicated collecting system. A mass effect, representing hydronephrosis, often involves the upper pole of the kidney and causes downward and lateral displacement of the lower portion of the collecting system.

Posterior urethral valves

Posterior urethral valves are thin transverse membranes, found almost exclusively in males, that cause bladder outlet obstruction and may lead to severe hydronephrosis and renal damage (Figure 5-9).

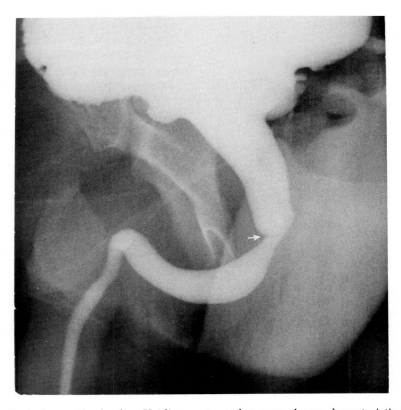

Figure 5-9 Posterior urethral valve. Voiding cystourethrogram shows characteristic thin transverse membrane of valve *(arrow)*. Distally, caliber of bulbous urethra is normal. *(From Friedland GW et al: Clin Radiol 27:367-373, 1976.)*

protinuric
hematuria
oliguria

INFLAMMATORY DISORDERS

Glomerulonephritis

← non pus-forming

Glomerulonephritis is a nonsuppurative inflammatory process involving the tufts of capillaries (glomeruli) that filter the blood within the kidney. It represents an antigen-antibody reaction that most commonly occurs several weeks after an acute upper respiratory or middle ear infection with certain strains of hemolytic streptococci. The inflammatory process causes the glomeruli to be extremely permeable, allowing albumin and red blood cells to leak into the urine (proteinuria, hematuria). Decreased glomerular filtration rate causes oliguria, a smaller-than-normal amount of urine.

Most cases of acute glomerulonephritis resolve completely and the kidney returns to normal. In some patients, however, chronic inflammation with periods of remission and exacerbation lead to a fibrotic reaction that results in shrinkage of the kidneys with loss of renal function and the development of uremia.

The excretory urographic findings in glomerulonephritis depend on the duration and severity of the disease process and on the level of renal function. In patients with acute glomerulonephritis the kidneys may be normal or diffusely increased in size with smooth contours and normal calyces. A loss of renal substance in chronic glomerulonephritis pro-

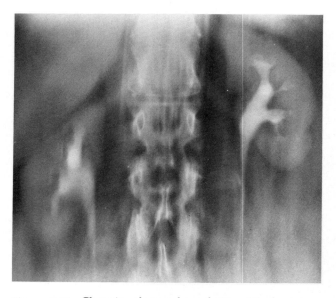

Figure 5-10 Chronic glomerulonephritis. Nephrotomogram shows bilateral small smooth kidneys. Uniform reduction in parenchymal thickness is particularly apparent in right kidney. Note that pelvocalyceal system is well opacified and without irregular contours and blunted calyces seen in chronic pyelonephritis.

duces bilateral small kidneys (Figure 5-10). The renal outline remains smooth and the collecting system is normal, unlike the irregular contours and blunted calyces seen in chronic pyelonephritis.

Pyelonephritis

Pyelonephritis is a suppurative inflammation of the kidney and renal pelvis caused by pyogenic (pus-forming) bacteria. Unlike glomerulonephritis, which primarily involves the parenchyma (glomeruli and tubules) of the kidney, the inflammatory process of pyelonephritis affects the interstitial tissue between the tubules. The infection is patchy in distribution, often involves only one kidney, and is asymmetric if both kidneys are involved. Although the infection may spread from the bloodstream or lymphatics, the infection usually originates in the bladder and ascends by means of the ureter to involve the kidneys. Pyelonephritis often occurs in women and children. The disease frequently develops in patients with obstruction of the urinary tract (enlarged prostate gland, kidney stone, congenital defect), which causes stagnation of the urine and provides a breeding ground for infection. Instrumentation or catheterization of the ureter is also an important contributing factor to the development of pyelonephritis.

Patients with pyelonephritis have high fever, chills, and sudden back pain that spreads over the abdomen. Painful urination (dysuria) usually occurs. Large amounts of pus may be detected in the urine (pyuria), and bacteria can be cultured from the urine or observed in the urinary sediment.

With the availability of antibiotic therapy, pyelonephritis generally heals without complication. However, fibrous scarring can cause irregular contraction of the kidney. Severe infection can destroy large amounts of renal tissue leading to uremia or septicemia as a result of diffuse spread of infection throughout the body.

In most patients with acute pyelonephritis, the excretory urogram is normal. Occasional abnormalities include generalized enlargement of the kidney on the symptomatic side, delayed calyceal opacification, and decreased density of the contrast material. A characteristic finding is linear striation in the renal pelvis, which probably represents mucosal edema. The urographic hallmark of chronic pyelonephritis is patchy calyceal clubbing with overlying parenchymal scarring (Figure 5-11). Initially, there is blunting of the calyces, which then become rounded or clubbed. Fibrotic scarring causes a cortical depression overlying the dilated calyx. Progressive cortical atrophy and thinning may be so extensive that the tip of the blunted calyx appears to lie directly beneath the renal capsule. The uro-

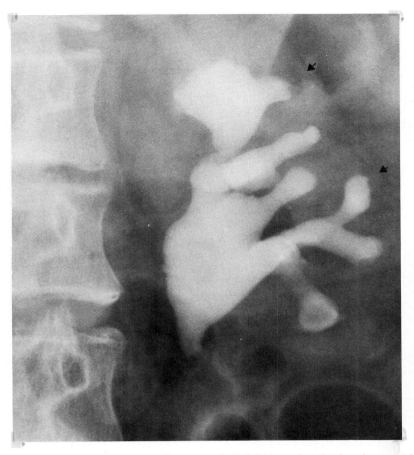

Figure 5-11 Chronic pyelonephritis. Diffuse rounded clubbing of multiple calyces with atrophy and thinning of overlying renal parenchyma. Arrows indicate outer margin of kidney.

graphic findings may be unilateral or bilateral and are often most pronounced at the poles. If calyceal changes are minimal, the overlying cortical depressions may simulate lobar infarctions or normal kidney lobulations. However, in chronic pyelonephritis the cortical depression lies directly over a calyx, rather than between calyces as in lobar infarctions or congenital lobulation. Chronic pyelonephritis may progress to end-stage renal disease with small, usually irregular, poorly functioning kidneys.

Emphysematous pyelonephritis

Emphysematous pyelonephritis is a severe form of acute parenchymal and perirenal infection with gas-forming bacteria that occurs virtually only in diabetic patients and causes an acute necrosis of the entire kidney. The presence of radiolucent gas shadows within and around the kidney is pathognomonic of emphysematous pyelonephritis (Figure 5-12), a surgical emergency that is lethal if treated medically.

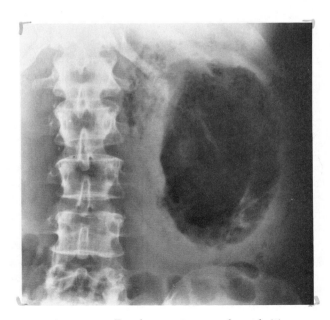

Figure 5-12 Emphysematous pyelonephritis.

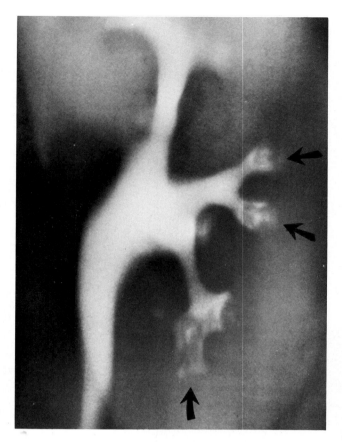

Figure 5-13 Tuberculosis. Early stage of papillary destruction *(arrows)*. *(From Tonkin AK and Witten DM: Semin Roentgenol 14:305-318, 1979.)*

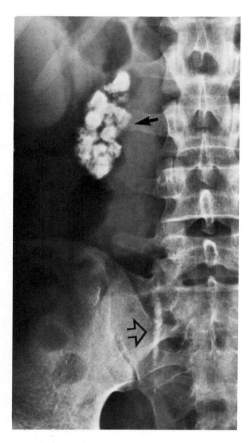

Figure 5-14 Tuberculous autonephrectomy. Plain film shows coarse irregular calcification that retains a kidney-like shape *(solid arrow)*. Note also tuberculous calcification of right distal ureter *(open arrow)*. *(From Tonkin AK and Witten DM: Semin Roentgenol 14:305-318, 1979.)*

Tuberculosis

The hematogenous spread of tuberculosis may lead to the development of small granulomas scattered in the cortical portion of the kidneys. Spread of infection to the renal pyramid causes an ulcerative, destructive process in the tips of the papillae with irregularity and enlargement of the calyces (Figure 5-13). Fibrosis and stricture formation lead to cortical scarring and parenchymal atrophy that may simulate the appearance of chronic bacterial pyelonephritis. Flecks of calcification may develop in multiple tuberculous granulomas. With progressive disease, gross amorphous and irregular calcifications can form. Eventually, the entire nonfunctioning renal parenchyma may be replaced by massive calcification (autonephrectomy) (Figure 5-14).

Tuberculosis can also involve the ureter and bladder. Initially, there are multiple ulcerations that result in a ragged, irregular appearance of the ureteral wall. As the disease heals, there are usually multiple areas in which the ureteral strictures alternate with dilated segments, producing a beaded, or corkscrew,

appearance. In advanced cases the wall of the ureter may become thickened and fixed with no peristalsis; this results in a pipestem ureter that runs a direct course toward the bladder (Figure 5-15). Tuberculous involvement of the urinary bladder may produce mural irregularities simulating carcinoma or, more commonly, a small, contracted bladder with a thickened wall.

Papillary necrosis

Papillary necrosis refers to a destructive process involving a varying amount of the medullary papillae and renal pyramids. It is most often seen in patients with diabetes, pyelonephritis, urinary tract infection or obstruction, sickle cell disease, or phenacetin abuse. The necrotic process causes cavitation of the central portion of the papillae or complete sloughing of the papillary tip (Figure 5-16). When a piece of medullary tissue has been completely separated from the rest of the renal parenchyma, an excretory urogram shows a characteristic ring of contrast material surrounding a triangular lucent filling defect representing the sloughed necrotic tissue. The remaining calyx has a round, saccular, or club-shaped configuration. The sloughed papilla may stay in place and become calcified, or it may pass down the ureter, where it may simulate a stone and even cause obstruction.

Cystitis

Inflammation of the urinary bladder is most common in women because of their shorter urethra. The major cause is the inadvertent spread of bacteria present in fecal material, which reaches the urinary opening and travels upward to the bladder. Instrumentation or catheterization of the bladder is another important cause of cystitis, which is the most common infection in hospitalized patients (nosocomial infection). Cystitis also can develop from sexual intercourse with the spread of infecting organisms from around the vaginal opening. Urinary frequency, urgency, and a burning sensation during urination are typical clinical findings. "Honeymoon Cystitis"

Although acute inflammation of the bladder generally does not produce changes detectable on excretory urography, chronic cystitis causes a decrease in bladder size that is often associated with irregu-

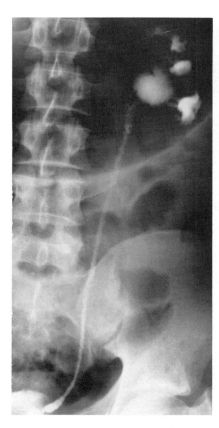

Figure 5-15 Ureteral tuberculosis.

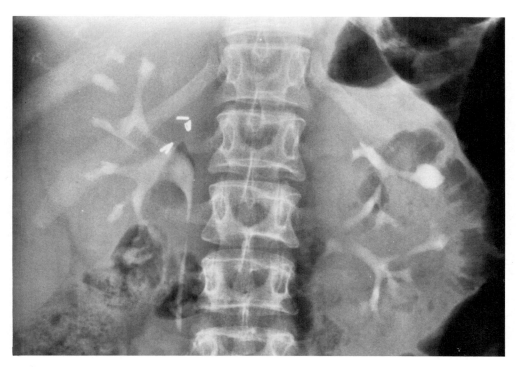

Figure 5-16 Papillary necrosis. Generalized saccular or club-shaped configuration of most calyces bilaterally in patient with sickle cell disease. Note surgical clips.

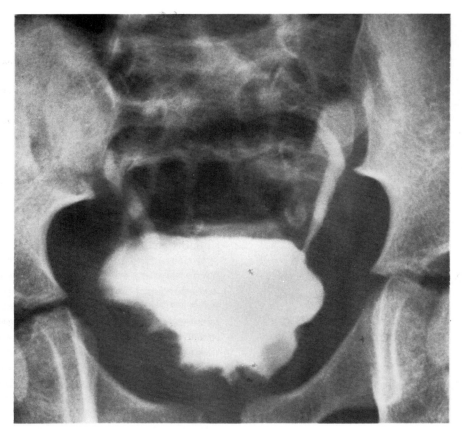

Figure 5-17 Cystitis. Excretory urogram shows irregular, lobulated filling defects (representing intense mucosal edema) at base of bladder.

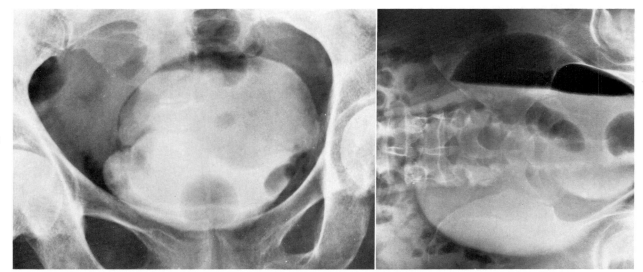

Figure 5-18 Emphysematous cystitis. **A,** Film from cystogram shows thin rim of lucency surrounding much of contrast-filled bladder. **B,** Right lateral decubitus view clearly shows long air-fluid level.

larity of the bladder wall (Figure 5-17). In candidal cystitis, fungus balls may produce lucent filling defects in the opacified bladder. Similar lucent filling defects in the bladder may reflect blood clots in patients with hemorrhagic cystitis and may complicate chemotherapy in the treatment of leukemia and lymphoma. A dramatic radiographic appearance is produced by emphysematous cystitis, an inflammatory disease of the bladder that most often occurs in diabetic patients and is caused by gas-forming bacteria. Characteristic plain film findings are a ring of lucent gas outlining all or a part of the bladder wall and the presence of gas within the bladder lumen (Figure 5-18).

KIDNEY STONES

Urinary calculi most commonly form in the kidney. They are asymptomatic until they lodge in the ureter and cause partial obstruction, resulting in extreme pain that radiates from the area of the kidney to the groin. The cause of kidney stones is varied and often reflects an underlying metabolic abnormality, such as hypercalcemia, resulting from hyperparathyroidism or any cause of increased calcium excretion in the urine. Urinary stasis and infection are also important factors in promoting stone formation.

More than 80% of symptomatic renal stones contain enough calcium to be radiopaque and detectable on plain abdominal radiographs (Figure 5-19). Completely radiolucent calculi contain no calcium and are composed of a variety of substances that are in excessive concentration in the urine. Excretory urography is used to detect these otherwise invisible nonopaque stones, which appear as filling defects in the contrast-filled collecting system. In patients with acute renal colic caused by an obstructing stone in the ureter, excretory urography may demonstrate the point of cutoff and dilation of the proximal ureter and pelvocalyceal system. With acute obstruction, the intrapelvic pressure may increase to such an extent that there is little or no glomerular filtration, resulting in a delayed but prolonged nephrogram and a lack of calyceal filling on the affected side.

Small renal stones may pass spontaneously in the urine. At times, a stone may completely fill the renal pelvis (staghorn calculus) (Figure 5-20), blocking the flow of urine. In the past, surgery was frequently necessary to remove large kidney stones. More recently, medication introduced into the upper urinary

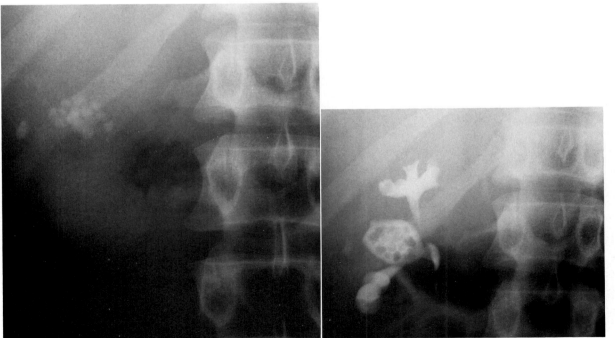

Figure 5-19 Cystine stones. **A,** Plain film shows multiple radiopaque calculi. **B,** Excretory urogram demonstrates stones as lucent filling defects in opacified renal pelvis. *(From Eisenberg, R.: Gastrointestinal radiology: a pattern approach, ed 2, Philadelphia, JB Lippincott Co, 1990.)*

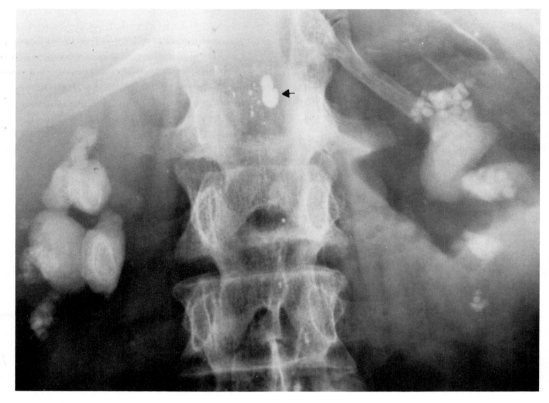

Figure 5-20 Staghorn calculi. Calculi fill renal pelves bilaterally. Of incidental note is residual contrast material (arrow) from prior myelogram.

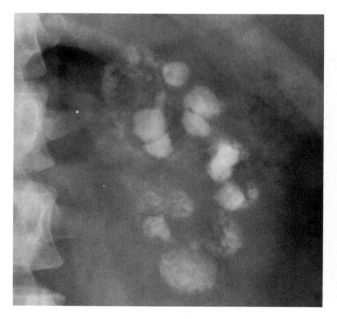

Figure 5-21 Nephrolithiasis. Multiple deposits are scattered throughout parenchyma of left kidney.

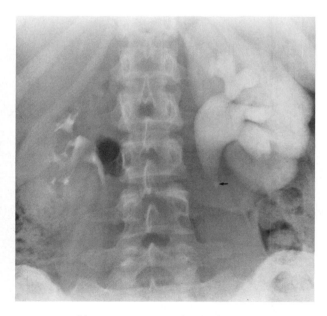

Figure 5-22 Obstructing ureteral calculus. Excretory urogram demonstrates prolonged nephrogram and marked dilation of collecting system and pelvis proximal to obstructing stone (arrow).

tract by means of a percutaneous catheter has been used to dissolve large kidney stones into smaller pieces that pass easily. A new technique is lithotripsy, in which the patient is immersed in a tank of water into which acoustic shock waves are introduced. These shock waves shatter the hard stones into sand-sized particles that are excreted in the urine.

Calcium can also deposit within the renal parenchyma (nephrocalcinosis) (Figure 5-21). This calcification varies from a few scattered punctate densities to very dense and extensive calcifications throughout both kidneys. The most common causes of nephrocalcinosis include hyperparathyroidism, increased intestinal absorption of calcium (sarcoidosis, hypervitaminosis D, milk-alkali syndrome), and renal tubular acidosis, a disorder in which the kidney is unable to excrete an acid urine (below pH 5.4).

Stones can also form in other portions of the genitourinary tract. Ureteral calculi almost invariably result from the downward movement of kidney stones (Figure 5-22). They are usually small, irregular, and poorly calcified and are therefore easily missed on abdominal radiographs that are not of good quality. Calculi most commonly lodge in the lower portion of the ureter, especially at the ureterovesical junction and at the pelvic brim (Figure 5-23). They are often oval, with their long axes paralleling the course of the ureter. Ureteral calculi must be differentiated from the far more common phleboliths, which are spherical and are located in the lateral portion of the pelvis below a line joining the ischial spines. In contrast, ureteral stones are situated medially above the interspinous line.

Stone formation in the bladder is primarily a disorder of elderly men with obstruction or infection of the lower urinary tract (Figure 5-24, A). Frequently associated lesions include bladder outlet obstruction, urethral strictures, neurogenic bladder, and bladder diverticula (Figure 5-24, B). At times, upper urinary tract stones migrate down the ureter and are retained in the bladder. Bladder calculi can be single or multiple. They vary in size from tiny

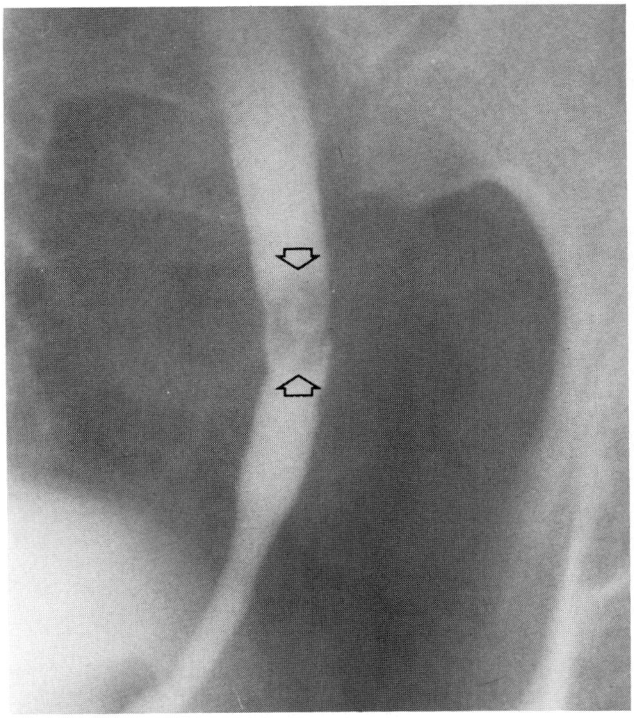

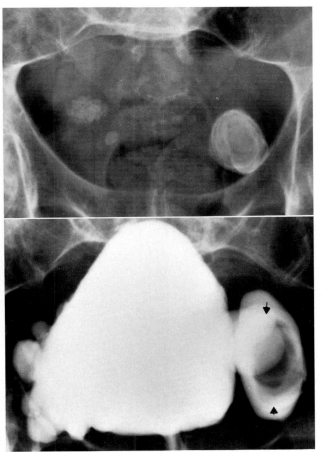

A

B

Figure 5-24 Bladder calculi. **A,** Plain radiograph of pelvis shows large laminated stone on left and multiple smaller calculi on right. **B,** Excretory urogram demonstrates large stone *(arrows)* in left-sided bladder diverticulum. Note that multiple smaller calculi on right have been obscured by overlying contrast material.

Figure 5-23 Ureteral calculus. Stone appears as nonopaque filling defect *(arrows)* in distal ureter.

concretions, each the size of a grain of sand, to an enormous single calculus occupying the entire bladder lumen. Most bladder calculi are circular or oval; however, almost any shape can be encountered. They can be amorphous, laminated (layered), or even spiculated. One unusual type with a characteristic radiographic appearance is the hard burr, or jackstone, variety, which gets its name from the many irregular prongs that project from its surface and simulate the child's toy.

renal colic - pain from kidney stone

URINARY TRACT OBSTRUCTION

Urinary tract obstruction produces anatomic and functional changes that vary with the rapidity of onset, the degree of occlusion, and the distance between the kidney and the obstructing lesion. In adults, urinary calculi, pelvic tumors, urethral strictures, and enlargement of the prostate gland are the major causes. In children, congenital malformations (ureteropelvic junction narrowing, ureterocele, retrocaval ureter, posterior urethral valve) are usually

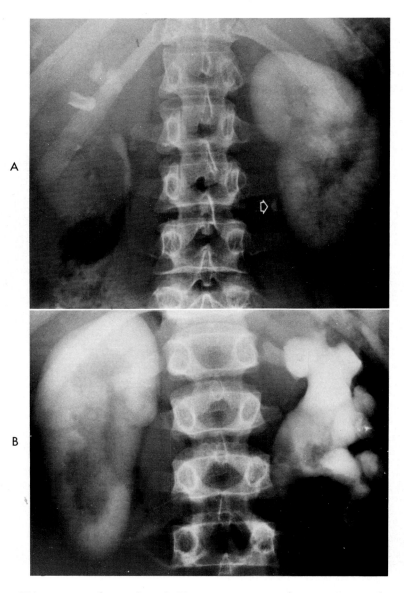

Figure 5-25   Urinary tract obstruction. **A,** Excretory urogram demonstrates prolonged nephrogram on left and no calyceal filling. Arrow points to obstructing stone in proximal left ureter. **B,** In another patient, there is prolonged and intensified obstructive nephrogram of right kidney. On left, there is marked dilation of pelvocalyceal system but no persistent nephrogram, reflecting intermittent chronic obstruction on this side.

responsible for mechanical obstruction. Normal points of narrowing, such as the ureteropelvic and ureterovesical junctions, the bladder neck, and the urethral meatus, are common sites of obstruction. Blockage above the level of the bladder causes unilateral dilation of the ureter (hydroureter) and renal pelvocalyceal system (hydronephrosis); if the lesion is at or below the level of the bladder, as in prostatic hypertrophy or tumor, bilateral involvement is the rule.

In acute urinary tract obstruction, diminished filtration of urographic contrast material results in delayed parenchymal opacification compared with the nonobstructed kidney. The nephrogram eventually becomes more dense than normal because of a decreased flow rate of fluid through the tubules, which results in enhanced water reabsorption by the nephrons and greater concentration of the contrast material (Figure 5-25). There is delayed and decreased pelvocalyceal filling because of dilation and elevated pressure in the collecting system. The radiographic study may have to be prolonged up to 48 hours after

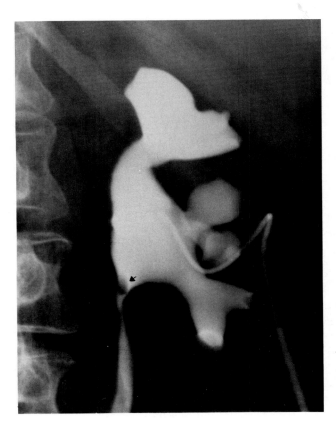

Figure 5-26 Hydronephrosis. Dilation of entire pelvocalyceal system proximal to obstructing *Cryptococcus* fungus ball *(arrow)* at ureteropelvic junction.

the administration of contrast material to determine the precise site of obstruction.

In the patient with acute urinary tract obstruction, the kidney is generally enlarged, and the calyces are moderately dilated. An uncommon but pathognomonic urographic finding in acute unilateral obstruction (usually due to ureteral stone) is opacification of the gallbladder 8 to 24 hours after the injection of contrast material. This "vicarious excretion" is related to increased liver excretion of contrast material that cannot be promptly excreted by the kidneys.

As an obstruction becomes more chronic, the predominant urographic finding is a markedly dilated pelvocalyceal system and ureter proximal to the obstruction (Figure 5-26). Prolonged increased pressure causes progressive papillary atrophy, leading to calyceal clubbing. Gradual enlargement of the calyces and renal pelvis with progressive destruction of renal parenchyma may continue until the kidney becomes a nonfunctioning hydronephrotic sac in which normal anatomy is obliterated.

Whenever possible, the site of obstruction should be demonstrated. Although excretory urography with delayed films may accomplish this purpose, antegrade pyelography is often required. In this procedure, a catheter or needle is placed percutaneously into the dilated collecting system under ultrasound or fluoroscopic guidance, and contrast material is then introduced. This approach has the added advantage of providing immediate and certain decompression of a unilateral obstructing lesion.

Ultrasound is of particular value in detecting hydronephrosis in patients with such severe urinary tract obstruction and renal dysfunction that there is no opacification of the kidneys and collecting systems on excretory urograms. The dilated calyces and pelvis become large, hydronephrotic, echo-free sacs separated by septa of compressed tissue and vessels (Figure 5-27, *A*). With increased duration and severity of hydronephrosis, the intervening septa may disappear, leaving a large fluid-filled sac with no evidence of internal structure and no normal parenchyma apparent at its margins (Figure 5-27, *B*).

A physiologic form of hydronephrosis often develops during pregnancy. The enlarging uterine mass and physiologic hormonal changes cause extrinsic pressure on the ureter, leading to progressive dilation of the proximal collecting systems (Figure 5-28). Often bilateral, the dilation usually is more prominent and develops earlier on the right side. After delivery, the urinary tract returns to normal within several weeks. In some women, however, persistent dilation of the ovarian vein can compress the ureter and result in prolonged postpartum hydronephrosis.

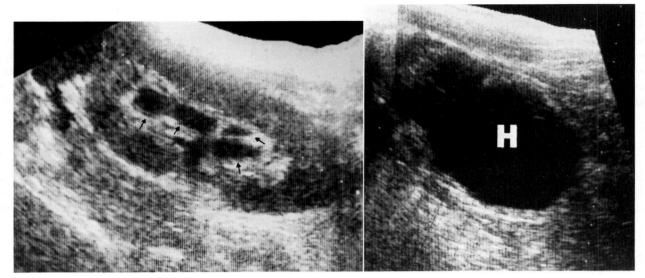

A

B

Figure 5-27 Hydronephrosis. **A,** In patient with moderately severe disease, dilated calyces and pelvis appear on ultrasound as echo-free sacs *(arrows)* separated by septa of compressed tissue and vessels. **B,** In patient with severe hydronephrosis, intervening septa have disappeared, leaving large fluid-filled sac *(H)* with no evidence of internal structure and no normal parenchyma apparent at its margins.

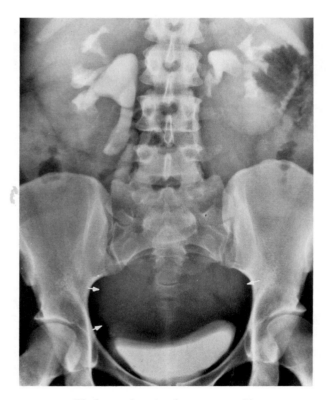

Figure 5-28 Hydronephrosis of pregnancy. Excretory urogram performed 3 days postpartum demonstrates bilateral large kidneys with dilation of ureters and pelvocalyceal systems, especially on right. Large pelvic mass *(arrows)* indenting superior surface of bladder represents uterus, which is still causing extrinsic pressure on ureters.

CYSTS AND TUMORS

Renal cyst

Simple renal cysts are the most common unifocal masses of the kidney. They are fluid-filled and usually unilocular, although septa sometimes divide the cyst into chambers that may or may not communicate with each other. Cysts vary in size, and they may occur at single or multiple sites in one or both kidneys. Thin curvilinear calcifications can be demonstrated in the wall of about 3% of simple cysts. However, this peripheral type of calcification is not pathognomonic of a benign process, since malignant kidney lesions can produce a similar pattern.

As a simple renal cyst slowly increases in size, its protruding portion elevates the adjacent edges of the cortex. The cortical margin appears on nephrotomography as a very thin, smooth radiopaque rim about the bulging lucent cyst (beak sign) (Figure 5-29). Although the beak sign is generally considered to be characteristic of benign renal cysts, it is merely a reflection of slow expansion of a mass and thus may occasionally be seen in slow-growing solid lesions, including carcinoma. Thickening of the rim about a lucent mass suggests bleeding into a cyst, cyst infection, or a malignant lesion. Renal cysts cause focal displacement of adjacent portions of the pelvocalyceal system. The displaced, attenuated collecting structures remain smooth, unlike the shag-

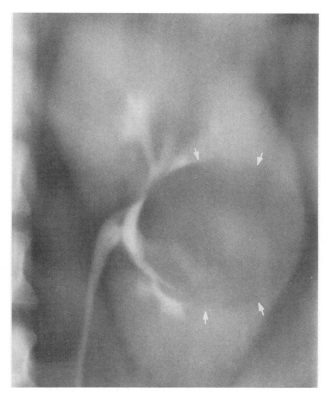

Figure 5-29 Renal cyst. Nephrotomogram shows smooth-walled, fluid-filled mass *(arrows)*.

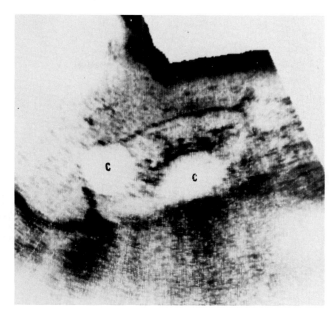

Figure 5-30 Renal cysts. Anechoic fluid-filled masses *(C)* with strongly enhancing posterior walls.

giness and obliteration that often occur when focal displacement is due to a malignant neoplasm.

Ultrasound is the modality of choice for distinguishing fluid-filled simple cysts from solid mass lesions. Fluid-filled cysts classically appear as echo-free structures with strongly enhanced posterior walls (Figure 5-30), in contrast to solid or complex lesions, such as tumors, that appear as echo-filled masses without posterior wall enhancement. CT is also highly accurate in detecting and characterizing simple renal cysts. On unenhanced scans, the cyst has a uniform attenuation value near that of water. After the injection of contrast material, a simple cyst becomes more apparent as the contrast material is concentrated by the normal surrounding parenchyma (Figure 5-31). The cyst itself shows no change in attenuation value, unlike a solid renal neoplasm, which always shows a small but definite increase in density. Because of the accuracy of CT and ultrasound, percutaneous cyst puncture is rarely necessary if these modalities provide unequivocal evidence of a simple cyst. However, because abscesses, cystic or necrotic tumors, and inflammatory or hemorrhagic cysts can mimic simple cysts, cyst puncture should be performed if there is an atypical appear-

ance or a strong clinical suspicion of abscess, or if the patient has hematuria or hypertension. Fluid aspirated from a renal cyst can be clearly differentiated from that obtained from an abscess or renal tumor. The introduction of contrast material or air after the cyst fluid has been removed demonstrates the smooth inner wall of the cyst and further decreases the possibility of missing a malignant neoplasm (Figure 5-32).

Polycystic kidney disease

Polycystic kidney disease is an inherited disorder in which multiple cysts of varying size cause lobulated

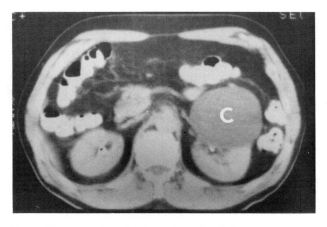

Figure 5-31 Renal cyst. Nonenhancing left renal mass *(C)* with sharply marginated border and thin wall.

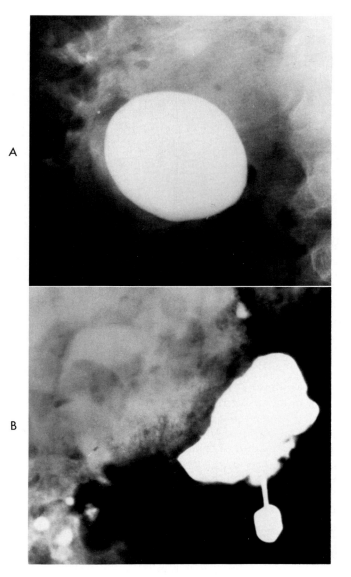

Figure 5-32 Renal cyst puncture. **A,** Instillation of contrast material shows smooth inner wall characteristic of benign cyst. **B,** In another patient, introduction of contrast material reveals markedly irregular inner border of necrotic renal cell carcinoma.

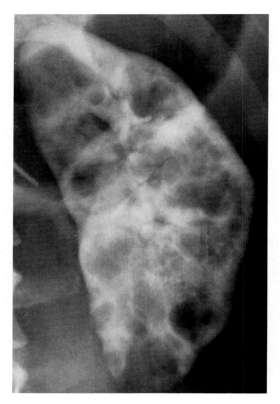

Figure 5-33 Polycystic kidney disease. Nephrogram phase from selective arteriography of left kidney demonstrates innumerable cysts ranging from pinhead size to 2 cm. Opposite kidney had identical appearance. *(From Bosniak MA and Ambos MA: Semin Roentgenol 10:133-143, 1975.)*

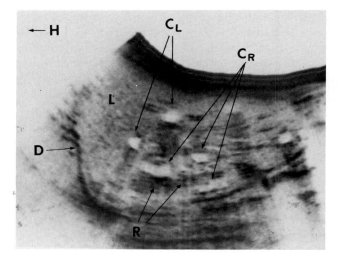

Figure 5-34 Polycystic kidney disease. Parasagittal sonogram shows multiple cysts (C_R, C_L) in right kidney *(R)* and liver *(L)*. D, Diaphragm; H, head. *(From Friedland GW et al., editors: Uroradiology: an integrated approach, New York, Churchill Livingstone, 1983.)*

enlargement of the kidneys and progressive renal impairment, which is presumably a result of cystic compression of nephrons that causes localized intrarenal obstruction. One third of patients with this condition have associated cysts of the liver, which do not interfere with hepatic function. About 10% have one or more saccular (berry) aneurysms of cerebral arteries, which may rupture and produce a fatal subarachnoid hemorrhage. Many patients with polycystic disease are hypertensive, a condition that may cause further deterioration of renal function and increase the likelihood that a cerebral aneurysm

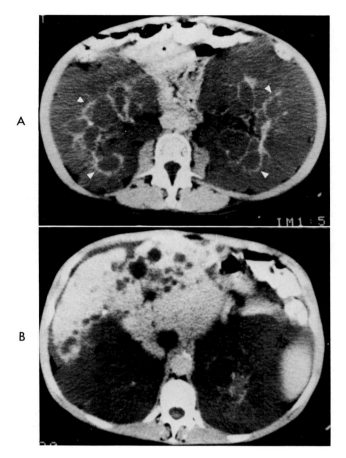

A

B

Figure 5-35 Polycystic kidney disease. **A,** CT scan shows contrast-enhancing rims *(arrowheads)* in severely thinned renal parenchyma about innumerable large renal cysts. **B,** CT scan at higher level also shows diffuse cystic involvement of liver.

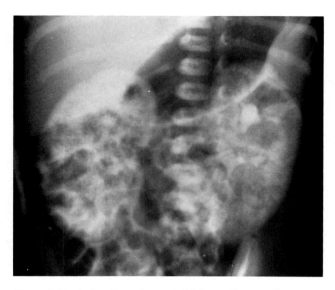

Figure 5-36 Infantile polycystic kidney disease. Excretory urogram in young boy with large, palpable abdominal masses demonstrates renal enlargement with characteristic streaky densities leading to calyceal tips. There is only minimal distortion of calyces.

will rupture. Because patients tend to be asymptomatic during the first three decades of life, early diagnosis is made either by chance or as a result of a specific search prompted by the discovery of a positive family history.

Excretory urography demonstrates enlarged kidneys with a multilobulated contour. The pelvic and infundibular structures are elongated, effaced, and often displaced around larger cysts to produce a crescentic outline. The nephrogram typically has a distinctive mottled or Swiss cheese pattern caused by the presence of innumerable lucent cysts of varying size throughout the kidneys (Figure 5-33). Plaques of calcification occasionally occur in cyst walls.

Ultrasound demonstrates grossly enlarged kidneys containing multiple cysts that vary markedly in size and are randomly distributed throughout the kidney (Figure 5-34). The demonstration of similar

hepatic cysts further strengthens the diagnosis. Ultrasound is also of value in screening family members of a patient known to have this hereditary disorder. In patients with bilateral kidney enlargement and poor renal function, ultrasound permits the differentiation of polycystic kidney disease from multiple solid masses.

The multiple cysts in polycystic kidney disease can also be detected on CT (Figure 5-35) and MRI. Although most individual cysts are histologically identical to simple cysts, intracystic hemorrhage is common. Unlike the low attenuation seen in simple renal cysts on CT, hemorrhagic cysts have high attenuation values. On MRI a hemorrhagic cyst has high signal intensity on both T1- and T2-weighted images, unlike the low signal intensity found on T1-weighted images of simple renal cysts.

A rare, usually fatal form of polycystic disease can present at birth with diffusely enlarged kidneys, renal failure, and maldevelopment of intrahepatic bile ducts. The margins of the kidneys are smooth in infantile polycystic disease, unlike the irregular renal contours in the adult form of polycystic disease that are due to the protrusion of innumerable cysts from the kidney surface. When renal function is sufficient, excretory urography results in a striking nephrogram in which a streaky pattern of alternating dense and lucent bands reflects contrast material puddling in elongated cystic spaces that radiate perpendicular to the cortical surface (Figure 5-36). Ultrasound shows distortion of the intraparenchymal architecture, although the individual cysts are too small to be visualized.

Renal carcinoma

Renal cell carcinoma (hypernephroma) is the most common renal neoplasm, predominantly occurring in patients older than 40 years and often presenting with painless hematuria. About 10% of hypernephromas contain calcification that is usually located in reactive fibrous zones about areas of tumor necrosis. In the differentiation of solid tumor fromfluid-filled benign cysts, the location of calcium within the mass is more important than the pattern of calcification. Of all masses containing calcium in a nonperipheral location, almost 90% are malignant. Although peripheral curvilinear calcification is much more suggestive of a benign cyst, hypernephromas can have a calcified fibrous pseudocapsule that results in an identical radiographic appearance.

Hypernephromas typically produce urographic evidence of localized bulging or generalized renal enlargement. The tumor initially causes elongation of adjacent calyces; progressive enlargement and infiltration lead to distortion, narrowing, or obliteration of part or all of the collecting system (Figure 5-37). Large tumors may partially obstruct the pelvis or upper ureter and cause proximal dilation. Complete loss of function on excretory urography usually indicates tumor invasion of the renal vein.

On nephrotomography, a hypernephroma generally appears as a mass with indistinct outlines and a density similar to that of normal parenchyma, unlike the classic radiolucent mass with sharp margins and a thin wall that represents a benign cyst. Necrotic neoplasms can also appear cystic, although they are usually surrounded by thick, irregular walls (Figure 5-38).

Ultrasound shows a renal carcinoma as a solid mass with numerous internal echoes and no evidence of the acoustic enhancement seen with renal cysts (Figure 5-39). On unenhanced CT scans, a hypernephroma appears as a solid neoplasm that is often not homogeneous and has an attenuation value near that of normal renal parenchyma, unlike a simple cyst, which has a uniform attenuation value near that of water. After the injection of contrast material, a simple cyst shows no change in attenuation value, whereas a solid renal neoplasm demonstrates a small but definite increase in density that is probably due primarily to vascular perfusion. However, this increased density is much less than that of surrounding normal parenchyma, which also tends to concentrate the contrast material, and thus renal neoplasms become more apparent on contrast-enhanced scans (Figure 5-40). CT is also an accurate method for detecting local and regional spread of hypernephroma. It can usually distinguish between neoplasms confined to the renal capsule and those

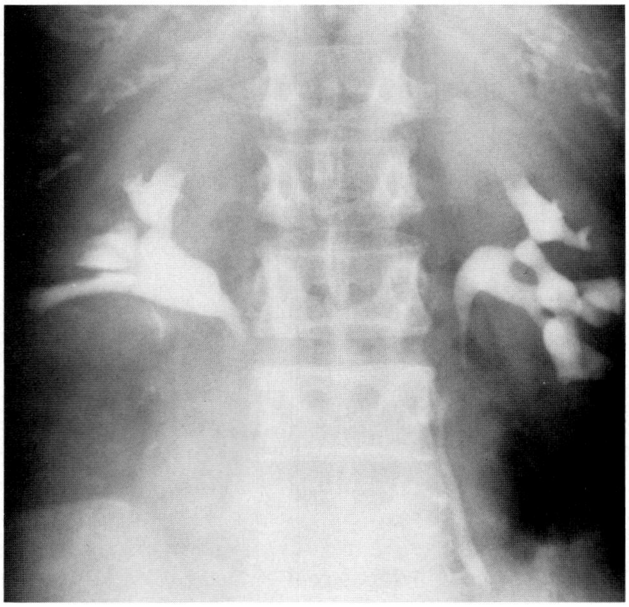

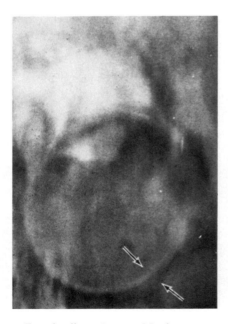

Figure 5-37 Renal cell carcinoma. Upward displacement of right kidney and distortion of collecting system by large lower pole mass.

Figure 5-38 Renal cell carcinoma. Nephrotomogram demonstrates lucent, well-demarcated renal mass with thick wall *(arrows). (From Bosniak MA and Faegenburg D: The thick wall sign, Radiology 84:692-698, 1965.)*

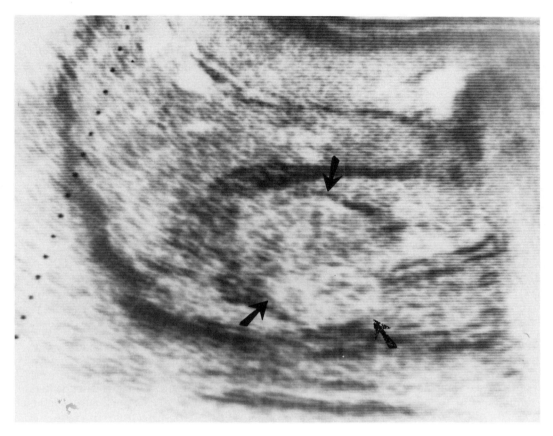

Figure 5-39 Renal cell carcinoma. Ultrasound shows echo-filled solid mass *(arrows)* with no posterior enhancement.

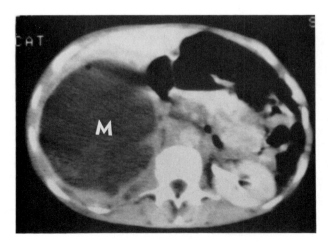

Figure 5-40 Necrotic renal cell carcinoma. CT shows huge nonenhancing, cystlike mass *(M)* that has irregular margins (especially on its medial and posterior aspects).

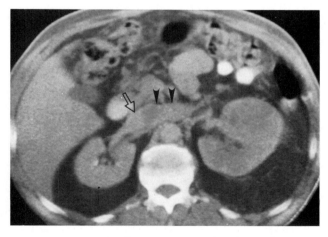

Figure 5-41 Renal cell carcinoma with left renal vein invasion. Postcontrast CT scan shows dilated left renal vein filled with tumor thrombus *(arrowheads)*. Thrombus extends to inferior vena cava *(arrow)*. *(From McClennan BL and Lee JKT: Kidney. In Lee JKT, Sagel SS, and Stanley RJ, editors: Computed body tomography, New York, Raven Press, 1983.)*

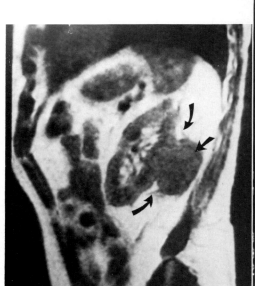
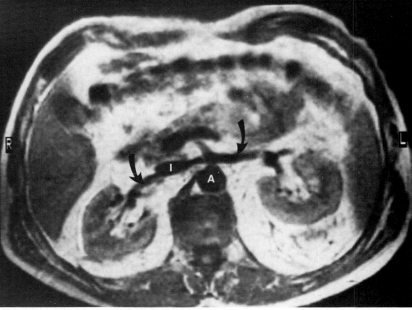

Figure 5-42   Renal cell carcinoma. **A,** Sagittal T1-weighted MR image through left kidney demonstrates large renal cell carcinoma *(straight arrow)* arising from posterior aspect of kidney and displacing Gerota's fascia outward *(curved arrows)*. **B,** Transverse MR image at level of renal veins *(arrows)* and inferior vena cava *(I)* demonstrates normal signal from flowing blood without evidence of tumor thrombus. This modality is especially useful for staging renal cell carcinoma because of its multiplanar capability and its ability to assess vascular invasion. *A,* Aorta.

that have extended beyond it. CT is also the most accurate method for detecting enlargement of para-aortic, paracaval, and retrocrural lymph nodes and spread to the ipsilateral renal vein and inferior vena cava (Figure 5-41).

MRI allows detailed demonstration of the renal anatomy and approaches the accuracy of CT in staging the abdominal extent of tumor in the patient with renal cell carcinoma (Figure 5-42, *A*) Advantages of MRI include its ability to determine the origin of the mass, to detect perihilar and perivascular lymph node metastases, and to demonstrate tumor invasion of adjacent organs. The superb delineation of blood vessels with MRI permits evaluation of tumor thrombus extension into the renal veins and inferior vena cava without the need for intravenous contrast material (Figure 5-42, *B*).

The most common sites of metastasis from renal cell carcinoma include the lungs, liver, bones, and brain.

Wilms' tumor (nephroblastoma)

Wilms' tumor is the most common abdominal neoplasm of infancy and childhood. The lesion arises from embryonic renal tissue, may be bilateral, and

tends to become very large and appear as a palpable mass.

Wilms' tumor must be differentiated from neuroblastoma, a tumor of adrenal medullary origin that is the second most common malignancy in children. Peripheral cystic calcification occurs in about 10% of Wilms' tumors, in contrast to the fine, granular, or stippled calcification seen in about half of the cases of neuroblastoma. At excretory urography, the intrarenal Wilms' tumor causes marked distortion and displacement of the pelvocalyceal system (Figure 5-43). The major effect of the extrarenal neuroblastoma is to displace the entire kidney downward and laterally. Because the kidney itself is usually not invaded, there is no distortion of the pelvocalyceal system.

Ultrasound is of value in distinguishing Wilms' tumor from hydronephrosis, another major cause of a palpable renal mass in a child. Wilms' tumors typically have a solid appearance with gross distortion of the renal structure (Figure 5-44), unlike the precise organization of symmetrically positioned fluid-filled spaces in hydronephrosis. Ultrasound can also demonstrate the intrarenal location of Wilms' tumor, in contrast to the extrarenal origin of a neuroblastoma.

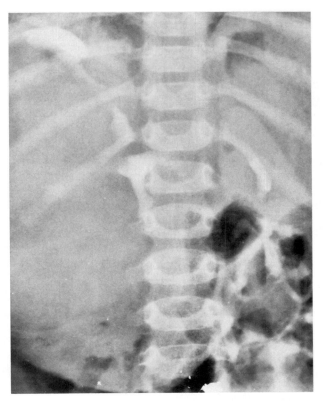

Figure 5-43 Wilms' tumor. Huge mass in right kidney distorts and displaces pelvocalyceal system. *(From Friedland GW et al, editors: Uroradiology: an integrated approach, New York, Churchill Livingstone, 1983.)*

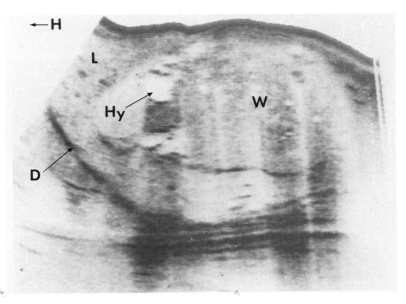

Figure 5-44 Wilms' tumor. Parasagittal supine sonogram demonstrates huge mass *(W)* involving lower pole of right kidney and resulting in hydronephrosis of upper collecting system *(Hy)*. Wilms' tumors tend to have moderately low internal echogenicity and, as in this patient, often contain multiple tiny cystic spaces. Large mass dramatically displaces liver *(L)*. D, Diaphragm; H, head. *(From Friedland GW et al, editors: Uroradiology: an integrated approach, New York, Churchill Livingstone, 1983.)*

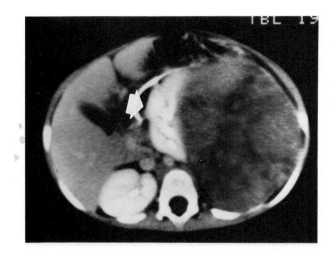

Figure 5-45 Wilms' tumor. Large low-density mass pushing functioning portion of left kidney *(arrow)* across midline.

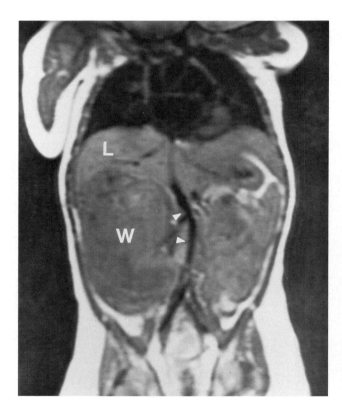

Figure 5-46 T1-weighted coronal MR scan shows sharply marginated infrahepatic mass *(W)* that is clearly distinct from liver. Inferior vena cava *(arrowheads)*, while displaced by mass, shows no evidence of tumor extension into it. L, Liver. *(From Merten DF and Kirks DR: In Eisenberg RL, editor: Diagnostic imaging: an algorithmic approach, Philadelphia, JB Lippincott Co, 1988.)*

Although it entails the use of ionizing radiation, CT can show the full extent of the tumor (including invasion of the inferior vena cava) and can detect any recurrence of the neoplasm after surgical removal (Figure 5-45). Coronal T1-weighted MR images can accurately differentiate Wilms' tumor from renal or hepatic lesions (Figure 5-46). This also is extremely useful in defining the extent of the lesion and showing possible tumor thrombus within the renal vein or inferior vena cava. Because MRI has no ionizing radiation, it is an ideal modality for follow-up evaluation after surgical removal of the tumor.

Carcinoma of the bladder

Bladder carcinoma is usually seen in men after age 50. A number of industrial chemicals have been implicated as factors in the development of carcinoma of the bladder. Cigarette smoking has also been associated with bladder tumors, presumably because of carcinogenic metabolites being excreted in the urine. The incidence of bladder cancer is especially high in Egypt, most likely related to the widespread prevalence of the parasitic infection schistosomiasis in that country.

Carcinoma of the bladder may produce fingerlike projections into the lumen or infiltrate the bladder wall. Plain radiographs may demonstrate punctate, coarse, or linear calcifications that are usually encrusted on the surface of the tumor but occasionally lie within it. On excretory urograms, bladder cancer appears as one or more polypoid defects arising from

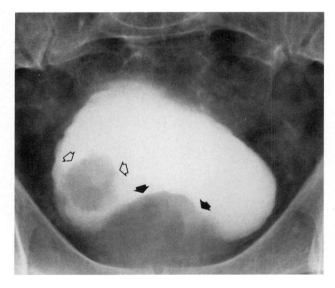

Figure 5-47 Carcinoma of bladder. Irregular tumor *(open arrows)* that is associated with large filling defect *(solid arrows)*, representing benign prostatic hypertrophy, at base of bladder.

the bladder wall or as focal bladder wall thickening (Figure 5-47). However, urography can detect only about 60% of bladder carcinomas because most are small when first symptomatic and are located on the trigone, where they can be difficult to visualize. Therefore all patients with lower urinary tract hematuria should undergo cystoscopy to exclude a bladder neoplasm.

CT with full distention of the bladder demonstrates a neoplasm as a mass projecting into the bladder lumen or as focal thickening of the bladder wall (Figure 5-48, *A*). This modality is the method of choice for preoperative staging because it can determine the presence and degree of extravesical extension, involvement of the pelvic sidewalls (Figure 5-48, *B*), and enlargement of pelvic or para-aortic lymph nodes.

Many carcinomas of the bladder have a low grade of malignancy, although they tend to recur repeatedly after surgical removal. More invasive tumors require removal of the entire bladder with transplantation of the ureters into a loop of ileum.

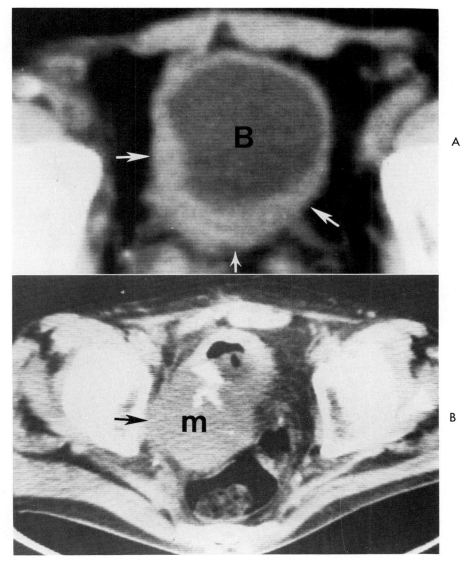

Figure 5-48 CT of bladder carcinoma *(B)*. **A,** Focal thickening of posterior wall *(arrows)*. **B,** In this patient, extensive bladder cancer *(m)* has extended to involve sidewall of pelvis *(arrow)*. *(From Friedland GW et al, editors: Uroradiology: an integrated approach, New York, Churchill Livingstone, 1983.)*

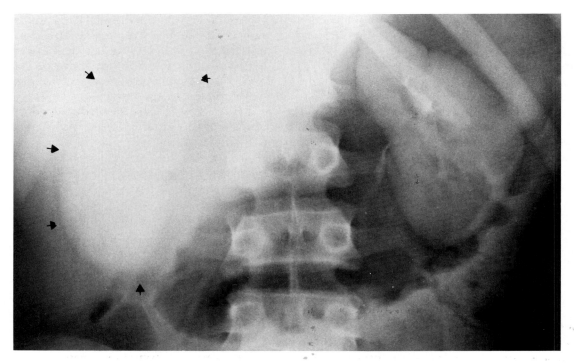

Figure 5-49 Acute renal vein thrombosis. Film of right kidney taken 5 minutes after injection of contrast material shows dense nephrogram *(arrows)* and absence of calyceal filling.

RENAL VEIN THROMBOSIS

Renal vein thrombosis occurs most frequently in children who are severely dehydrated. In the adult, thrombosis is most often a complication of another renal disease (chronic glomerulonephritis, amyloidosis, pyelonephritis), trauma, the extension of a thrombus from the inferior vena cava, or direct invasion or extrinsic pressure resulting from renal tumors.

Renal vein thrombosis may be unilateral or bilateral. The clinical and radiographic findings are greatly influenced by the rapidity with which venous occlusion occurs. Sudden total occlusion causes striking kidney enlargement with minimal or no opacification on excretory urograms (Figure 5-49). If unresolved, this acute venous occlusion leads to the urographic appearance of a small, atrophic, nonfunctioning kidney.

When venous occlusion is partial or accompanied by adequate collateral formation, the kidney is large and smooth but with some degree of contrast excretion. There is stretching and thinning of the collecting system as a result of surrounding interstitial edema. Enlargement of collateral pathways for renal venous outflow (gonadal and ureteric veins) produces characteristic notching of the upper ureter.

The confirmation of renal vein thrombosis re-

quires venographic demonstration of vessel occlusion or a localized filling defect (Figure 5-50). An examination of the inferior vena cava with a catheter placed well below the renal veins is often performed initially to exclude caval thrombosis with proximal

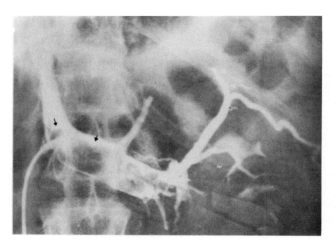

Figure 5-50 Renal vein thrombosis. Renal venogram demonstrates large filling defect in left renal vein *(arrows)* that extends into vena cava. *(From Cohn LH, et al: The treatment of bilateral renal vein thrombosis and nephrotic syndrome, Surgery 64:387-396, 1968.)*

extension before the renal veins are catheterized directly.

ACUTE RENAL FAILURE

Acute renal failure refers to a rapid deterioration in kidney function that is sufficient to result in the accumulation of nitrogen-containing wastes in the blood and a characteristic odor of ammonia on the breath. In prerenal failure, there is decreased blood flow to the kidneys caused by low blood volume (e.g., hemorrhage, dehydration, surgical shock), cardiac failure, or obstruction of both renal arteries. Postrenal failure is caused by obstruction of the urine outflow from both kidneys, most commonly a result of prostatic disease or functional obstruction of the bladder neck. Acute renal failure may also be the result of specific kidney diseases, such as glomerulonephritis, bilateral acute pyelonephritis, and malignant (severe) hypertension. Other causes of acute renal failure include nephrotoxic agents (antibiotics, radiographic contrast material, anesthetic agents, heavy metals, organic solvents), intravascular hemolysis, and large amounts of myoglobin (muscle protein) in the circulation resulting from muscle trauma or ischemia.

Because it is independent of renal function, ultrasound is especially useful in the evaluation of patients with acute renal failure. In addition to demonstrating dilation of the ureters and pelves caused by postobstructive hypernephrosis, ultrasound can assess renal size and the presence of focal kidney lesions or diffuse renal cystic disease. In the patient with prerenal failure, ultrasound can aid in distinguishing low blood volume from right-sided heart failure. In the latter there is dilation of the inferior vena cava and hepatic veins that does not occur in patients with low circulating blood volume.

Plain film tomography can often demonstrate renal size and contours. Bilaterally enlarged, smooth kidneys suggest acute renal parenchymal dysfunction; small kidneys usually indicate chronic, preexisting renal disease. Plain film tomograms can also demonstrate bilateral renal calcification, which may suggest either secondary hyperparathyroidism caused by chronic renal disease or bilateral stones that have obstructed both ureters to produce postrenal failure.

Excretory urography in the patient with acute renal failure demonstrates bilateral renal enlargement with a delayed but prolonged nephrogram (Figure 5-51); vicarious excretion of contrast material by the

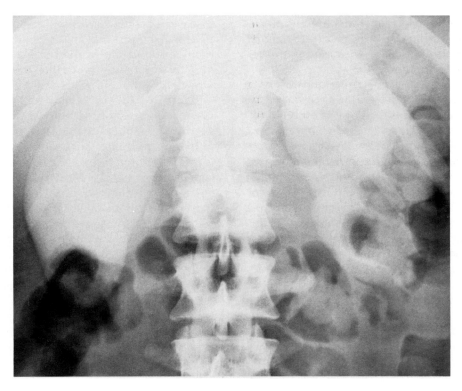

Figure 5-51 Acute renal failure. Film from excretory urogram 20 minutes after injection of contrast material shows bilateral persistent nephrograms with no calyceal filling.

liver occasionally results in opacification of the gall-bladder. However, in most instances excretory urography is unnecessary in the patient with acute renal failure, especially since many authors believe that intravenous contrast material can cause further damage to the kidneys in this condition.

CHRONIC RENAL FAILURE

Like acute renal failure, chronic kidney dysfunction may reflect prerenal, postrenal, or intrinsic kidney disease. Therefore underlying causes of chronic renal failure include bilateral renal artery stenosis, bilateral ureteral obstruction, and intrinsic renal disorders such as chronic glomerulonephritis, pyelonephritis, and familial cystic diseases.

A failure to adequately clear nitrogen-containing wastes from the circulation leads to the accumulation of excessive blood levels of urea and creatinine (waste products of protein metabolism) in the blood. This condition is called **uremia** and produces toxic effects on many body systems. Irritation of the gastrointestinal tract produces nausea, vomiting, and diarrhea. In the nervous system, uremia causes drowsiness, dim vision, decreased mental ability, convulsions, and eventually coma. A decreased ability of the kidney to synthesize erythropoietin, which helps regulate the production of red blood cells, leads to the development of anemia. In the skin, uremia causes intense itching (pruritus) and a sallow, yellow coloring resulting from the combined effects of anemia and retention of a variety of pigmented metabolites (urochromes).

Because of the kidney's role in maintaining water balance and regulating acid-base balance and electrolyte levels, chronic renal failure causes abnormalities involving all of these vital functions. Retention of sodium leads to increased water retention and the development of generalized edema and congestive heart failure. An elevated serum potassium level is potentially life threatening because of its direct effect on cardiac muscle contractility and the possibility of causing an arrhythmia or cardiac arrest. A reduction of serum calcium can produce the muscle twitching commonly seen in uremic patients. Low calcium levels also lead to increased activity of the parathyroid glands, which results in the removal of calcium from bones and a high incidence of renal stones.

Because it is independent of renal function, ultrasound is often the initial procedure in the eval-

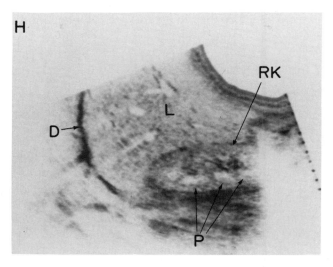

Figure 5-52 Chronic renal failure. Parasagittal sonogram of right kidney *(RK)* shows irregular echo pattern with echogenicity of renal cortical tissue increased to such an extent that it is greater than that of hepatic parenchyma *(L)*. Renal medullary pyramids *(P)* are clearly visible in right kidney. (*H*, head; *D*, diaphragm). *(From Friedland GW et al, editors: Uroradiology: an integrated approach, New York, Churchill Livingstone, 1983.)*

uation of patients with chronic renal failure (Figure 5-52). It is of special value in diagnosing treatable diseases such as hydronephrosis and intrarenal or perirenal infections. This modality can also assess renal size and the presence of focal kidney lesions or diffuse renal cystic disease and can localize the kidneys for percutaneous renal biopsy.

Even in patients with chronic renal failure and uremia, excretory urography with tomography may produce sufficient opacification of the kidneys to be of diagnostic value. However, excretory urography is infrequently required because similar information can be provided by ultrasound or retrograde pyelography. An initial plain abdominal radiograph may demonstrate bilateral renal calcifications (nephrocalcinosis) or obstructing ureteral stones. Small kidneys with smooth contours suggest chronic glomerulonephritis, nephrosclerosis, or bilateral renal artery stenosis. Small kidneys with irregular contours, thin cortices, and typical clubbing of the calyces are consistent with chronic pyelonephritis. Large kidneys suggest obstructive disease, infiltrative processes (lymphoma, myeloma, amyloidosis), renal vein thrombosis, or polycystic kidney disease.

QUESTIONS

1. The imaging criteria for a pyelogram are the same as for an abdominal radiograph but must include all of the _____ to the _____.
   A. Diaphragm: kidneys
   B. Kidneys; pelvis
   C. Kidneys; superior pubis
   D. A and B

2. What organ of the body plays an essential role in maintaining the acid-base balance of the blood and body fluids, as well as the electrolyte balance.
   A. Nephron
   B. Glomerulus
   C. Bladder
   D. Kidney

3. A bacterial inflammation of the kidney and renal pelvis is termed _____.
   A. Renitis
   B. Pyelonephritis
   C. Glomerulitis
   D. None of the above

4. The medical term used to describe dilated calyces and renal pelvis is _____.
   A. Hydronephrosis
   B. Pyelonephritis
   C. Nephrosis
   D. None of the above

5. What is the name for the most common abdominal neoplasm of infants and children?
   A. Polycystic disease
   B. Pyelonephritis
   C. Wilms' tumor
   D. Hypernephroma

6. What is the name of the most common fusion anomaly of the kidneys?
   A. Complete fusion
   B. Crossed ectopia
   C. Pelvic kidney
   D. Horseshoe kidney

7. What is the name for a cystic dilation of the distal ureter near the bladder?
   A. Compensatory hypertrophy
   B. Renal agenesis
   C. Ureterocele
   D. Hypoplastic

8. Name the first portion of the kidney to visualize after injection of a contrast agent.
   A. Nephron
   B. Glomerulus
   C. Bowman's capsule
   D. Calyces

9. What term is used to describe a kidney not in the normal area of the abdomen?
   A. Horseshoe
   B. Duplex
   C. Ectopic
   D. Ectopic ureterocele

10. The medical term for painful urination is _____.
    A. Dysuria
    B. Anuria
    C. Micturition
    D. Exacerbation

BIBLIOGRAPHY

Davidson AJ: Radiology of the kidney, Philadelphia, WB Saunders Co, 1985.
Ney C and Friedenberg RM: Radiographic atlas of the genitourinary system, Philadelphia, JB Lippincott Co, 1981.
Witten DM, Myers GH, and Utz DC: Emmett's clinical urography, ed 4, Philadelphia, WB Saunders Co, 1977.

Urinary retention - urine is produced but held in the bladder

Urinary suppression - ↓ urine production

Anuria - w/out urine

Oliguria - scanty urine

Polyuria - excessive urine

Nocturia - night urinating

Enuresis - bed wetting

Diuretic - ↑ urine production

Antidiuretic - ↓ urine production

Renal colic - pain due to stones

hemodialysis - blood filtered by a machine

CHAPTER 6

Cardiovascular System

PREREQUISITE KNOWLEDGE

The student should have a basic knowledge of the anatomy and physiology of the cardiovascular system. In addition, proper learning and understanding of the material will be facilitated if the student has some clinical experience in chest radiography and film evaluation, including a concept of the changes in technique required to compensate for density differences produced by the underlying pathologic conditions. Previous experience in a cardiac catheterization laboratory would be beneficial.

GOALS

To acquaint the student radiographer with the pathophysiology and radiographic manifestations of all of the common and some of the unusual disorders of the cardiovascular system

OBJECTIVES

1. Describe the physiology of the cardiovascular system
2. Identify anatomic structures on both diagrams and radiographs of the cardiovascular system
3. Be able to define terminology relating to the cardiovascular system
4. Be able to describe the various pathologic conditions affecting the cardiovascular system and their radiographic manifestations
5. Be familiar with the special procedures that are indicated for imaging of particular pathologic conditions

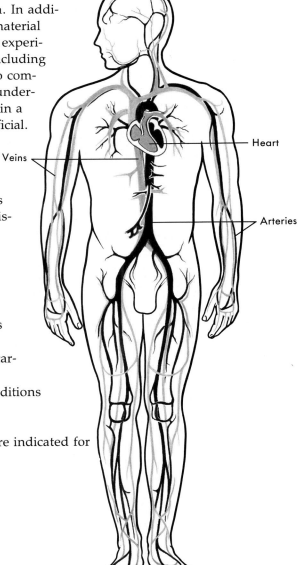

Veins — Heart

Arteries

RADIOGRAPHER NOTES

Plain chest radiography and fluoroscopy of the cardiovascular system are used to identify abnormalities in the size and shape of the heart and to detect calcification of heart valves, coronary arteries, or the pericardium. The presence and extent of functional disorders are better achieved using angiography, ultrasound, radionuclide imaging, and magnetic resonance.

As with all chest radiographs, it is essential that the radiographer perform cardiovascular studies with the patient positioned correctly and using proper technical factors. To this end, it would be helpful for the reader to review the radiographer notes at the beginning of the chapter on the respiratory system. An abnormality identified on a chest radiograph may be the first evidence of cardiovascular disease in an asymptomatic patient.

Radiographers now can specialize in invasive diagnostic and therapeutic cardiovascular procedures and be employed by heart catheterization laboratories. Angiocardiography is a diagnostic procedure performed to identify the exact anatomic location of an intracardiac disorder. Coronary angioplasty is a therapeutic procedure in which a narrowed coronary artery is dilated by inflating a balloon that is attached to a catheter and manipulated fluoroscopically to the site of the stenosis. Because both angiocardiography and angioplasty involve the use of contrast material in patients who often have severe pre-existing medical conditions, it is essential that the radiographer be continually alert to the possibility of cardiac or respiratory arrest and be prepared to immediately assist with basic and advanced life support.

The injection of contrast material into arteries (arteriograms) and veins (venograms) can be performed in almost any portion of the body. As in the heart, these invasive studies use potentially dangerous substances so that the radiographer must be alert for possible complications and be prepared to assist in cardiorespiratory emergencies. In addition, all of these examinations require that the radiographer be trained in sterile technique and be familiar with the various types of catheters that are inserted into the vascular system for the delivery of contrast material.

PHYSIOLOGY OF THE CARDIOVASCULAR SYSTEM

The function of the cardiovascular system is to maintain an adequate supply of blood to all the tissues of the body. This is accomplished by the rhythmic contractions of the heart, the rate of which is controlled by the autonomic nervous system. The vagus nerve slows heart action by transmitting the chemical acetylcholine, whereas the sympathetic nervous system stimulates the release of epinephrine that accelerates the heart rate and increases the force of its contractions.

The heart consists of four chambers whose walls are composed of smooth muscle (myocardium), and it is lined with a smooth delicate membrane (endocardium) that is continuous with the inner surface of the blood vessels. The heart consists of two atria and two ventricles, with a partition (septum) separating the right and left sides of the heart. The ventricles are considerably larger and thicker walled than the atria because they have a substantially heavier pumping load. Between each atrium and its associated ventricle are the right and left atrioventricular valves that permit blood to flow in only one direction. These valves consist of flaps (cusps) of endocardium that are anchored to the papillary muscles of the ventricles by cordlike structures called chordae tendineae. The **mitral,** or bicuspid, **valve** between the left atrium and left ventricle has two cusps, whereas the **tricuspid valve** between the right atrium and right ventricle has three cusps. The semilunar valves separate the ventricles from the great vessels leaving the heart. The **pulmonary valve** lies between the right ventricle and pulmonary artery, whereas the **aortic valve** separates the aorta from the left ventricle.

Deoxygenated venous blood is returned to the heart from the body through the superior and inferior venae cavae, which empty into the right atrium. Blood flows from the right atrium across the triscuspid valve into the right ventricle, which in turn pumps blood through the pulmonary valve into the pulmonary artery. Within the capillaries of the lungs, the red blood cells take up oxygen and release carbon dioxide. The freshly oxygenated blood then passes through the pulmonary veins into the left atrium, from which it flows across the mitral valve into the left ventricle. Contraction of the left venticle forces oxygenated blood through the aortic valve into the aorta and the rest of the arterial tree to provide oxygen and nourishment to tissues throughout the body. The general circulation of the body is termed the **systemic circulation,** whereas the circulation of blood through the lungs is called the **pulmonary circulation.** Because greater pressure is needed to pump blood through the systemic circulation than through the pulmonary circulation, the wall of the left ventricle is considerably thicker than that of the right ventricle.

The atria and ventricles alternately contract and relax. The contracting phase is called **systole,** whereas the heart chambers relax and fill with blood during **diastole.** The normal cardiac impulse that stimulates mechanical contraction of the heart arises in the sinoatrial (SA) node, or pacemaker, which is situated in the right atrial wall near the opening of the superior vena cava. The impulse passes slowly through the atrioventricular (AV) node, which is located in the right atrium along the lower part of the interatrial septum, and then spreads quickly throughout the ventricles by way of the fibrous bundle of His, which terminates in Purkinje's fibers that can conduct impulses throughout the muscle of both ventricles and stimulate them to contract almost simultaneously. Specialized pacemaker cells in the SA node possess an **intrinsic rhythm,** so that even without any stimulation by the autonomic nervous system the node itself initiates impulses at regular intervals (about 70 to 75 beats per minute). If the SA node for some reason is unable to generate an impulse, pacemaker activity shifts to some other excitable component of the conduction system. These **ectopic pacemakers** also generate impulses rhythmically, although at a much slower rate. For example, if the AV node controls pacemaker activity, the heart would beat 40 to 60 times per minute. If the conduction system of the heart is unable to maintain an adequate rhythm, the patient may receive an artificial pacemaker that electrically stimulates the heart either at a set rhythm or only when the heart rate decreases below a preset minimum.

The heart muscle is supplied with oxygenated arterial blood by way of the right and left coronary arteries. These small vessels arise from the aorta just above the aortic valve. Unoxygenated blood from the myocardium drains into the coronary veins, which lead into the coronary sinus before opening into the right atrium.

The heart is surrounded by a double membranous sac termed the **pericardium**. The pericardium has a well-lubricated lining that protects against friction and permits the heart to move easily during contraction.

ACQUIRED HEART DISEASE

Coronary artery disease

Narrowing of the coronary arteries causes oxygen deprivation of the myocardium and ischemic heart disease. In most patients narrowing of the lumen of one or more of the coronary arteries is due to the deposition of fatty material on the inner arterial wall (atherosclerosis). Factors predisposing to the development of coronary artery disease include hypertension, obesity, smoking, a high-cholesterol diet, and lack of exercise.

The speed and degree of luminal narrowing determines whether an atherosclerotic lesion causes significant and clinically evident ischemia. Temporary oxygen insufficiency causes angina pectoris, a feeling of severe chest pain that may radiate to the neck, jaw, and left arm and is often associated with the sensation of chest tightness or suffocation. Attacks of angina pectoris are often related to a sudden increase in the demand of the myocardium for oxygen, such as following strenuous exercise, a heavy meal, emotional stress, or exposure to severe cold. The placing of a nitroglycerin tablet under the tongue causes dilation of the coronary arteries, which permits an adequate flow to the myocardium.

Occlusion of a coronary artery deprives an area of myocardium of its blood supply and leads to the death of muscle cells (myocardial infarction) in the area of vascular distribution. The size of the coronary artery that is occluded determines the extent of heart muscle damage. The greater the area affected, the poorer the prognosis. A favorable prognostic factor is the development of collateral circulation, through which blood from a surrounding area is channeled into the damaged tissue. If the patient survives, the infarcted region heals with fibrosis. Long-term complications include the development of thrombi on the surface of the damaged area and the production of a local bulge (ventricular aneurysm) at the site of the weakness of the myocardial wall.

Radionuclide thallium perfusion scanning is the major noninvasive study for assessing regional blood flow to the myocardium (Figure 6-1). Focal decreases in thallium uptake that are observed immediately after exercise but are no longer identified on delayed scans usually indicate transient ischemia associated with significant coronary artery stenosis or spasm. After exercise, focal defects that are unchanged on delayed scans more frequently reflect scar formation. A normal thallium exercise scan makes the diagnosis of myocardial ischemia un-

Anterior   Left anterior oblique   Left lateral

Exercise

Redistribution

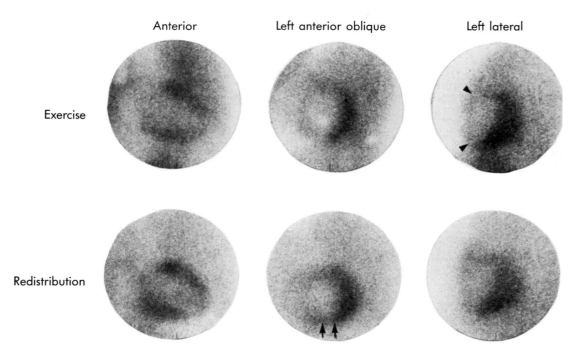

Figure 6-1 Radionuclide thallium perfusion scan in myocardial infarction. On images obtained immediately after exercise, extensive regions of reduced isotope uptake can be seen on all three projections. This reduced uptake is most marked in anterior wall *(arrowheads)*, as seen on left lateral view. Virtually no redistribution into this region occurred at 4 hours *(bottom row)*, a finding suggestive of extensive scar formation. Note small region at apex *(double arrows)* in which redistribution of thallium did occur. This suggests presence of transiently ischemic yet viable myocardium in this area. *(From Ashburn WL and Tubau J: Radiol Clin North Am 18:467-486, 1980.*

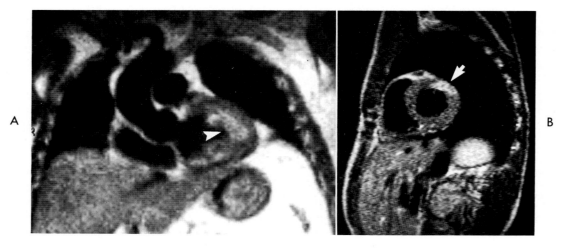

Figure 6-2 MRI of acute myocardial infarction. **A,** T2-weighted coronal image obtained in patient 10 days after acute myocardial infarction demonstates area of increased signal intensity (indicating edema associated with muscle necrosis) in subendocardial regions of lateral wall *(arrowhead)*. **B,** Short-axis view of another patient shows acute transmural infarction *(arrow)* of anterolateral wall. *(From Stark DD and Bradley WG, editors: Magnetic resonance imaging, St. Louis, The CV Mosby Co, 1988.)*

likely, although in about 10% of patients with significant obstructive disease the presence of sufficient collateral vessels can prevent the radionuclide demonstration of regional ischemia.

Radionuclide scanning using technetium pyrophosphate or other compounds that are taken up by acutely infarcted myocardium is a new noninvasive technique for detecting, localizing, and classifying myocardial necrosis. On CT, areas of myocardial ischemia appear as regions of decreased attenuation value because of the increased water content caused by intramyocardial cellular edema. Initial studies have suggested that MRI will also be of value in detecting early signs of muscular necrosis in myocardial infarction (Figure 6-2).

Plain chest radiographs are usually normal or nonspecific in most patients with ischemic heart disease. Calcification of a coronary artery, although infrequently visualized on routine chest radiographs and usually requiring cardiac fluoroscopy, strongly suggests the presence of hemodynamically significant coronary artery disease (Figure 6-3). Plain chest radiographs are also entirely normal in many, if not most, patients after myocardial infarction. They are primarily of value in detecting evidence of pulmonary venous congestion in patients who develop congestive heart failure as a result of an inability of the remaining heart muscle to adequately propel blood through the circulation.

Coronary arteriography is generally considered the definitive test for determining the presence and

assessing the severity of coronary artery disease. About 30% of significant stenoses involve a single vessel, most commonly the anterior descending artery. Two vessels are involved in 30%, and significant stenosis of the three main vessels can be demonstrated in the remaining 40%.

Aortocoronary bypass grafting, usually using sections of saphenous vein, is an increasingly popular procedure in patients with ischemic heart disease. Arteriography has been the procedure of choice in demonstrating the patency and functional efficiency of aortocoronary bypass grafts. Patent functioning grafts demonstrate prompt clearing of contast material and good filling of the grafted artery. Stenotic or malfunctioning grafts demonstrate areas of narrowing, filling defects and slow flow with delayed washout of contrast material.

Percutaneous transluminal angioplasty using a balloon catheter is now a recognized procedure for the treatment of patients with narrowing of one or more coronary arteries (Figure 6-4). As in other types of percutaneous transluminal angioplasty, a catheter is placed using fluoroscopic guidance into the affected coronary artery, and an arteriogram is performed for localization. The angioplasty balloon is then positioned at the level of the stenosis and inflated. After dilation, coronary arteriography is repeated to show the subsequent appearance of the stenosis and to detect any complications of the procedure. Symptomatic improvement occurs in 50% to 70% of dilations. About 3% to 8% of patients who

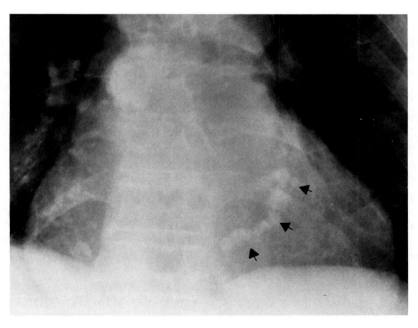

Figure 6-3 Ischemic heart disease. Frontal projection of chest demonstrates cardiomegaly with typical linear calcification in coronary artery (arrows).

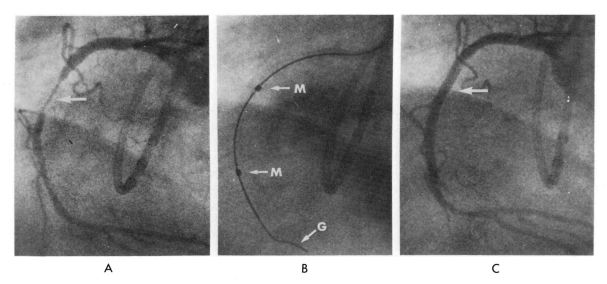

A   B   C

Figure 6-4   Percutaneous transluminal coronary angioplasty. **A,** Initial right coronary angiogram shows severe narrowing *(arrow)* of midportion of right coronary artery. **B,** During percutaneous transluminal coronary angioplasty, steerable wire guide *(G)* has been passed down coronary artery and through coronary stenosis. Tip lies within distal right coronary artery. Radiopaque markers *(M)* identify balloon portion of dilating catheter that has been advanced over wire guide through coronary stenosis. **C,** Immediately after angioplasty, previous site of stenosis *(arrow)* is now patent. *(From Fischell TA and Block PC: Cardiovasc Reviews Reports 6:89-99, 1985.)*

undergo percutaneous angioplasty develop either persistent coronary insufficiency or sudden occlusion of a coronary artery at the site of dilation at the time of the procedure. Therefore the procedure should be done at a time when an operating room, an anesthetist, and a cardiac surgeon are available so that immediate coronary bypass surgery can be performed if necessary. The mortality rate of coronary angioplasty is less than 1%.

Congestive heart failure

Congestive heart failure refers to the inability of the heart to propel blood at a sufficient rate and volume to provide an adequate supply to the tissues. It may be caused by an intrinsic cardiac abnormality or by hypertension or any obstructive process that abnormally increases the peripheral resistance to blood flow.

Left-sided heart failure produces a classic radiographic appearance of cardiac enlargement, redistribution of pulmonary venous blood flow (enlarged superior pulmonary veins and decreased caliber of the veins draining the lower lungs), interstitial edema, alveolar edema (irregular, poorly defined patchy densities), and pleural effusions (Figure 6-5). In acute left ventricular failure resulting from coronary thrombosis, however, there may be severe

pulmonary congestion and edema with very little cardiac enlargement. The major causes of left-sided heart failure include coronary heart disease, valvular disease, and hypertension.

In right-sided heart failure, dilation of the right ventricle and right atrium is present (Figure 6-6). The transmission of increased pressure may cause dilation of the superior vena cava, widening of the right superior mediastinum, and edema of the lower extremities. The enlargement of a congested liver may elevate the right hemidiaphragm. Common causes of right-sided heart failure include pulmonary valvular stenosis, emphysema, and pulmonary hypertension resulting from pulmonary emboli.

Pulmonary edema

Pulmonary edema refers to an abnormal accumulation of fluid in the extravascular pulmonary tissues. The most common cause of pulmonary edema is an elevation of the pulmonary venous pressure. This is most often due to left-sided heart failure but may also be caused by pulmonary venous obstruction (mitral valve disease, left atrial tumor) or lymphatic blockade (fibrotic, inflammatory, or metastatic disease involving the mediastinal lymph nodes). Other causes of pulmonary edema include uremia, narcotic overdose, exposure to noxious

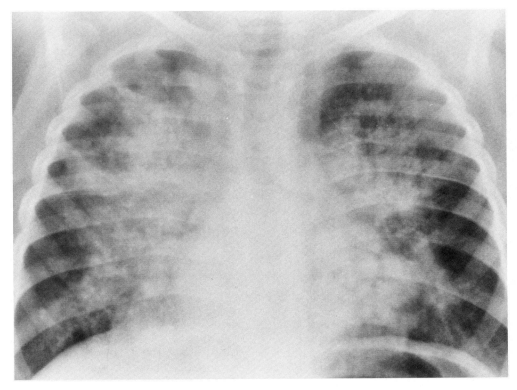

Figure 6-5 Left-sided heart failure. Diffuse perihilar alveolar densities.

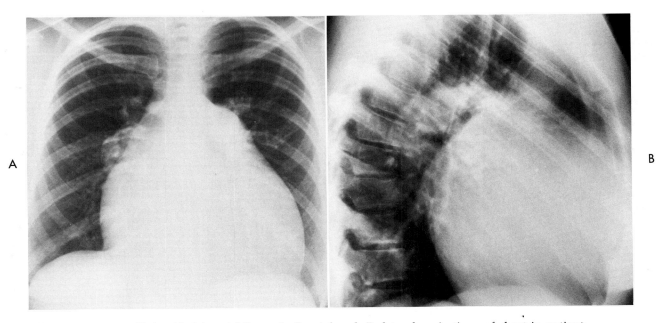

Figure 6-6 Right-sided heart failure. **A,** Frontal and, **B,** lateral projections of chest in patient with primary pulmonary hypertension show marked globular cardiomegaly with prominence of pulmonary trunk and central pulmonary arteries. Peripheral pulmonary vascularity is strikingly reduced. Right ventricular enlargement has obliterated retrosternal air space on lateral projection.

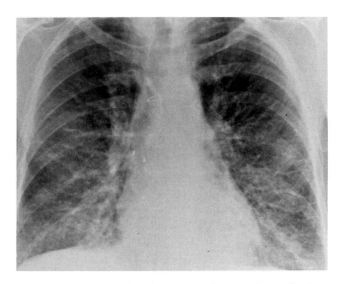

Figure 6-7 Interstitial pulmonary edema. Edema fluid in interstitial space causes loss of normal sharp definition of pulmonary vascular markings and perihilar haze. At bases, note thin horizontal lines of increased density (Kerley-B lines) that represent fluid in interlobular septa.

fumes, excessive oxygen, high altitudes, fat embolism, adult respiratory distress syndrome, and various neurologic abnormalities.

Transudation of fluid into the interstitial spaces of the lungs is the earliest stage of pulmonary edema. However, in patients with congestive heart failure or pulmonary venous hypertension, increased pulmonary venous pressure first appears as a redistribution of blood flow from the lower to the upper lung zones. This phenomenon, probably caused by reflex venous spasm, causes prominent enlargement of the superior pulmonary veins and decreased caliber of the veins draining the inferior portions of the lung. Edema fluid in the interstitial space causes a loss of the normal sharp definition of pulmonary vascular markings (Figure 6-7). Accentuation of the vascular markings about the hila produces a perihilar haze. Fluid in the interlobular septa produces characteristic thin horizontal lines of increased density at the axillary margins of the lung inferiorly (Kerley-B lines).

A further increase in pulmonary venous pressures leads to the development of alveolar or pleural transudates. Alveolar edema appears as irregular, poorly defined patchy densities scattered throughout the lungs. The classic radiographic finding of alveolar pulmonary edema is the butterfly (or bat's-wing) pattern, a diffuse, bilaterally symmetric, fan-shaped infiltration that is most prominent in the central portion of the lungs and fades toward the periphery (Figure 6-8).

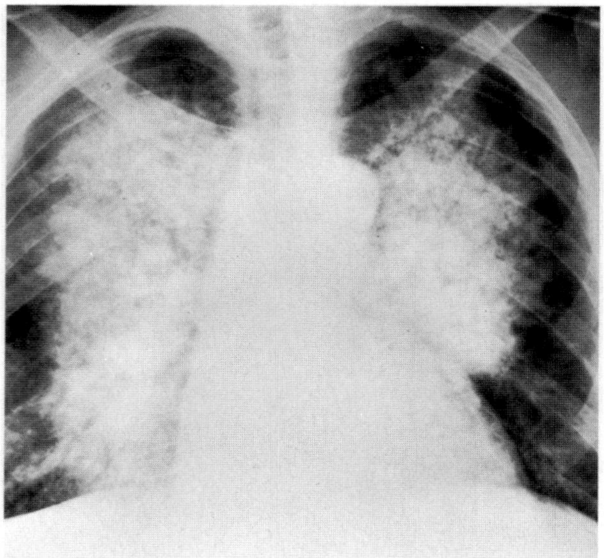

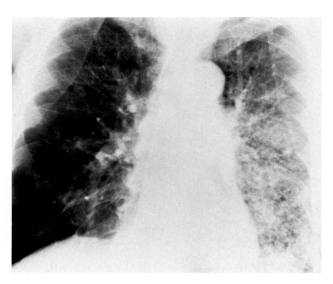

Figure 6-8 Butterfly pattern of severe pulmonary edema. Diffuse bilateral symmetric infiltration of central portion of lungs along with relative sparing of periphery produces butterfly pattern. *(From Fraser RG and Pare JAP: Diagnosis of diseases of the chest, Philadelphia, WB Saunders Co, 1979.)*

Figure 6-9 Unilateral pulmonary edema. Diffuse alveolar pattern limited to left lung because of effect of gravity on patient lying on left side.

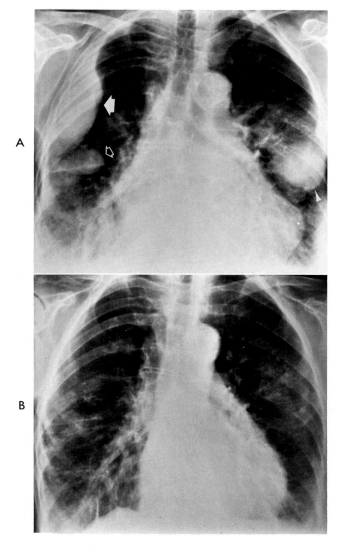

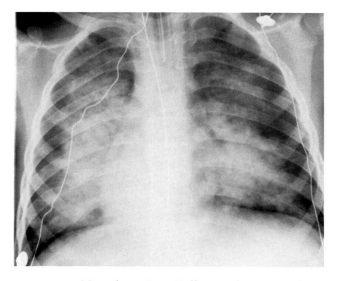

Figure 6-11 Near-drowning. Diffuse pulmonary edema pattern with normal-sized heart.

Figure 6-10 Loculated pleural fluid (phantom tumors). **A,** Frontal chest radiograph taken during episode of congestive heart failure demonstrates marked cardiomegaly with bilateral pleural effusions. Note fluid collections along lateral chest wall *(solid arrow)*, in minor fissure *(open arrow)*, and in left major fissure *(arrowhead)*. **B,** With improvement in patient's cardiac status, phantom tumors have disappeared. Bilateral small pleural effusions persist.

Pleural effusion associated with pulmonary edema usually occurs on the right side (Figure 6-9). When bilateral, the effusion tends to be more marked on the right. There is often an associated thickening of the interlobar fissures.

After adequate treatment of pulmonary edema, the interstitial, alveolar, and pleural abnormalities may disappear within several hours. Loculated pleural fluid within a fissure (especially the minor fis-

sure) may resorb more slowly and appear as a sharply defined, elliptical or circular density that simulates a solid parenchymal mass (Figure 6-10).

Most patients with pulmonary edema caused by congestive failure or other heart disease have evidence of cardiomegaly. In noncardiogenic causes of pulmonary edema the heart often remains normal in size (Figure 6-11).

Hypertension

Hypertension, or high blood pressure, is the leading cause of strokes and congestive heart failure. The blood pressure is a function of cardiac output, the amount of blood pumped per minute by the heart, and the total peripheral resistance, which reflects the condition of the walls of the blood vessels throughout the body. Although the peripheral resistance and cardiac output may fluctuate rapidly, depending on such factors as whether a person sits or stands and is quiet or excited, the systemic blood pressure remains remarkably constant in a normal person.

A blood pressure reading consists of two parts. The systolic pressure is the highest pressure in the peripheral arteries that occurs when the left ventricle contracts. The diastolic pressure is the pressure in the peripheral arteries when the left ventricle is relaxing and filling with blood from the left atrium. High blood pressure is defined as elevation of the systolic pressure above 140 millimeters of mercury (mm Hg) and of the diastolic pressure above 90 mm Hg. In patients older than 40 years of age the systolic pressure may be somewhat higher and still be considered within normal limits. As a rough rule of thumb, a person is allowed an additional 10 mm Hg in the systolic pressure for each decade over age 40.

Most patients with elevated blood pressure have essential, or idiopathic, hypertension. The benign form of essential hypertension is characterized by a gradual onset and a prolonged course, often of many years. In the much less common malignant form the elevated blood pressure has an abrupt onset, runs a rapid course, and often leads to renal failure or cerebral hemorrhage.

About 6% of patients have secondary hypertension resulting from another disease. Although some patients in this group have adrenal abnormalities (Cushing's syndrome, primary aldosteronism, pheochromocytoma) in which there is an abnormality of the regulation of salt and water content (and thus the blood volume) or the secretion of a substance that increases vascular tone and peripheral arterial resistance, most have renal parenchymal or vascular disease as the underlying cause of hypertension.

The standard screening test for renovascular hypertension has been the rapid-sequence (hypertensive) excretory urogram, in which radiographs are

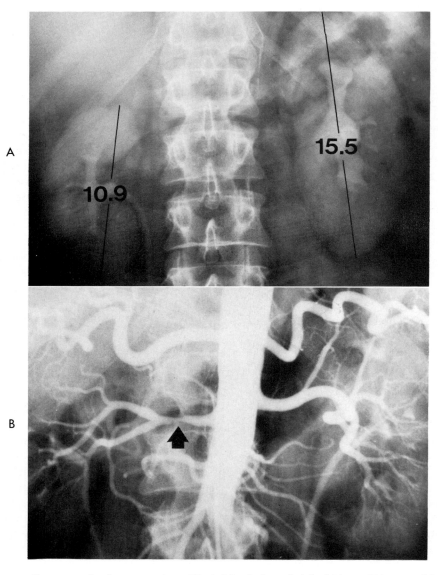

Figure 6-12 Renovascular hypertension. Diminished size of right kidney **(A)** caused by renal artery stenosis **(B)**. *Arrow, Stenosis. (From Burko H et al: In Eisenberg RL and Amberg JR, editors: Critical diagnostic pathways in radiology: an algorithmic approach, Philadelphia, JB Lippincott Co, 1981.)*

obtained at each of the first 5 minutes after the rapid injection of contrast material. Features suggesting renal ischemia include (1) unilateral delayed appearance and excretion of contrast material; (2) difference in kidney size greater than 1.5 cm (Figure 6-12, *A*); (3) irregular contour of the renal silhouette, suggesting segmental infarction or atrophy; (4) indentations on the ureter or renal pelvis caused by dilated, tortuous ureteral arterial collaterals; and (5) hyperconcentration of contrast material in the collecting system of the smaller kidney on delayed films. Although up to 25% of patients with renovascular hypertension have a normal rapid-sequence excretory urogram, this modality is also of value in detecting other less frequent causes of hypertension such as tumor, polynephritis, polycystic kidneys, or renal infarction.

Arteriography is the most accurate screening examination for detecting renovascular lesions. The most common cause of renal artery obstruction is arteriosclerotic narrowing, which usually occurs in the proximal portion of the vessel close to its origin from the aorta (Figure 6-12, *B*) Bilateral renal artery stenoses are noted in up to one third of the patients. Oblique projections, which demonstrate the vessel origins in profile, are often required to demonstrate renal artery stenosis.

The other major cause of renovascular hypertension is fibromuscular dysplasia. This disease is most frequent in young adult women and is often bilateral. The most common radiographic appearance of fibromuscular dysplasia is the string-of-beads pattern, in which there are alternating areas of narrowing and dilation (Figure 6-13). Smooth, concentric stenoses occur less frequently.

The mere presence of a renovascular lesion does not mean that it is the cause of hypertension; indeed, many patients with normal blood pressure have severe renal artery disease. Therefore bilateral renal vein catheterization for the measurement of plasma renin activity is used to assess the functional significance of any stenotic lesion. A renal vein renin concentration on the abnormal side that is more than 50% greater than the renin level in the renal vein on the normal side indicates the functional significance of a lesion with an accuracy rate of about 85%.

Surgery has been the traditional treatment for a patient with arteriographically demonstrated renal artery studies and confirmatory renal vein renin studies. Recently, percutaneous transluminal angioplasty has been shown to be effective in dilating renal artery stenoses (Figure 6-14). Although insufficient time has elapsed to compare the long-term results of renal transluminal angioplasty with corrective surgical procedures, initial studies demonstrate the improvement or cure of hypertension in about 80% of patients treated with angioplasty.

Prolonged high blood pressure forces the heart to

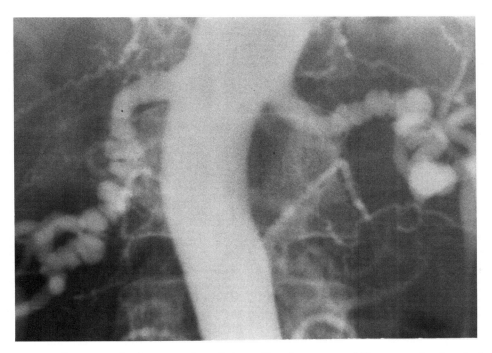

Figure 6-13 Renovascular hypertension. String-of-beads pattern of fibromuscular dysplasia bilaterally.

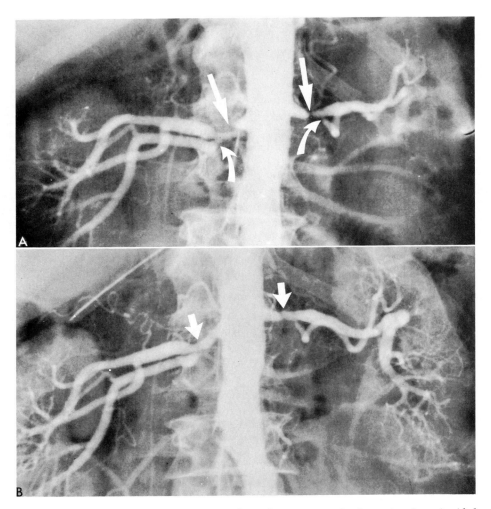

Figure 6-14 Percutaneous transluminal angioplasty for renovascular hypertension. **A,** Abdominal aortogram demonstrates severe bilateral stenoses of main renal arteries *(straight arrows)* and stenoses at origins of early bifurcations *(curved arrows)*. **B,** Aortogram after angioplasty of both renal arteries shows irregularities in areas of previous atherosclerotic narrowing *(arrows)* but improved residual lumen in both main renal arteries. After procedure, patient's previous severe hypertension was controllable to normal levels with only minimal dosages of diuretic medication. *(From Waltman AC: In Athanasoulis CA et al, editors: Interventional radiology, Philadelphia, WB Saunders Co, 1982.)*

overwork, causing the left ventricle to enlarge and eventually fail. Since the high blood pressure affects all arteries of the body, including the coronary and carotid vessels, this condition increases the risk of coronary occlusion and myocardial infarction, as well as carotid narrowing leading to a stroke.

Decreased function of the kidneys leads to the retention of water and salt, which increases the blood volume and elevates the blood pressure. Long-standing hypertension causes atherosclerosis of the renal artery, which reduces blood flow to the kidneys and further damages them.

Hypertensive heart disease

Long-standing high blood pressure causes narrowing of systemic blood vessels and an increased resistance to blood flow. The left ventricle is forced to assume an increased work load, which initially causes hypertrophy and little if any change in the radiographic appearance of the cardiac silhouette. Eventually, the continued strain on the heart leads to dilation and enlargement of the left ventricle (Figure 6-15) along with downward displacement of the cardiac apex, which often projects below the left hemidiaphragm. Aortic tortuosity with prominence

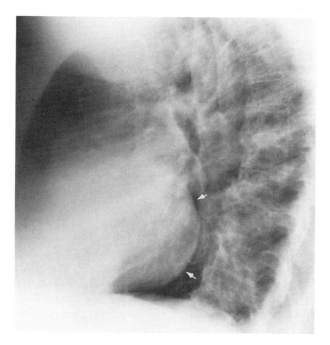

Figure 6-15 Hypertensive heart disease. Lateral projection of chest shows marked prominence of left ventricle *(arrows)*.

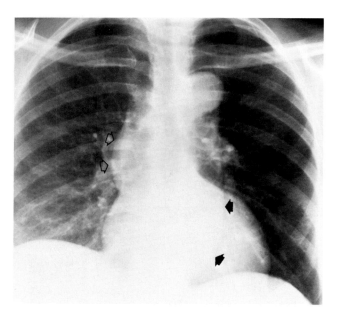

Figure 6-16 Hypertensive heart disease. Generalized tortuosity and elongation of ascending aorta *(open arrows)* and descending aorta *(solid arrows)*.

of the ascending portion commonly occurs (Figure 6-16). Failure of the left ventricle leads to increased pulmonary venous pressure and congestive failure.

Aneurysm

An aneurysm is a localized dilation of an artery that most commonly involves the aorta, especially its abdominal portion. A **saccular** aneurysm involves only one side of the arterial wall, whereas bulging of the entire circumference of the vessel wall is termed **fusiform.** An aneurysm represents a weakness in the wall of a blood vessel caused by atherosclerosis, syphilis or other infection, trauma, or a congenital defect such as Marfan's syndrome. Multiple small aneurysms suggest a generalized arterial inflammation (arteritis). In the abdominal aorta, most aneurysms occur below the origin of the renal arteries, and thus the aneurysm can be surgically replaced by a prosthetic graft without injuring the kidneys. The danger of an aneurysm is its tendency to increase in size and rupture, leading to massive hemorrhage that may be fatal if it involves a critical organ such as the brain.

Although plain abdominal radiographs can demonstrate curvilinear calcification in the wall of an aneurysm (Figure 6-17), ultrasound is the modality of choice for detecting an abdominal aortic aneurysm. The sonographic definition of aneurysmal dilation of the abdominal aorta is an enlargement of

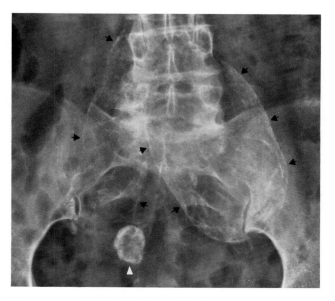

Figure 6-17 Calcification in walls of aneurysms of lower abdominal aorta and both common iliac arteries *(arrows)*. Of incidental note is calcified uterine fibroid *(arrowhead)* in pelvis. *(From Eisenberg, R: Gastrointestinal radiology: a pattern approach, ed 2, Philadelphia, JB Lippincott, Co, 1990.)*

the structure to a diameter greater than 3 cm. Ultrasound can demonstrate an intraluminal clot (Figure 6-18, *A*), and the noninvasive nature of ultrasound permits an evaluation of the enlargement of an aneurysm on serial studies. CT and MRI also can demonstrate the location and extent of an aneurysm. The major value of arteriography in patients with abdominal aortic aneurysm is as a presurgical road map to define the extent of the lesion and whether the renal arteries or other major branches are involved. Because the lumen of an aneurysm may be filled with clot, aortography often underestimates the extent of aneurysmal dilation.

In the chest, CT after the intravenous injection of contrast material is the most efficient technique for demonstrating the size and extent of an aortic aneurysm and for differentiating this vascular lesion from a solid mediastinal mass. Unlike aortography, CT is relatively noninvasive and can directly identify an intraluminal thrombus (seen as a soft-tissue density separating the contrast-filled portion of the lumen from the aortic wall), which can only be inferred on contrast examination (Figure 6-18, *B*). CT can also demonstrate aortic mural calcification and effects of the aneurysm on adjacent structures, such as displacement of the mediastinum or bone erosion. Because of its ability to demonstrate flowing blood as a signal void and clot as a heterogeneous collection of signal intensities, MRI can provide information about an aneurysm that is comparable to that obtained from CT without the need for intravenous contrast material (Figure 6-19).

Traumatic rupture of the aorta

Traumatic rupture of the aorta is a potentially fatal complication of closed chest trauma (rapid deceleration, blast, compression). In almost all cases the

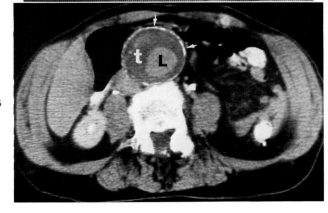

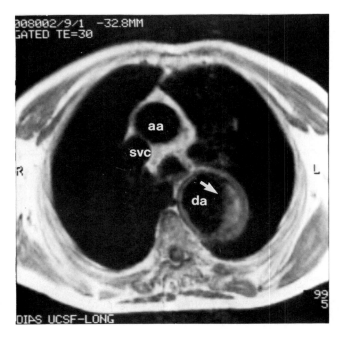

Figure 6-18 Abdominal aortic aneurysm. **A,** Ultrasound shows large aneurysm *(arrows)* with echogenic thrombus *(t)* filling anterior half of sac. **B,** CT scan of abdominal aortic aneurysm in another patient shows low-density thrombus *(t)* surrounding blood-filled lumen *(L).* Wall of aneurysm contains high-density calcification *(arrows).*

Figure 6-19 MRI of aortic aneurysm. Transverse scan with cardiac gating permits differentiation of large mural thrombus *(arrow)* from signal void of rapidly flowing intraluminal blood. *da,* Descending aorta; *aa,* ascending aorta; *svc,* superior vena cava. *(From Thoeni RF and Margulis AR: In Eisenberg RL, editor: Diagnostic imaging: an algorithmic approach, Philadelphia, JB Lippincott Co, 1988.)*

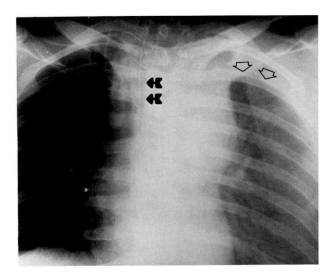

Figure 6-20 Traumatic aneurysm of aorta. There is widening of mediastinum and deviation of nasogastric tube to right *(solid arrows)*. Open arrows point to collection of fluid over left apex (apical pleural cap) in this patient after severe blunt chest trauma. *(From Fisher RG, Hadlock FP, and Ben-Menachem Y: Radiol Clin North Am 19:91-112, 1981.)*

aortic tear occurs just distal to the left subclavian artery at the site of the ductus arteriosus. On plain chest radiographs, hemorrhage into the mediastinum causes widening of the mediastinal silhouette and loss of a discrete aortic knob shadow. Associated rib or sternal fractures may be apparent. However, because nonspecific mediastinal widening is a frequent finding, especially on the supine, AP portable radiographs taken after trauma, other plain film signs are of diagnostic importance (Figure 6-20). These include displacement of an opaque nasogastric tube to the right (because of a hematoma that displaces the esophagus), widening of the right paratracheal stripe (Figure 6-21), and a collection of blood over the apex of the left lung (apical pleural cap sign). Emergency aortography is the definitive examination for the evaluation of possible laceration or rupture of the aorta.

Dissection of the aorta

Dissection of the aorta is a potentially life-threatening condition in which disruption of the intima (inner layer) permits blood to enter the wall of the aorta and separate its layers. Most aortic dissections occur in patients with arterial hypertension. Some are a result of trauma, whereas others are due to a congenital defect such as Marfan's syndrome. An acute dissection typically causes sudden sharp or excruciating pain in the chest or abdomen. Although

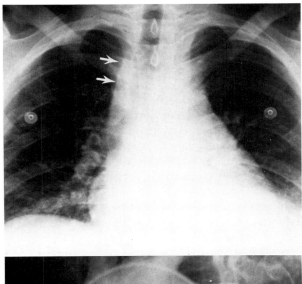

A

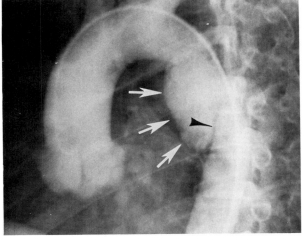

B

Figure 6-21 Traumatic aneurysm of aorta. **A,** Supine chest radiograph in patient with blunt chest trauma shows thickening of right paratracheal stripe *(arrows)*, which measures 1 cm in width. **B,** Aortogram demonstrates pseudoaneurysm at level of aortic isthmus *(arrows)*. Arrowhead indicates intimal flap. *(From Woodring JH, Pulmano CM and Stevens RK: The right paratracheal stripe in blunt chest trauma, Radiology 143:605-608, 1982.)*

the pain passes, death frequently occurs some days later from rupture of the aneurysm into the chest or abdominal cavity.

Most aortic dissections begin as a tear in the intima immediately above the aortic valve. In two thirds of these (type I) the dissection continues into the descending aorta, often extending as far as the level of the iliac bifurcation. In the remainder (type II) the dissection is limited to the ascending aorta and stops at the origin of the innominate artery. In type III disease the dissection begins in the thoracic aorta distal to the subclavian artery and extends for a variable distance proximal and distal to the original site.

On plain chest radiographs, aortic dissection causes progressive widening of the aortic shadow, which may have an irregular or wavy outer border (Figure 6-22). However, this is a nonspecific appearance and a definite diagnosis of dissection must be made on the basis of aortography or CT. In the patient with a suspected acute dissection of thoracic aorta, aortography is the procedure of choice. The diagnosis of aortic dissection depends on the demonstration of two channels separated by a thin radiolucent intimal flap (Figure 6-23). The false channel may be filled with clot and be impossible to opacify with contrast material. In this case, the diagnosis can be made by demonstrating narrowing and compression of the true channel. When both the true and false lumens fill with contrast material, it is important to demonstrate the distal re-entry point where the false lumen joins the true lumen. If the dissection extends below the diaphragm, arteriography can provide presurgical information about which major vessel branches from the aorta are blocked and which remain patent.

In the patient in whom nonacute aortic dissection is considered in the differential diagnosis of chest pain, CT and MRI offer low-risk alternative diagnostic methods to aortography. CT demonstrates an aortic dissection as a double channel with an intimal flap. With dynamic scanning and the rapid injection of a bolus of contrast material, differential filling of the true and false channels can be observed as with aortography. The major limitation of CT in the patient with suspected acute dissection is that only a single level can be evaluated on a given slice, as opposed to the rapid series of images covering a large portion of the aorta that can be obtained with aortography.

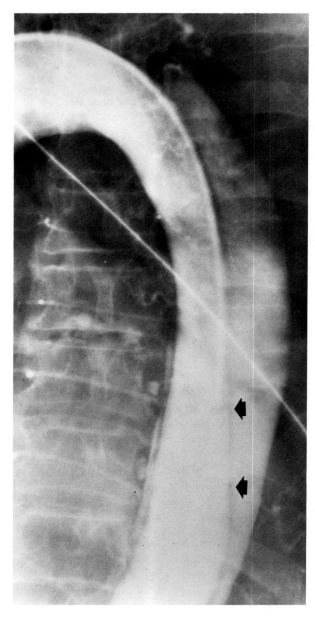

Figure 6-23 Aortic dissection. Aortogram demonstrates thin radiolucent intimal flap *(arrows)* separating true and false aortic channels.

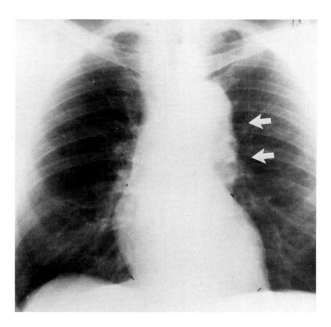

Figure 6-22 Aortic dissection. Plain chest radiograph shows diffuse widening of descending aorta with irregular, wavy outer border *(arrows)*. *(From Ovenfors CO and Godwin JD: In Eisenberg RL, editor: Diagnostic imaging: an algorithmic approach, Philadelphia, JB Lippincott Co, 1988.)*

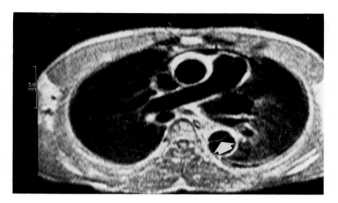

Figure 6-24 MRI of aortic dissection. Axial scan at level of main and right pulmonary arteries clearly shows intimal flap *(arrow)* in descending aorta. *(From Ovenfors CO and Godwin JD: In Eisenberg RL, editor: Diagnostic imaging: an algorithmic approach, Philadelphia, JB Lippincott Co., 1988.)*

The high contrast between rapidly flowing blood, vessel wall, and adjacent soft-tissue structures permit identification of vessels by MRI without the need for intravenous injection of contrast material. This technique can demonstrate aortic dissections and show their extent. The intimal flap is usually detected as a linear, medium-intensity structure separating the true and false lumens (Figure 6-24). Rapidly flowing blood in these lumens appears as a signal void. If the false lumen is thrombosed, or even if it is open but the flow is slow, the intimal flap may

not be visualized. In this situation aortic dissection is difficult to differentiate from an aortic aneurysm with mural thrombus, and aortography may be required to make this distinction.

Atherosclerosis

The major cause of vascular disease of the extremities is atherosclerosis, in which fatty deposits called plaques develop in the intima and produce progressive narrowing and often complete occlusion of large and medium-sized arteries. In the abdomen the disease primarily involves the aorta and the common iliac arteries, often sparing the external iliac vessels. In the lower extremities arteriosclerotic narrowing most commonly affects the superficial femoral artery just above the knee. Plaque formation and luminal narrowing often involve the coronary and cerebral arteries, thus decreasing the blood flow to the heart muscle and the brain and leading to a myocardial infarction or stroke (cerebrovascular accident).

Arteriosclerotic plaques often calcify and appear on plain radiographs as irregularly distributed densities along the course of an artery (Figure 6-25). Small vessel calcification, especially in the hands and feet, is often seen in patients with accelerated arteriosclerosis, especially those with diabetes mellitus.

Doppler ultrasound is an effective noninvasive technique for screening patients with clinically suspected peripheral arteriosclerotic disease. Definitive diagnosis requires arteriographic demonstration of the peripheral vascular tree. Evidence of arterioscle-

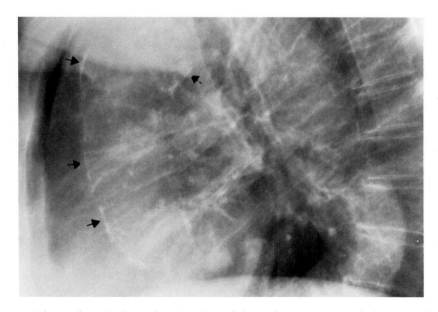

Figure 6-25 Atherosclerosis. Lateral projection of chest demonstrates calcification of anterior and posterior walls of ascending aorta *(arrows)*. Descending thoracic aorta is tortuous.

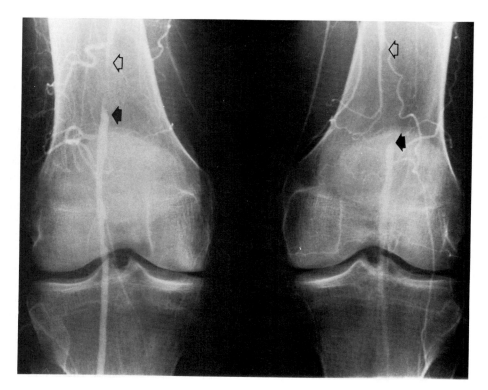

Figure 6-26 Bilateral atherosclerotic occlusion of superficial femoral arteries. Arteriogram demonstrates occlusion of both distal superficial femoral arteries *(open arrows)* with reconstitution by collateral vessels *(solid arrows)*.

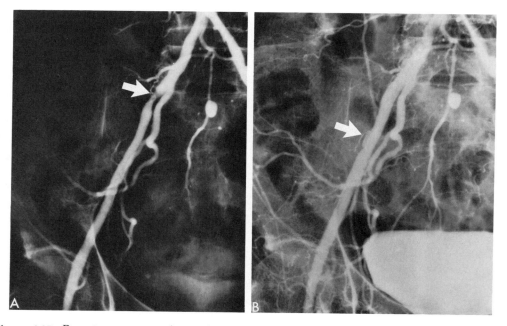

Figure 6-27 Percutaneous transluminal angioplasty of right external iliac artery stenosis. **A,** Initial film in patient with claudication demonstrates narrowing of proximal right external iliac artery *(arrow)*. **B,** After angioplasty, there is relief of stenosis *(arrow)* and of symptoms. *(From Waltman AC: In Athanasoulis CA et al, editors: Interventional radiology, Philadelphia, WB Saunders Co, 1982.)*

rosis includes diffuse vascular narrowing, irregularity of the lumen, and filling defects. In patients with severe stenosis or obstruction, arteriography demonstrates the degree and source of collateral circulation and the status of the vessels distal to an area of narrowing (Figure 6-26).

Percutaneous transluminal angioplasty using a balloon catheter is now a recognized procedure for the alleviation of symptoms of peripheral ischemia in patients with arteriosclerosis (Figure 6-27). It is of special value in patients who are extremely ill and those who would not benefit from reconstructive arterial surgery.

Thrombosis and embolism

The blood-clotting mechanism is the major protective device of the body in response to the escape of blood from a vessel (hemorrhage). This same mechanism can occur in intact blood vessels, leading to the development of an intravascular clot called a thrombus. Three factors lead to the development of intravascular thrombosis. Clots tend to form where blood flow is slow, and thus develop much more commonly in veins than in arteries. Thrombi especially occur in areas of stasis (slow circulation) in patients who are inactive or immobilized, such as after abdominal surgery.

Changes in the wall of blood vessels can lead to thrombosis. Normally, the inner wall of a blood vessel has a very smooth lining (endothelium), and platelets cannot stick, or adhere, to it. However, when the endothelium is destroyed by injury or inflammation, platelets rapidly adhere to the rough spot, and a clot begins to form from the blood as it flows past. Arteriosclerosis is the major cause of endothelial irregularity and subsequent thrombosis. Nodules of vegetation on heart valves caused by rheumatic heart disease are also important predisposing factors for thrombus formation.

Changes in the blood itself can lead to thrombosis. A low level of oxygen within the blood, as in some forms of heart disease, forces the body to compensate by increasing the number of red blood cells (polycythemia). This causes the blood to become more viscous and increases the risk of thrombosis. Changes in the clotting and fibrinolytic mechanism also may increase the risk of thrombus formation.

Anticoagulants such as heparin and coumadin are often used to prevent intravascular cotting. Heparin prevents platelets from sticking together and to the vessel wall, so that a thrombus is not formed. Coumadin acts by antagonizing the action of vitamin K, which is necessary for blood clotting. However, these medications also interfere with the person's normal ability to stop bleeding and may lead to severe hemorrhage from relatively minor trauma or to potentially fatal bleeding in the brain and gastrointestinal tract. Recent reports have suggested the value of aspirin to prevent intravascular clotting because of its inhibition of platelet aggregation.

Once a thrombus is formed, it may follow one of three courses. The thrombus may contract or become canalized so that blood can once again flow through the lumen. The thrombus may continually enlarge or become converted into fibrous tissue, resulting in permanent occlusion of the vessel. A potentially catastrophic event is the production of an embolus, which refers to part or all of a thrombus that becomes detached from the vessel wall and enters the bloodstream. Embolization is especially likely to occur if there is infected tissue around the thrombus or if there is a sudden movement caused by rough handling of the involved area. Depending on the size of the vessels through which it travels, an embolism may lodge at any of several points. Since veins become larger as they approach the heart, an embolism arising from a thrombus in a leg vein flows easily to the heart and typically gets stuck in a pulmonary artery (pulmonary embolism). An embolism arising from a mitral valve damaged by rheumatic heart disease flows through the left ventricle and aorta and lodges in a smaller artery in the brain, kidney, or other organ. A septic embolism contains infected material from pyogenic bacteria, whereas tumor emboli are groups of cancer cells that have invaded a vein, become detached, and are then carried to the lungs or other organs where they form metastases. Fat emboli are the result of trauma, especially leg fractures, in which marrow fat enters torn peripheral veins and is trapped by the pulmonary circulation. An air embolism refers to bubbles of air introduced into a vein during surgery, trauma, or improperly an administered intravenous injection.

Regardless of its type or source, an embolism blocks the vascular lumen and cuts off the blood supply to the organ or parts supplied by that artery. The effect of an embolism depends on the size of the embolus and on the extent of collateral circulation, which can bring blood to an affected part by way of an alternate route.

Acute embolic occlusion of an artery most commonly affects the lower extremities. The success of therapy depends on the rapid recognition of the clinical problem and the institution of appropriate treatment. Arteriography is the procedure of choice to confirm the clinical diagnosis and to demonstrate the extent of occlusion, the degree of collateral circulation, and the condition of the distal vessels. Embolic occlusion typically appears as an abrupt ter-

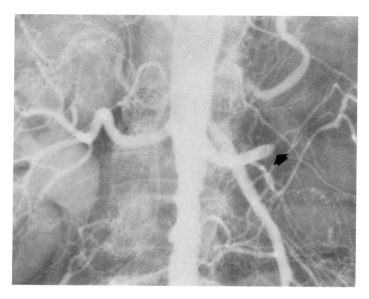

Figure 6-28 Acute embolic occlusion of left renal artery. There is abrupt termination of contrast column *(arrow)*. Note irregular infrarenal aortic contour, which represents atherosclerotic disease.

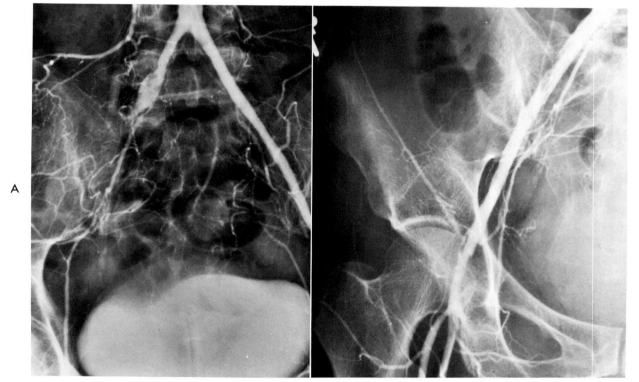

Figure 6-29 Streptokinase therapy for acute arterial occlusion. **A,** After angioplasty of right external iliac artery, there was loss of right common femoral pulse. Repeat arteriogram from left femoral approach shows complete occlusion of external iliac artery at its origin. **B,** After 8 hours of streptokinase administration, arteriogram demonstrates lysis of thrombus and reestablishment of lumen. One year after angioplasty, patient had normal femoral pulse and patent artery. *(From Katzen BT and van Breda A: AJR 136:1171-1178, 1981.)*

mination of the contrast column along with a proximal curved margin reflecting the nonopaque embolus protruding into the contrast-filled lumen (Figure 6-28). In acute occlusion, there is usually little, if any, evidence of collateral circulation.

Although emergency surgery to remove the embolus (embolectomy) has been the traditional treatment for acute arterial occlusion, the intra-arterial infusion of streptokinase by means of a catheter placed immediately proximal to the occlusion is becoming a more common alternative therapy, especially in patients who are poor surgical risks (Figure 6-29). The tissue plasminogen activator (TPA) Activase, produced by recombinant DNA technology, has been administered intravenously to lyse thrombi obstructing coronary arteries in the treatment of acute myocardial infarction.

CONGENITAL HEART DISEASE

Left-to-right shunts

The most common congenital cardiac lesions are left-to-right shunts, which permit mixing of blood in the systemic and pulmonary circulations. Because blood is preferentially shunted from the high-pressure systemic circulation to the relatively low-pressure pulmonary circulation, the lungs become overloaded with blood. The magnitude of the shunt depends on the size of the defect and the differences in pressure on both sides of it. An increased load on the

heart produces enlargement of specific cardiac chambers, depending on the location of the shunt.

The most common congenital cardiac lesion is **atrial septal defect**, which permits free communication between the two atria. Because the left atrial pressure is usually higher than the pressure in the right atrium, the resulting shunt is from left to right and causes increased pulmonary blood flow and overloading of the right ventricle. This produces a radiographic appearance of enlargement of the right ventricle, right atrium, and the pulmonary outflow tract (Figure 6-30).

In a **ventricular septal defect** the resulting shunt is also from left to right because the left ventricular pressure is usually higher than the pressure in the right ventricle. The shunt causes increased pulmonary blood flow and, consequently, increased pulmonary venous return (Figure 6-31). This leads to diastolic overloading and enlargement of the left atrium and left ventricle. Because shunting occurs primarily in systole and any blood directed to the right ventricle immediately goes into the pulmonary artery, there is no overloading of the right ventricle and no right ventricular enlargement is seen.

The third major type of left-to-right shunt is **patent ductus arteriosus**. The ductus arteriosus is a

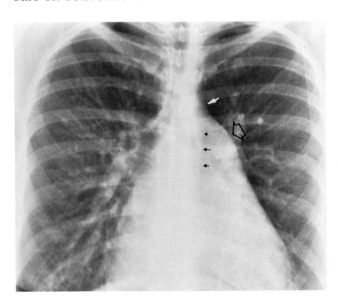

Figure 6-30 Atrial septal defect. Frontal projection of chest demonstrates cardiomegaly along with increase in pulmonary vascularity reflecting left-to-right shunt. Small aortic knob (*white arrow*) and descending aorta (*small arrows*) are dwarfed by enlarged pulmonary outflow tract (*open arrow*).

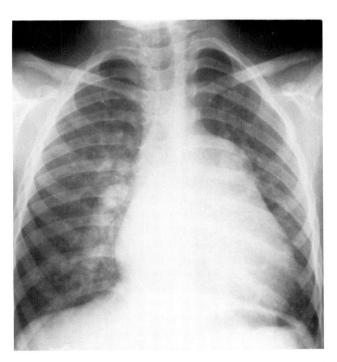

Figure 6-31 Ventricular septal defect. Heart is enlarged and somewhat triangular, and there is increase in pulmonary vascular volume. Pulmonary trunk is very large and overshadows normal-sized aorta, which seems small by comparison. (*From Cooley RN and Schreiber MH: Radiology of the heart and great vessels, Baltimore, Williams & Wilkins Co, 1978.*)

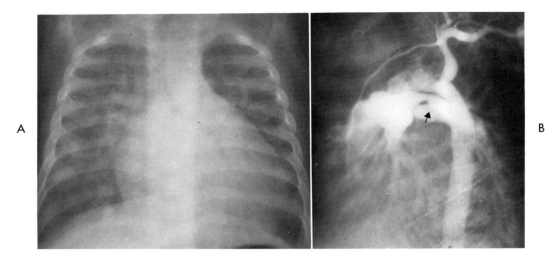

Figure 6-32 Patent ductus arteriosus. **A,** Frontal chest radiograph demonstrates cardiomegaly with enlargement of left atrium, left ventricle, and central pulmonary arteries. There is diffuse increase in pulmonary vascularity. **B,** In another patient, aortogram shows patency of ductus arteriosus *(arrow). (From Cooley RN and Schreiber MH: Radiology of the heart and great vessels, Baltimore, Williams & Wilkins Co, 1978.)*

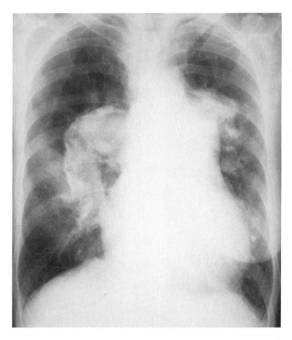

Figure 6-33 Eisenmenger's syndrome in atrial septal defect. There is slight but definite cardiomegaly and great increase in size of pulmonary trunk. Right and left pulmonary artery branches are huge, but peripheral pulmonary vasculature is relatively sparse. Long-standing pulmonary hypertension has produced degenerative changes in walls of pulmonary arteries, which have become densely calcified. *(From Cooley RN and Schreiber MH: Radiology of the heart and great vessels, Baltimore, Williams & Wilkins Co, 1978.)*

vessel that extends from the bifurcation of the pulmonary artery to join the aorta just distal to the left subclavian artery. It serves to shunt blood from the pulmonary artery into the systemic circulation during intrauterine life. Persistence of the ductus arteriosus, which normally closes soon after birth, results in a left-to-right shunt. The flow of blood from the higher-pressure aorta to the lower-pressure pulmonary artery causes increased pulmonary blood flow, and an excess volume of blood is returned to the left atrium and left ventricle. Radiographically, there is enlargement of the left atrium, the left ventricle, and the central pulmonary arteries, along with a diffuse increase in pulmonary vascularity (Figure 6-32). The increased blood flow through the aorta proximal to the shunt produces a prominent aortic knob, in contrast to the small or normal-sized aorta seen in atrial and ventricular septal defects.

All left-to-right shunts can be complicated by the development of pulmonary hypertension (**Eisenmenger's syndrome**). This is caused by increased vascular resistance within the pulmonary arteries related to chronic increased flow through the pulmonary circulation. Pulmonary hypertension appears radiographically as an increased fullness of the central pulmonary arteries with abrupt narrowing and pruning of peripheral vessels (Figure 6-33). The elevation of pulmonary arterial pressure tends to balance or even reverse the left-to-right shunt, thus easing the volume overloading of the heart.

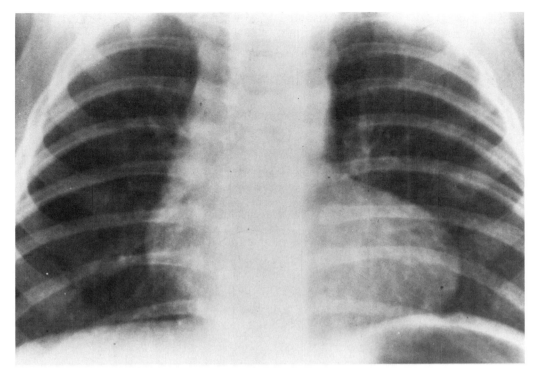

Figure 6-34 Tetralogy of Fallot. Plain chest radiograph demonstrates characteristic lateral displacement and upward tilting of prominent cardiac apex. There is also decreased pulmonary vascularity and flat pulmonary outflow tract.

Tetralogy of Fallot

Tetralogy of Fallot is the most common cause of cyanotic congenital heart disease and consists of four (tetra) abnormalities: (1) high ventricular septal defect, (2) pulmonary stenosis, (3) overriding of the aortic orifice above the ventricular defect, and (4) right ventricular hypertrophy. Pulmonary stenosis causes an elevation of pressure in the right ventricle and hypertrophy of that chamber. Because of the narrow opening of the pulmonary valve, an inadequate amount of blood reaches the lungs to be oxygenated. The ventricular septal defect and the overriding of the aorta produce right-to-left shunting of unoxygenated venous blood into the right ventricle and then into the systemic circulation, thus increasing the degree of cyanosis.

Enlargement of the right ventricle causes upward and lateral displacement of the apex of the heart (Figure 6-34). This results in the classic **coeur en sabot** appearance resembling the curved-toe portion of a wooden shoe. In about one fourth of patients with tetralogy of Fallot the aorta is on the right side.

Coarctation of the aorta

Coarctation refers to a narrowing, or constriction, of the aorta that most commonly occurs just beyond the branching of the blood vessels to the head and arms. Although the blood supply and pressure to the upper extremities is normal, there is decreased blood flow through the constricted area to the abdomen and legs. Classically, the patient has normal blood pressure in the arms but very low blood pressure in the legs.

The relative obstruction of aortic blood flow leads to the progressive development of collateral circulation, the enlargement of normally tiny vessels in an attempt to compensate for the inadequate blood supply to the lower portion of the body. This is often seen radiographically as rib notching (usually involving the posterior fourth to eighth ribs) resulting from pressure erosion by dilated and pulsating intercostal collateral vessels that run along the inferior margins of these ribs (Figure 6-35, *A*). Notching of the posterior border of the sternum may be produced by dilation of mammary artery collaterals.

Coarctation of the aorta often causes two bulges in the region of the aortic knob that produce a characteristic figure-3 sign on plain chest radiographs (Figure 6-35, *B*) and a reverse figure-3 or figure-E impression on the barium-filled esophagus (Figure 6-35, *C*). The more cephalad bulge represents dilation of the proximal aorta and the base of the subclavian artery (prestenotic dilation); the lower bulge reflects poststenotic aortic dilation.

Aortography can accurately localize the site of obstruction, determine the length of the coarctation, and identify any associated cardiac malformations. More recently, MRI has been used to demonstate aortic narrowing (Figure 6-36) and to check the appearance of the aorta after corrective surgery.

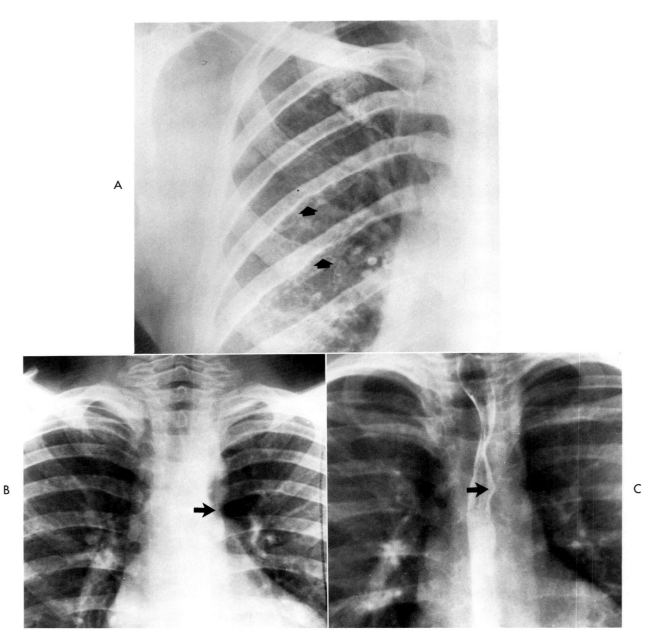

Figure 6-35 Coarctation of aorta. **A,** Rib notching. There is notching of posterior fourth through eighth ribs (arrows point to examples). **B,** Plain chest radiograph demonstrates figure-3 sign (arrow points to center of 3). Upper bulge represents prestenotic dilation; lower bulge represents poststenotic dilation. **C,** Esophagram demonstrates reverse figure-3 sign (arrow points to center of reverse figure-3). *(From Swischuk LE: Plain film interpretation in congenital heart disease, Baltimore, Williams & Wilkins Co, 1979.)*

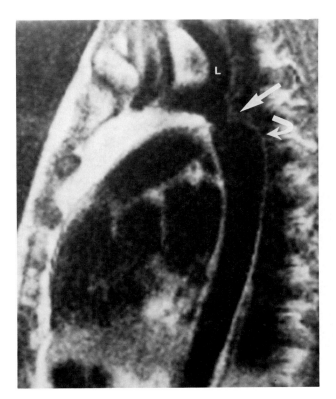

Figure 6-36 Coarctation of aorta. Sagittal MRI demonstrates coarctation *(straight arrow)* of thoracic aorta with associated poststenotic dilation of proximal descending thoracic aorta *(curved arrow). L,* Left subclavian artery.

RHEUMATIC HEART DISEASE

Rheumatic fever is an autoimmune disease that results from a reaction of the patient's antibodies against antigens from a previous streptococcal infection. The disease is much less common today because of the frequent use of antibiotics to treat streptococcal throat or ear infections. The symptoms of rheumatic fever (fever, inflamed and painful joints, rash) typically develop several weeks after the streptococcal infection.

The major damage of rheumatic fever is to the valves of the heart, especially the mitral and aortic valves. The allergic response causes inflammation of the valves. Deposits of blood platelets and fibrin from blood flowing over the valve produce small nodules (**vegetations**) along the margin of the valve cusps. The thickened valves may stick together, remaining permanently narrowed (**stenosis**) rather than opening properly when blood flows through the valvular opening. Conversely, fibrous scarring may cause retraction of the valve cusps so that the cusps are unable to meet when the valve tries to

close (**insufficiency**). In this case, there is leakage of blood across the valve.

VALVULAR DISEASE

The valves of the heart permit blood to flow in only one direction through the heart. When the valve is closed, a heart chamber fills with blood; when the valve opens, blood can move forward and exit the chamber. There are four heart valves. The **tricuspid valve** separates the right atrium and right ventricle, and the **mitral valve** separates the left atrium and left ventricle. The **pulmonary valve** lies between the right ventricle and pulmonary artery, and the **aortic valve** is situated between the left ventricle and the aorta.

The malfunction of a heart valve alters the normal blood flow through the heart. Too small an opening (stenosis) does not permit sufficient blood flow. In contrast, too large an opening or failure of the valve to properly close permits back flow of blood (regurgitation) and the condition of valvular insufficiency. Both stenosis and insufficiency of valves cause heart murmurs with characteristic sounds that indicate the nature of the defect. Although valvular heart disease used to invariably force a patient to restrict activity and was associated with a limited life span, surgical reconstruction or replacement of a diseased valve (Figure 6-37) can offer a patient the prospect of a normal life.

Mitral stenosis

Stenosis of the mitral valve, almost always a complication of rheumatic disease, results from diffuse thickening of the valve by fibrous tissue, calcific deposits, or both. The obstruction to blood flow from the left atrium into the left ventricle during diastole causes increased pressure in the left atrium and enlargement of this chamber (Figure 6-38). The enlarged left atrium produces a characteristic anterior impression on and posterior displacement of the barium-filled esophagus that is best seen on lateral and right anterior oblique projections. Other radiographic signs of the left atrial enlargement include posterior displacement of the left main stem bronchus, widening of the tracheal bifurcation (carina), and a characteristic "double contour" configuration caused by the projection of the enlarged left atrium through the normal right atrial silhouette. The increased left atrial pressure is transmitted to the pulmonary veins and produces the appearance of chronic venous congestion.

Calcification of the mitral valve or left atrial wall (Figure 6-39), best demonstrated by fluoroscopy, can

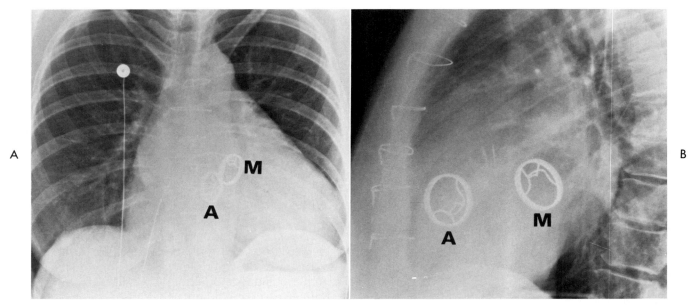

Figure 6-37 Prosthetic aortic and mitral valves. **A,** Frontal and, **B,** lateral projections of chest show anteromedially located prosthetic aortic valve *(A)* and posterolaterally situated prosthetic mitral valve *(M)*.

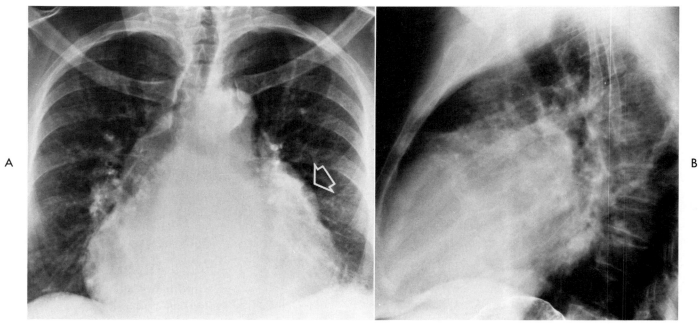

Figure 6-38 Mitral stenosis. **A,** Frontal and, **B,** lateral projections of chest demonstrate cardiomegaly with enlargement of right ventricle and left atrium. Right ventricular enlargement causes obliteration of retrosternal air space, whereas left atrial enlargement produces convexity of upper left border of heart *(arrow)*.

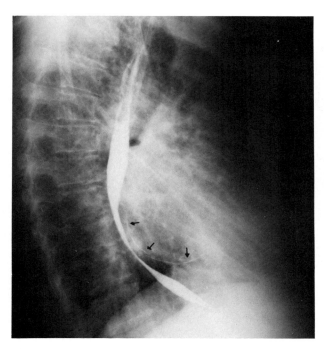

Figure 6-39 Left atrial calcification in mitral stenosis. Lateral projection with barium in esophagus shows enlargement of left atrium and calcification of wall of its chamber *(arrows)*. *(From Vickers SCW et al: Left atrial calcification, Radiology 72:569-575, 1959.)*

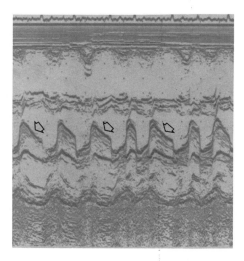

Figure 6-40 Echocardiogram of mitral stenosis. There is thickening of mitral valve with decreased slope *(arrows)*.

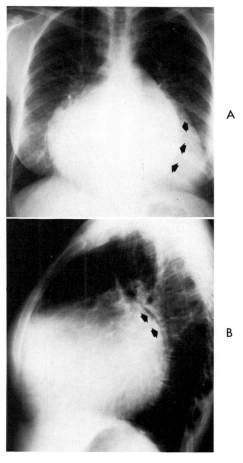

Figure 6-41 Mitral insufficiency. **A,** Frontal and, **B,** lateral projections of chest demonstrate gross cardiomegaly with enlargement of left atrium and left ventricle. Note striking double-contour configuration *(arrows)* on frontal film and elevation of left main-stem bronchus *(arrows)* on lateral film, characteristic signs of left atrial enlargement.

develop in patients with long-standing severe mitral stenosis. A thrombus may form in the dilated left atrium and be the source of emboli to the brain or elsewhere in the systemic circulation.

Echocardiography is the most sensitive and most specific noninvasive method for diagnosing mitral stenosis (Figure 6-40). More recently, MRI has been used to show the abnormal pattern of flow between the left atrium and left ventricle in this condition.

Mitral insufficiency

Although most often caused by rheumatic heart disease, mitral insufficiency may also be caused by rupture of chordae tendineae or by dysfunction of the papillary muscles that are attached to the underside of the valve cusps and normally prevent them from swinging up into the atrium when the ventricles contract. Regurgitation of blood into the left atrium during ventricular systole causes overfilling and dilation of this chamber (Figure 6-41). In most cases, the left atrium is considerably larger in mitral insufficiency than in mitral stenosis; occasionally, an enormous left atrium can form both the right and left borders of the heart on frontal projections. An increased volume of blood flowing from the dilated left atrium to the left ventricle in diastole increases

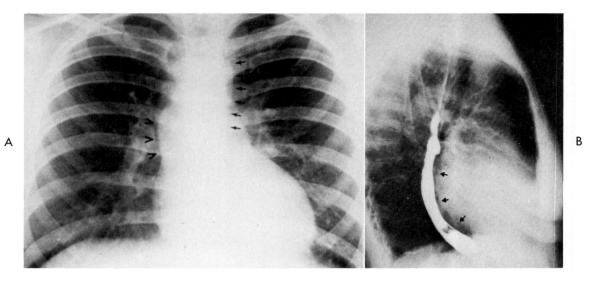

Figure 6-42 Aortic stenosis. **A,** Frontal projection shows downward displacement of cardiac apex with poststenotic dilation of ascending aorta *(arrowheads)*. Aortic knob and descending aorta *(arrows)* are normal. **B,** On lateral projection in another patient, bulging of lower half of posterior cardiac silhouette causes broad indentation on barium-filled esophagus *(arrows)*.

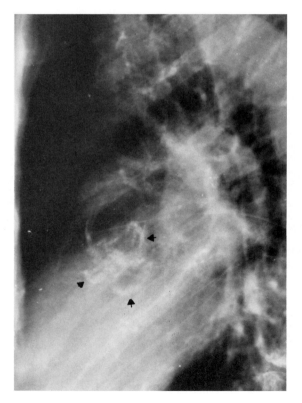

Figure 6-43 Aortic stenosis. Calcification in three leaflets of aortic valve *(arrows)*.

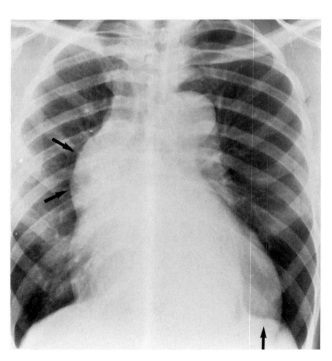

Figure 6-44 Aortic insufficiency. Frontal chest radiograph shows left ventricular enlargement with downward and lateral displacement of cardiac apex. Note that cardiac shadow extends below dome of left hemidiaphragm *(small arrow)*. Ascending aorta is strikingly dilated *(large arrows)*, suggesting some underlying aortic stenosis.

the left ventricular work load and leads to dilation and hypertrophy of this chamber. This causes downward displacement of the cardiac apex and rounding of the lower left border of the heart.

Aortic stenosis

Aortic stenosis may be caused by rheumatic heart disease, a congenital valvular deformity (especially a bicuspid valve), or a degenerative process of aging (idiopathic calcific stenosis). The obstruction to left ventricular outflow in aortic stenosis increases the work load of the left ventricle. Initially, this results in left ventricular hypertrophy without dilation that produces only some rounding of the cardiac apex on frontal chest radiographs and slight backward displacement on lateral projections. The overall size of the heart remains within normal limits until left ventricular failure develops. Significant aortic stenosis is usually associated with lateral bulging (poststenotic dilation) of the ascending aorta caused by the jet of blood forced under high pressure through the narrowed valve (Figure 6-42). Aortic valve calcification, best demonstrated on fluoroscopic examination, is a common finding and indicates that the aortic stenosis is severe (Figure 6-43).

Aortic insufficiency

Although most commonly caused by rheumatic heart disease, aortic insufficiency may be due to syphilis, infective endocarditis, dissecting aneurysm, or Marfan's syndrome. Reflux of blood from the aorta during diastole causes volume overloading of the left ventricle and dilation of this chamber. This causes downward, lateral, and posterior displacement of the cardiac apex (Figure 6-44). Marked left ventricular dilation causes relative mitral insufficiency, which leads to left atrial enlargement and signs of pulmonary edema.

Infective endocarditis

Infective endocarditis refers to the development of nodules or vegetations forming on heart valves. Unlike the smaller nodules in rheumatic fever, the vegetations of infective endocarditis are filled with bacteria and tend to break apart easily (friable) to enter the bloodstream and form septic emboli that travel to the brain, kidney, lung, or other vital organs. Emboli lodging in the skin may cause rupture of small blood vessels and characteristic tiny hemorrhagic red spots (petechiae).

Plain radiography is of little value in patients with infective endocarditis. The cardiac silhouette may be normal or demonstrate evidence of previous valvular heart disease or congestive heart failure. Echo-

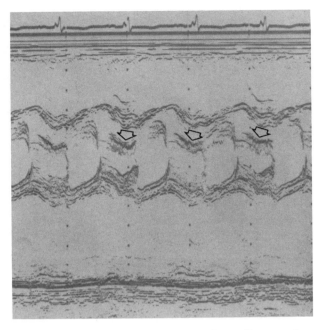

Figure 6-45 Infective endocarditis. Echocardiogram demonstrates vegetations as masses of shaggy echoes producing irregular thickening of aortic valve *(arrows)*.

cardiography is the only noninvasive procedure that can detect the valvular vegetations that are the hallmark of infective endocarditis. On the echocardiogram, these vegetations appear as masses of shaggy echoes producing an irregular thickening of the affected valves (Figure 6-45).

PERICARDIAL EFFUSION

Pericardial effusion refers to the accumulation of fluid within the pericardial space surrounding the heart. Echocardiography is the most effective imaging technique for demonstrating pericardial effusions and has largely replaced other methods. As little as 50 ml of fluid can be detected by this modality. On plain chest radiographs, a pericardial effusion causes enlargement of the cardiac silhouette (Figure 6-46). However, at least 200 ml of fluid must be present before a pericardial effusion can be detected by this technique. Rapid enlargement of the cardiac silhouette, especially in the absence of pulmonary vascular engorgement indicating congestive heart failure, is highly suggestive of pericardial effusion.

Angiocardiography, intravenous carbon dioxide injection, and a pericardial tap with air injection have been used in the past to demonstrate pericardial effusion by showing an excessive distance (greater than 5 mm) between the contrast- or air-

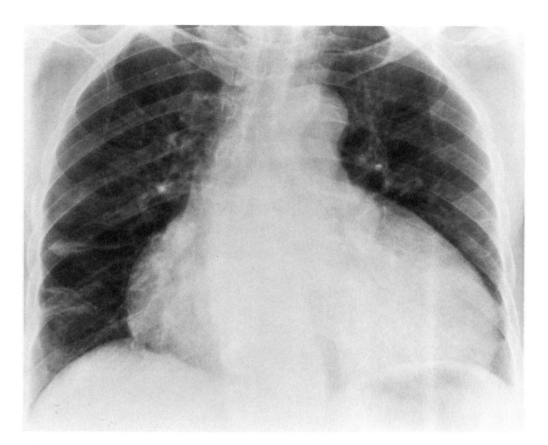

Figure 6-46   Pericardial effusion. Globular enlargement of cardiac silhouette.

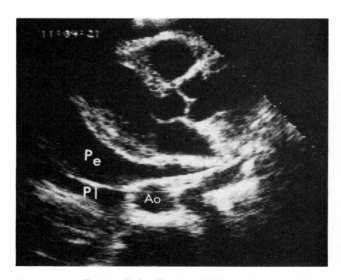

Figure 6-47 Pericardial effusion. Echocardiogram demonstrates both pericardial *(Pe)* and pleural *(P1)* effusions. Descending aorta *(Ao)* is separated from heart by pericardial effusion. *(From Miller SW and Gillam LD: In Eisenberg RL, editor: Diagnostic imaging: an algorithmic approach, Philadelphia, JB Lippincott Co, 1988.)*

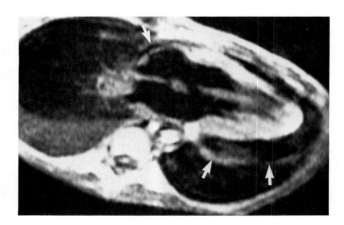

Figure 6-48   MRI of pericardial effusion. Pericardium *(arrows)* is displaced away from heart by huge pericardial effusion that has very little signal intensity. Effect of gravity is seen in posterior location of both pericardial and right pleural effusions. *(From Miller et al: Radiol Clin North Am 23:756-764, 1985.)*

filled atrium and the outer border of the cardiac silhouette. However, echocardiography has effectively replaced these invasive techniques (Figure 6-47).

Gated MRI (Figure 6-48) shows a pericardial effusion as a region of decreased signal intensity between the myocardium and the fat on the surface of the parietal pericardium (which is usually invisible when it is in direct contact with the heart).

VENOUS DISEASE

Deep venous thrombosis

Deep venous thrombosis, which primarily involves the lower extremities, is the major source of potentially fatal pulmonary embolism. Precipitating factors in the development of venous thrombosis include trauma, bacterial infection, prolonged bed rest, and oral contraceptives. At times, deep vein thrombosis may be the earliest symptom of an un-

suspected malignancy of the pancreas, lung, or gastrointestinal system.

A precise diagnosis of deep vein thrombosis requires contrast venography, which can demonstrate the major venous channels and their tributaries from the foot to the inferior vena cava. The identification of a constant filling defect, representing the actual thrombus, is conclusive evidence of deep vein thrombosis (Figure 6-49). Venographic findings that are highly suggestive of, although not conclusive for, the diagnosis of deep vein thrombosis include the abrupt ending of the opaque column in a vein, the nonfilling of one or more veins that are normally opacified, and extensive collateral venous circulation.

Because venography is an invasive technique, other modalities have been developed for detecting deep vein thrombosis. Duplex Doppler ultrasound demonstrates changes in the velocity of venous

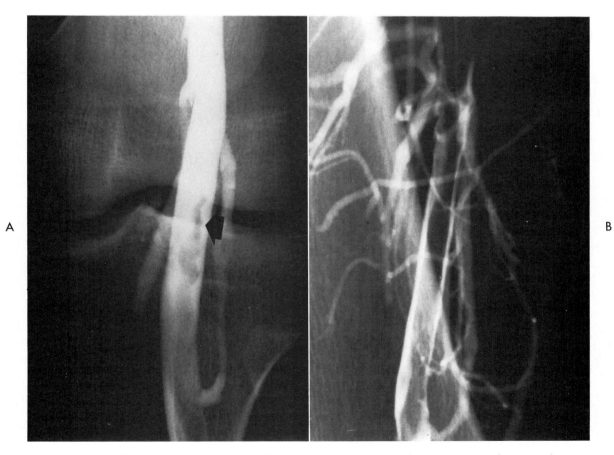

Figure 6-49 Deep vein thrombosis. **A,** Initial contrast venogram demonstrates early nonocclusive thrombus extending from valve cusp. Arrow points to thrombus tail, the portion most likely to embolize. **B,** Subsequent contrast venogram demonstrates growth and proximal extension of thrombus, which has resulted in occlusion of popliteal vein at adductor hiatus. *(From Holden RW, Mail JT and Becker GJ: In Eisenberg RL editor: Diagnostic imaging: an algorithmic approach, Philadelphia, JB Lippincott Co, 1988.)*

blood flow. It is of special value in showing thrombotic occlusion of major venous pathways in the popliteal and femoral regions. An abnormal Doppler ultrasound examination is not specific for thrombosis, since similar changes in venous blood flow may be caused by congestive heart failure, extensive leg edema, local soft-tissue masses, and decreased inflow of arterial blood into the extremity.

Varicose veins

Varicose veins are dilated, elongated, and tortuous vessels that most commonly involve the superficial veins of the leg just under the skin (Figure 6-50). If the venous dilation becomes extreme, the valves that normally prevent back flow of blood because of gravity become incompetent and cease to function, thus increasing the volume of blood in these slow-flowing vessels.

Although heredity plays some role in the development of varicose veins, which often run in a family, the underlying cause is increased pressure in an affected vein. Varicose veins can be an occupational hazard for people who stand or sit for long periods.

Normally, the action of leg muscles helps move blood upward toward the heart from one venous valve to the next. If this "milking action" of the muscles is absent, the blood puts pressure on the closed valves and the thin walls of the veins resulting in venous dilation, incompetence of the valves, and stasis of blood in the stagnant lower extremity veins. Increased pressure on a vein can also be due to a pregnant uterus or a pelvic tumor.

Stasis of blood within varicose veins may lead to the development of phleboliths, calcified clots within a vein that appear radiographically as rounded densities that often contain lucent centers (Figure 6-51). Chronic venous stasis may also lead to periosteal new bone formation along the tibial and fibular shafts and development of plaquelike calci-

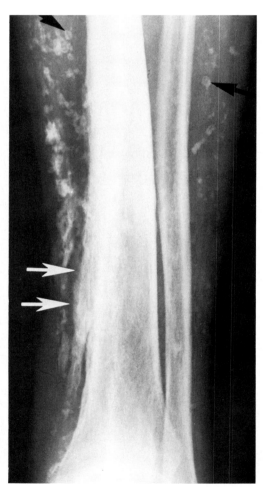

Figure 6-51 Varicose veins. Multiple round and oval calcifications in soft tissues (phleboliths) representing calcified thrombi, some of which have characteristic lucent centers *(black arrows)*. Extensive new bone formation along medial aspect of tibial shaft *(white arrows)* is caused by long-standing venous stasis.

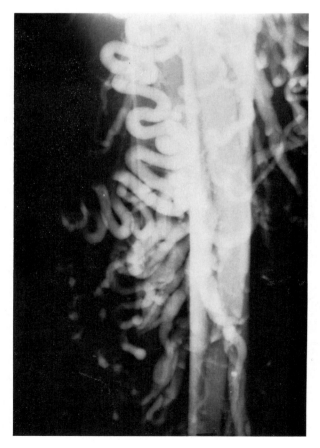

Figure 6-50 Varicose veins. Lower extremity venogram shows multiple tortuous, dilated venous structures.

fications in the chronically congested subcutaneous tissues. The poor venous flow can lead to the development of superficial ulcers, and the distended veins can rupture, causing hemorrhage into the surrounding tissues.

Although the diagnosis of varicose veins is primarily based on the clinical observation of the multiple bluish nodules just under the skin, venography is of value in demonstrating the patency of the deep venous system and the degree of collateral circulation from the superficial to the deep veins, especially if there is consideration of surgical intervention (tying off and removing the superficial veins). After the application of a tourniquet to occlude superficial flow, the peripheral injection of contrast material opacifies the deep venous system. Filling of the superficial veins indicates that the perforating veins above the level of the tourniquet are incompetent.

QUESTIONS

1. The heart rate is controlled by the _____ nervous system.
   - A. Psychogenic
   - B. Central
   - C. Peripheral
   - D. Autonomic

2. The _____ valve is located between the left atrium and the left ventricle, whereas the _____ valve is located between the right atrium and right ventricle.
   - I. Tricuspid
   - II. Mitral
   - III. Pulmonary
   - IV. Aortic
   - A. II, I
   - B. III, I
   - C. IV, I
   - D. I, II

3. The general circulation of the body is termed the _____ circulation.
   - A. Pulmonary
   - B. Systemic
   - C. General
   - D. Autonomic

4. The contracting phase of the heart is termed _____, whereas the relaxation phase is termed _____.
   - I. Autonomic
   - II. Diastole
   - III. Systemic
   - IV. Systole
   - A. I, III
   - B. II, IV
   - C. II, III
   - D. IV, II

5. Contraction of which chamber of the heart forces oxygenated blood into the aorta?
   - A. Right atrium
   - B. Right ventricle
   - C. Left atrium
   - D. Left ventricle

6. Oxygenated blood reaches the heart muscle by way of the _____.
   - I. Right coronary artery
   - II. Left coronary artery
   - III. Left coronary vein
   - IV. Right coronary vein
   - A. I, III
   - B. IV, I
   - C. II, I
   - D. II, III

7. The heart has a specialized pacemaker named the _____.
   - A. Bundle of His
   - B. Sinoatrial node
   - C. Purkinje fibers
   - D. Atrioventricular node

8. Factors that lead to coronary artery disease are _____.
   - A. Lack of exercise
   - B. Obesity, hypertension
   - C. Smoking, high-cholesterol diet
   - D. All of the above

9. Temporary oxygen insufficiency to the heart muscle causes severe chest pain termed _____.
   - A. Angina pectoris
   - B. Myocardial occlusion
   - C. Myocardial pectoris
   - D. Angina occlusion

10. Arterial disease caused by fatty deposits on the inner arterial wall is termed _____.
    - A. Arteriosclerosis
    - B. Myocardial infarction
    - C. Aneurysm
    - D. Myocardial ischemia

11. What radiographic procedure is used to determine the presence of coronary artery disease?
    - A. Angioplasty
    - B. Chest film
    - C. Coronary arteriogram
    - D. CT

12. The procedure of using a balloon to dilate narrowed coronary arteries is named _____.
    - A. Aortocoronary bypass
    - B. Coronary arteriography
    - C. Percutaneous transluminal angioplasty
    - D. Fluoroscopy

13. The term _____ refers to an inability of the heart to propel blood at a sufficient rate and volume.
    - A. Congestive heart failure
    - B. Pulmonary edema
    - C. Valvular disease
    - D. Valvular stenosis

14. An elevation of the pulmonary venous pressure is the most common cause of _____.
    - A. Congestive heart failure
    - B. Pulmonary edema
    - C. Valvular disease
    - D. Valvular stenosis

15. The leading cause of strokes and congestive heart failure is _____.
    A. Hypertension
    B. Low blood pressure
    C. Hypotension
    D. Cor pulmonale

16. A localized bulging or dilation of an artery is termed _____.
    A. Edema
    B. Effusion
    C. Aneurysm
    D. Fat emboli

17. What is the modality of choice for demonstration of an abdominal aortic aneurysm?
    A. MRI
    B. Ultrasonography
    C. CT
    D. Plain film radiography

18. A congenital narrowing or constriction of the thoracic aorta is referred to as _____.
    A. Embolism
    B. Plaque
    C. Coarctation
    D. Tetralogy

19. The _____ of the heart is the major site of damage from rheumatic fever.
    A. Myocardium
    B. Valves
    C. Septum
    D. Endocardium

20. The most sensitive and specific noninvasive method of diagnosing mitral stenosis is _____.
    A. Ultrasonagraphy
    B. Echocardiography
    C. Cardiac arteriography
    D. CT

21. The accumulation of fluid within the pericardial space surrounding the heart is termed _____.
    A. Pericardial thrombosis
    B. Pericardial effusion
    C. Pulmonary edema
    D. Pulmonary effusion

22. The invasive procedure for determining deep vein thrombosis is _____.
    A. Doppler ultrasound
    B. Venography
    C. CT
    D. Arteriography

23. The most accurate screening procedure for assessing renovascular lesions is _____.
    A. Doppler ultrasound
    B. Venography
    C. CT
    D. Arteriography

24. A potentially life-threatening condition that usually begins as a tear in the intima above the aortic valve is an _____.
    A. Aortic stenosis
    B. Aortic coarctation
    C. Aortic thrombosis
    D. Aortic dissection

BIBLIOGRAPHY

Swischuk LE: Plain film interpretation in congenital heart disease, Baltimore, Williams & Wilkins, 1979.

Cooley RN and Schreiber MH: Radiology of the heart and great vessels, Baltimore, Williams & Wilkins, 1978.

CHAPTER 7

Nervous System Disease

PREREQUISITE KNOWLEDGE

The student should have a basic knowledge of the anatomy and physiology of the skull and nervous system. In addition, proper learning and understanding of the material will be facilitated if the student has some clinical experience in skull radiography and film evaluation, including a concept of newer imaging modalities (CT, MRI).

GOALS

To acquaint the student radiographer with the pathophysiology and radiographic manifestations of all of the common and some of the unusual disorders of the skull and nervous system

OBJECTIVES

1. Describe the physiology of the nervous system
2. Identify anatomic structures on both diagrams and images of the skull and nervous system
3. Be able to define terminology relating to the skull
4. Be able to describe the various pathologic conditions affecting the skull and nervous system and their radiographic manifestations

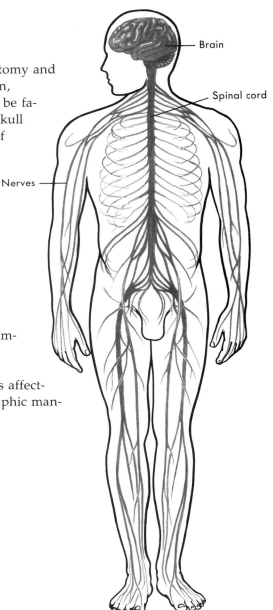

Brain

Spinal cord

Nerves

RADIOGRAPHER NOTES

Proper positioning is critical in skull and spine radiography to ensure bilateral symmetry and to permit an evaluation of the complex anatomy and structural relationships. The demonstration of asymmetry or a shift in the normal location of a structure in a patient who is positioned correctly may be indicative of an underlying pathologic condition. Proper positioning and correct angulation of the central ray may allow visualization of otherwise superimposed structures. When evaluating such anatomic areas as the sinuses or facial bones, it is often necessary to place the patient in the erect position (either standing or sitting) and to use a horizontal beam to demonstrate an air-fluid level indicative of underlying inflammatory disease or fracture. If the patient's condition prohibits placement in an erect position, air-fluid levels can only be demonstrated by obtaining a cross-table lateral projection using a horizontal beam with the patient in a dorsal decubitus position.

Exposure factors should produce a scale of contrast that provides for maximal detail (definition), especially when imaging vascular structures and subtle changes in bone density such as fractures of the skull or spine. Advanced stages of certain patho-

logic conditions can result in the need for technical changes to maintain the proper level of penetration, contrast, and visibility of detail (Table 1-1). If contrast material is used, the kVp level must remain in the low to mid range to provide enough radiographic contrast to properly show the contrast-filled vessels.

The administration of radiographic contrast material is an essential component of many examinations of the skull and nervous system. Therefore it is essential that the radiographer be familiar with the use of these agents and be extremely alert to the development of possible allergic reactions. After contrast administration, the radiographer is often left alone in the room with the patient and thus must be able to immediately recognize an allergic reaction to contrast material and be able to initiate and maintain basic life support until advanced life support personnel have arrived. Depending on departmental policy, it is usually the radiographer's responsibility to assist during resuscitation procedures. Therefore it is essential that the radiographer be familiar with the contents of the emergency cart and be responsible for ensuring that the cart is completely stocked with all appropriate medications.

PHYSIOLOGY OF THE NERVOUS SYSTEM

The divisions of the nervous system can be classified by location or by the type of tissue they supply. The **central nervous system** (CNS) consists of the brain and spinal cord. The remaining neural structures, including 12 pairs of cranial nerves, 31 pairs of spinal nerves, autonomic nerves, and ganglia make up the **peripheral nervous system** (PNS). The PNS consists of afferent and efferent neurons. Afferent **(sensory)** neurons conduct impulses from peripheral receptors to the CNS. Efferent **(motor)** neurons conduct impulses away from the CNS to peripheral effectors. The **somatic nervous system** supplies the striated skeletal muscles, whereas the **autonomic nervous system** supplies smooth muscle, cardiac muscle, and glandular epithelial tissue.

The basic unit of the nervous system is the **neuron,** or nerve cell. A neuron consists of a cell body and two types of long threadlike extensions. A single **axon** leads from the nerve cell body, and one or more **dendrites** lead toward it. Axons are insulated by a

fatty covering called the **myelin sheath,** which increases the rate of transmission of nervous impulses. Deterioration of this fatty myelin sheath (demyelination) is a characteristic abnormality in multiple sclerosis.

The impulse conduction route to and from the CNS is termed a **reflex arc.** The basic reflex arc consists of an afferent or sensory neuron that conducts impulses to the CNS from the periphery and an efferent or motor neuron that conducts impulses from the CNS to peripheral effectors (muscles or glandular tissue).

Impulses are passed from one neuron to another at a junction called the **synapse.** Transmission at the synapse is a chemical reaction in which the terminal ends of the axon release a neurotransmitter substance that produces an electrical impulse in the dendrites of the next axon. Once the neurotransmitter has accomplished its task, its activity is rapidly terminated so that subsequent impulses can be conducted along this same route.

The largest part of the brain is the **cerebrum,** which consists of two cerebral hemispheres. The surface of the cerebrum is highly convoluted with elevations called **gyri** and shallow grooves called **sulci.** Deeper grooves called fissures divide each cerebral hemisphere into lobes. The outer portion of the cerebrum is termed the **cortex,** which consists of a thin layer of gray matter where the nerve cell bodies are concentrated. The inner area consists of white matter, which is composed of the nerve fiber tracts.

The cerebral cortex is responsible for receiving sensory information from all parts of the body and for triggering impulses that govern all motor activity. Just posterior to the central sulcus, the cerebral cortex has specialized areas to receive and precisely localize sensory information from the PNS. Visual impulses are transmitted to the posterior part of the brain; olfactory (smell) and auditory impulses are received in the lateral parts. The primary motor cortex is just anterior to the central sulcus. Because efferent motor fibers cross over from one side of the body to the other at the level of the medulla and spinal cord, stimulation on one side of the cerebral cortex causes contraction of muscles on the opposite side of the body. The premotor cortex, which lies anterior to the primary motor cortex, controls coordinate movements of muscles by stimulating groups of muscles that work together. This region also contains the portion of the brain responsible for speech, which is usually on the left side in right-handed people. The cerebral cortex also is the site of all higher functions, including memory and creative thought.

The two cerebral hemispheres are connected by a mass of white matter called the **corpus callosum.** These extensive bundles of nerve fibers lie in the midline just above the roofs of the lateral ventricles.

Deep within the white matter are a few islands of gray matter that are collectively called the **basal ganglia.** These structures help control position and automatic movements and consist of the caudate nuclei, globus pallidum, and putamen.

Between the cerebrum and spinal cord lies the brainstem, which is composed (from top down) of the **midbrain** (mesencephalon), **pons,** and **medulla.** In addition to performing sensory, motor, and reflex functions, the brainstem contains the nuclei of the 12 cranial nerves and the vital centers controlling cardiac, vasomotor, and respiratory function. Centers in the medulla are responsible for such nonvital reflexes as vomiting, coughing, sneezing, hiccuping, and swallowing.

The **cerebellum,** the second largest part of the brain, is located just below the posterior portion of the cerebrum. It is composed of two large lateral masses, the cerebellar hemispheres, and a central section **(vermis)** that resembles a worm coiled on itself. The cerebellum acts with the cerebral cortex to produce skilled movements by coordinating the activities of groups of muscles. It coordinates skeletal muscles in maintaining equilibrium and posture by functioning below the level of consciousness to make movements smooth rather than jerky, steady rather than trembling, and efficient and coordinated rather than ineffective and awkward. Therefore cerebellar disease produces such characteristic symptoms as ataxia (muscle incoordination), tremors, and disturbances of gait and equilibrium.

The **diencephalon** lies between the cerebrum and the midbrain. It consists of several structures located around the third ventricle, primarily the thalamus and hypothalamus. The **thalamus** primarily functions as a relay station that receives and processes sensory information of almost all kinds of sensory impulses before sending this information on to the cerebral cortex. The tiny **hypothalamus** is an extremely complex structure that functions as a link between the mind and body and is the site of "pleasure" or "reward" centers for such primary drives as eating, drinking, and mating. It plays a major role in regulating the body's internal environment by coordinating the activities of the autonomic nervous system and secreting the **releasing hormones** that control the secretion of hormones by the anterior and posterior portions of the pituitary gland. The hypothalamus is also important in helping to maintain a normal body temperature and keeping the individual in a waking state.

The spinal cord lies within the vertebral column and extends from its junction with the brainstem at the foramen magnum to approximately the lower border of the first lumbar vertebra. It consists of an inner core of gray matter surrounded by white matter tracts. The basic function of the spinal cord is to conduct impulses up the cord to the brain (ascending tracts) and down the cord from the brain to spinal nerves (descending tracts). It also serves as the center for spinal reflexes, involuntary responses such as the knee jerk (patellar reflex).

The delicate, yet vital, brain and spinal cord are protected by two layers of coverings. The outer bony coverings are the cranial bones of the skull encasing the brain and the vertebrae surrounding the spinal cord. The inner coverings consist of three distinct layers of **meninges.** The innermost layer adhering to the outer surface of the brain and spinal cord is the transparent **pia mater,** and the tough outermost covering is termed the **dura mater.** Between these layers is the delicate, cobweblike **arachnoid mem-**

brane. Inflammation of these three protective layers is called **meningitis.**

Three extensions of the dura mater separate portions of the brain. The **falx cerebri** projects downward into the longitudinal fissure to separate the cerebral hemispheres. Similarly, the **falx cerebelli** separates the two cerebellar hemispheres. The **tentorium cerebelli** forms a tentlike covering over the cerebellum that separates it from the occipital lobe of the cerebrum.

In addition to bony and membranous coverings, the brain and spinal cord are further protected by a cushion of fluid both around them and within them. The ventricles are four spaces within the brain that contain cerebrospinal fluid (CSF). There are two large lateral ventricles, one located in each cerebral hemisphere. The slitlike third ventricle lies between the right and left thalamus. The anterior parts of the lateral ventricles (frontal horns) are connected by a Y-shaped canal that extends downward to open into the upper part of the third ventricle at the foramen of Monro. The fourth ventricle is a diamond-shaped space between the cerebellum posteriorly and the medulla and pons anteriorly. It is continuous inferiorly with the central canal of the spinal cord. The third and fourth ventricles are connected by the aqueduct of Sylvius, a narrow canal that runs through the posterior part of the midbrain.

CSF is formed by filtration of plasma from blood in the choroid plexuses, networks of capillaries that project from the pia mater into the lateral ventricles and into the roofs of the third and fourth ventricles. After flowing through the ventricular system, the fluid circulates in the subarachnoid space around the brain and spinal cord before being absorbed into venous blood through arachnoid villi. Obstruction of CSF circulation results in hydrocephalus.

TRAUMATIC DISEASES OF THE BRAIN

In the patient with head trauma the purpose of radiographic imaging is to detect a surgically correctable hematoma. Emergency CT has virtually replaced all other radiographic investigations in patients with suspected neurologic dysfunction resulting from head injury. Because the presence or absence of a skull fracture does not correlate with intracranial abnormalities, plain radiographs of the skull are no longer indicated in the patient with head trauma.

Because of medicolegal reasons and the fear of missing a skull fracture, CT scans (and plain skull radiographs) are often overused. The following indications have been established for the use of radiographic procedures in the patient with head trauma:

1. Unexplained focal neurologic signs
2. Unconsciousness (including the unarousable alcoholic)
3. Documented decreasing level of consciousness or progressive mental deterioration

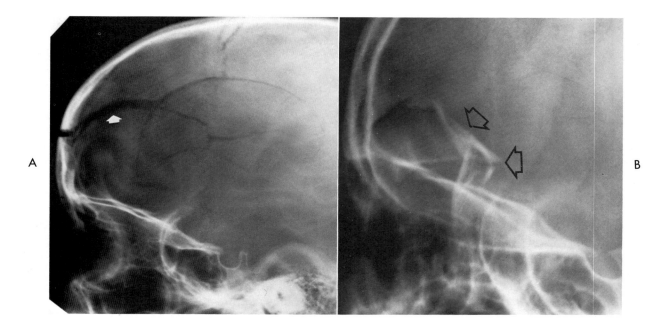

Figure 7-1 Skull fracture. **A,** Lateral projection of skull shows widely separated fracture *(arrow)* extending to star-shaped array of linear fractures. **B,** In another patient, lateral projection shows severely depressed skull fracture *(arrows).*

4. History of previous craniotomy with shunt tube in place
5. Skull depression or subcutaneous foreign body palpable or identified by a probe through a laceration or puncture wound
6. Hemotympanum or fluid discharge from the ear
7. Discharge of CSF from the nose
8. Ecchymosis over the mastoid process (Battle's sign)
9. Bilateral orbital ecchymoses (raccoon eyes)

Skull fracture

A linear skull fracture appears on a plain radiograph as a sharp lucent line that is often irregular or jagged and occasionally branches (Figure 7-1). The fracture must be distinguished from suture lines, which generally have serrated edges and tend to be bilateral and symmetric, and vascular grooves, which usually have a smooth curving course and are not as sharp or distinct as a fracture line. The location of a linear skull fracture can indicate possible complications. A fracture that crosses a dural vascular groove may cause vessel laceration leading to an epidural hematoma. A fracture involving the sinuses or mastoid air cells may result in post-traumatic pneumocephalus, with air seen in the ventricles on plain radiographs. A diastatic fracture refers to a linear fracture that intersects a suture and courses along it, causing sutural separation.

More severe trauma, especially if localized to a small area of the skull, may force a fragment of bone to be separated and depressed into the cranial cavity (Figure 7-2). The underlying dura is frequently torn, and there is a relatively high incidence of cerebral parenchymal injury. Depressed fractures are often stellate (star-shaped), with multiple fracture lines radiating outward from a central point. When the fracture is viewed en face, the overlap of fragments makes the fracture line appear denser than the normal bone. Tangential views are required to determine the amount of depression.

Fractures limited to the base of the skull are often hidden by the complex basal anatomy and may be very difficult to visualize on plain radiographs. A finding suggestive of a basilar skull fracture is an air-fluid level in the sphenoid sinus seen on an erect or cross-table lateral projection of the skull obtained with a horizontal x-ray beam. CT can demonstrate the presence of blood or fluid in the basilar cisterns and show some basilar skull fractures that are not visible on routine skull radiographs. Potential complications of basal skull fractures include leakage of CSF, meningitis, and damage to the facial nerve or auditory apparatus within the petrous bone.

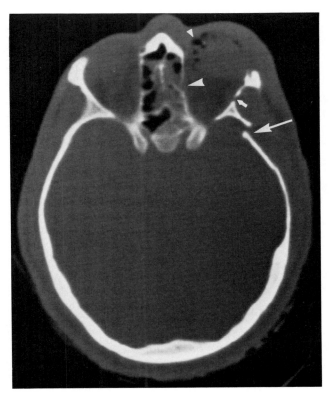

Figure 7-2 Skull fracture. CT bone window image demonstrates depressed temporal fracture (*long arrow*). Note also lateral orbital wall fracture (*short arrow*), medial orbital wall fracture (*large arrowhead*), and ethmoid opacification caused by hemorrhage. There is also air in orbital soft tissues (*small arrowhead*) resulting from medial fracture into ethmoids. (*From Pressman BD: In Eisenberg RL, editor: Diagnostic imaging: an algorithmic approach, Philadelphia, JB Lippincott Co, 1988.*)

It must be stressed that the presence or absence of a skull fracture does not correlate with intracranial abnormalities. Indeed, serious treatable intracranial hematomas can be present without skull fractures.

Epidural hematoma

Epidural hematomas are caused by acute arterial bleeding and most commonly form over the parietotemporal convexity. Because of a high arterial pressure, epidural hematomas rapidly cause significant mass effect and acute neurologic symptoms. Because the dura is very adherent to the inner table of the skull, an epidural hematoma typically appears as a biconvex (lens-shaped), peripheral high-density lesion (Figure 7-3). There usually is a shift of the midline structures toward the opposite side unless a contralateral balancing hematoma is present. If not promptly recognized, an epidural hematoma can lead to rapid progressive loss of consciousness, dilation of the ipsilateral pupil, compression of the

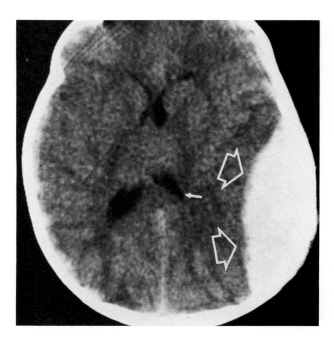

Figure 7-3 Acute epidural hematoma. CT scan of 4-year-old involved in motor vehicle accident shows characteristic lens-shaped epidural hematoma *(open arrows)*. Substantial mass effect associated with hematoma distorts lateral ventricle *(solid arrow)*.

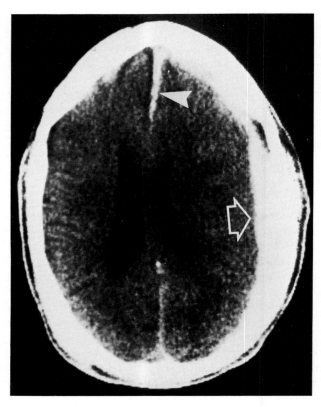

Figure 7-4 Acute subdural hematoma. High-density, crescent-shaped lesion *(arrow)* adjacent to inner table of skull. Hematoma extends into interhemispheric fissure *(arrowhead)*.

upper midbrain, and eventually compression of the entire brainstem and death.

Subdural hematoma

Subdural hematomas reflect venous bleeding, most commonly from ruptured veins between the dura and meninges. Symptoms may occur within the first few minutes; however, because of the low pressure of venous bleeding, patients with subdural hematomas tend to have a chronic course with symptoms of headache, agitation, confusion, drowsiness, and gradual neurologic deficits.

An acute subdural hematoma typically appears on CT scans as a peripheral zone of increased density that follows the surface of the brain and has a crescentic shape adjacent to the inner table of the skull (Figure 7-4). There usually is an associated mass effect with displacement of midline structures and obliteration of sulci over the affected hemisphere. The absence of displacement away from the side of a lesion suggests the not infrequent presence of bilateral subdural hematomas. On MRI scans, a sub-

dural hematoma is detectable within a few days as an extra-axial mass of high signal intensity representing the accumulation of methemoglobin (Figure 7-5).

Serial CT scans demonstrate a gradual decrease in the attenuation value of a subdural hematoma over a period of weeks. With absorption and lysis of the blood clot, the hematoma becomes isodense with normal brain tissue, and the lesion may be identified only because of its mass effect. At this stage, scanning after the administration of contrast material may be of value because of enhancement of the membrane around the subdural hematoma and identification of the cortical veins. MRI scanning of a CT-isodense lesion may show medial displacement of the superficial cerebral veins, an indication of an extracerebral mass, as well as the entire extent of the hematoma over the cerebral convexity. A chronic subdural hematoma has a density similar to that of spinal fluid (Figure 7-6). At times, the small bridging veins associated with a chronic subdural hematoma may bleed and produce the difficult prob-

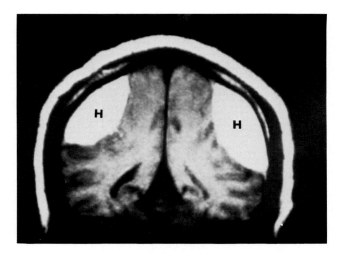

Figure 7-5 Bilateral subdural hematoma. Axial MR image shows high signal intensity of bilateral subdural collections *(H)*.

lem of an acute subdural hematoma superimposed on a chronic one.

Cerebral contusion

Cerebral contusion is an injury to brain tissue caused by movement of the brain within the calvarium after blunt trauma to the skull. Contusions occur when the brain contacts rough skull surfaces such as the superior orbital roof and petrous ridges. The patient loses consciousness and cannot remember the traumatic event. Cerebral contusions typically appear on CT scans as low-density areas of edema and tissue necrosis, with or without nonhomogeneous-density zones reflecting multiple small areas of hemorrhage (Figure 7-7). After the administration of intravenous contrast material, contusions generally enhance for several weeks after the injury because of a breakdown of the blood-brain barrier. On MRI scans, the cerebral edema causes high signal intensity on T2-weighted images; associated areas of hemorrhage may produce high signal intensity regions on T1-weighted scans.

Intracerebral hematoma

Traumatic hemorrhage into the brain parenchyma can result from shearing forces to intraparenchymal arteries, which tend to occur at the junction of the gray and white matter. Injury to the intima of intracranial vessels can cause the development of traumatic aneurysms, which can rupture. On CT scans, an intracerebral hematoma appears as a well-circumscribed, homogeneous, high-density region that usually is surrounded by areas of low-density edema

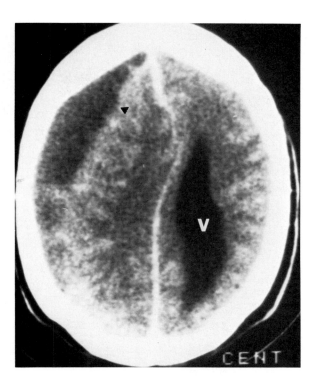

Figure 7-6 Chronic right subdural hematoma. Crescent-shaped, low-density region in right frontoparietal area *(arrows)*. Herniation of brain tissue across midline underneath falx is present. *V,* Dilated left lateral ventricle.

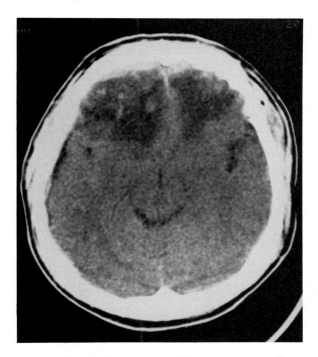

Figure 7-7 Cerebral contusion. CT scan shows small punctate hemorrhages (high density) within extensive areas of edema (low density). *(From Pressman BD: In Eisenberg RL, editor: Diagnostic imaging: an algorithmic approach, Philadelphia, JB Lippincott Co, 1988.)*

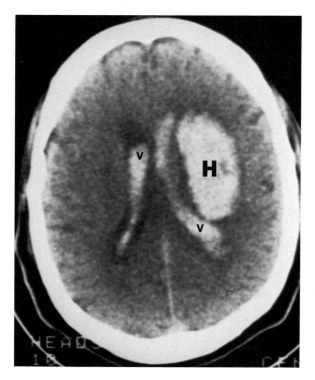

Figure 7-8 Intracerebral hematoma. Large homogeneous high-density area *(H)* with acute bleeding into lateral ventricles *(V)*.

(Figure 7-8). As the blood components within the hematoma disintegrate, the lesion eventually becomes isodense with normal brain (usually 2 to 4 weeks after injury). On MRI scans, the hematoma has high signal intensity. A chronic hematoma filled with hemosiderin will appear black on T2-weighted images.

Although most intracerebral hematomas develop immediately after head injury, delayed hemorrhage is common. This is especially frequent after the evacuation of acute subdural hematomas that are compressing (tamponading) potential bleeding sites. Therefore a repeat CT (or MRI) scan is often performed within 48 hours in patients who have undergone decompressive surgery.

Subarachnoid hemorrhage

Injury to surface veins, cerebral parenchyma, or cortical arteries can produce bleeding into the ventricular system. On a CT scan, a subarachnoid hemorrhage appears as increased density within the basilar cisterns, cerebral fissures, and sulci. Identification of the falx cerebri, straight sinus, or superior sagittal sinus on noncontrast CT scans is often considered an indication of subarachnoid blood in the interhemispheric fissure. However, with high-res-

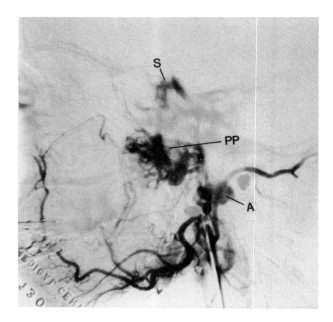

Figure 7-9 Carotid injury. From Eisenberg RL: Diagnostic imaging in surgery, New York, McGraw-Hill Book Co., 1987.

olution scanners, this appearance may be seen in patients with a normal or calcified falx.

Carotid artery injury

The extracerebral carotid arteries can be injured by penetrating trauma to the neck as from gunshot wounds or stabbing. Angiography can demonstrate laceration of the artery or intimal damage that may result in either dissection or thrombotic occlusion (Figure 7-9). Hyperextension injuries from motor vehicle accidents can cause intimal damage to the carotid or vertebral arteries that may result in pseudoaneurysm formation. Traumatic arteriovenous fistulas usually arise between the internal carotid artery and the cavernous sinus. In this condition carotid arteriography demonstrates opacification of the cavernous sinus during the arterial phase. Reverse flow from the cavernous sinus may rapidly opacify a markedly dilated ophthalmic vein. The placement of a detachable balloon catheter within the fistula using angiographic guidance may eliminate the need for surgical intervention.

Facial fractures

Although it is padded by overlying skin and fat and the muscles of expression, the face consists of thin and poorly supported bone that can easily break in response to a traumatic force. The purpose of radiographic imaging in the patient with a facial injury is to demonstrate major disruptions of the facial skeleton and displacement of fracture fragments that

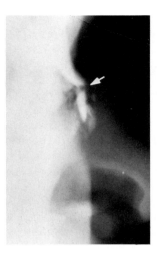

Figure 7-10 Depressed nasal fracture *(arrow)*.

will affect the surgical reduction and stabilization of the fracture.

Plain radiographs of the face are usually performed as an initial screening procedure, especially in a severely traumatized patient with substantial injuries to multiple organ systems. Whenever possible, films should be obtained with the patient in the erect position to show any air-fluid levels within the sinuses that could indicate recent hemorrhage and raise the suspicion of an underlying fracture. Complex-motion (pluridirectional) tomography can

blur unrelated overlying structures and thus display details of injury that are obscure or only suspected on plain radiographs. CT can demonstrate soft-tissue abnormalities, such as intraorbital or retrobulbar hematomas, that are impossible to detect by conventional means. In addition bone detail and displacement can be exquisitely demonstrated when CT window and level settings are adjusted to optimize bony structures.

Fractures of the nasal bone are the most common facial fractures. Isolated nasal fractures vary from simple, nondisplaced linear fractures to comminuted lesions with depression of the septum and lateral splaying of the fracture fragments (Figure 7-10). These fractures are best demonstrated on an underexposed (soft-tissue) lateral projection, which also can define interruption of the anterior nasal spine—the anterior projection of the maxilla at the base of the cartilaginous nasal septum. Most fractures are transverse and tend to depress the distal portion of the nasal bones.

A blowout fracture is caused by a direct blow to the front of the orbit that causes a rapid increase in intraorbital pressure. The fracture occurs in the thinnest, weakest portion of the orbit, which is the orbital floor just above the maxillary sinus. Plain radiographs (modified Waters' method) and thin-section tomography can demonstrate most blowout fractures (Figure 7-11), although CT may be necessary for better visualization and for detecting en-

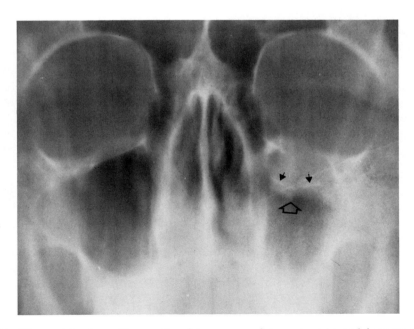

Figure 7-11 Blowout fracture. Conventional tomogram shows comminuted fracture of floor of left orbit with inferior displacement of fracture fragments *(solid arrows)*. Note characteristic soft-tissue shadow *(open arrow)* protruding through floor into superior portion of maxillary sinus.

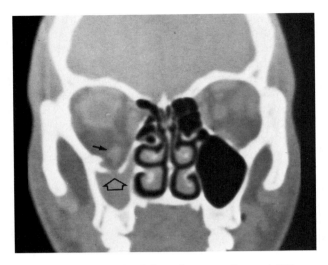

Figure 7-12 CT of orbital floor fracture. Coronal CT scan using bone window shows fractured orbital floor as double-hinged trap door with separation in center *(open arrow).* There is opacification of right maxillary sinus. Note displacement of inferior rectus muscle *(solid arrow)* in this patient who had limited upward gaze. *(Courtesy Kenneth D. Dolan, MD.)*

trapment of the extraocular muscles in the upper portion of the adjacent maxillary sinus (Figure 7-12). The fracture segment can be comminuted, with a sagging, hammocklike appearance, or be of the trap-door variety, with a displaced segment hanging into the antrum by a periosteal hinge. Herniation of orbital fat and extraocular muscles into the fractured orbital floor produces a characteristic soft-tissue shadow protruding through the floor into the superior portion of the maxillary sinus. Opacification of the sinus caused by hemorrhage and mucosal edema is an indirect sign of orbital floor fracture. The presence of air within the orbit (orbital emphysema) indicates that there is a communication with a paranasal sinus, usually the ethmoid, as a result of an associated fracture of the medial wall of the orbit through the lamina papyracea.

The zygomatic arch is vulnerable to a blow from the side of the face, which produces a fracture with inward displacement of the fragments centrally and outward displacement of the fragments at the zygomatic and temporal ends of the arch (Figure 7-13). Zygomatic arch fractures are best demonstrated on underexposed films taken in the basal (submentovertex) projection ("jug handle" view).

A tripod fracture consists of fractures of the zygomatic arch and the orbital floor or rim combined with separation of the zygomaticofrontal suture (Figure 7-14). It is so named because it reflects separation of the zygoma from its three principal attachments. The resulting free-floating zygoma may

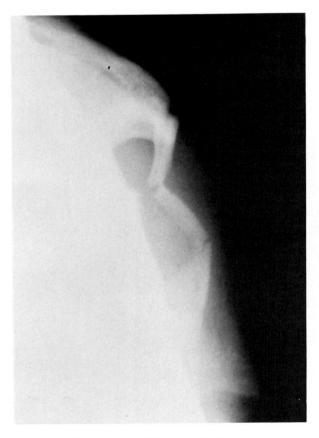

Figure 7-13 Zygomatic arch fracture. Submentovertex projection demonstrates three fractures on left with depression of zygomatic arch. *(Courtesy Kenneth D. Dolan, MD.)*

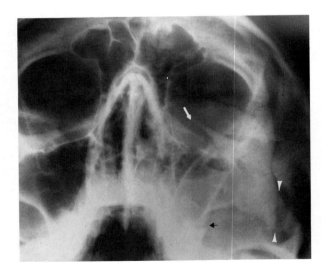

Figure 7-14 Tripod fracture. Interruption of orbital rim *(white arrow),* lateral maxillary fracture *(black arrow),* and undisplaced zygomatic arch fracture *(arrowheads)* are present. *(From Dolan K, Jacoby C, and Smoker W: The radiology of facial features, RadioGraphics 4:576-663, 1984.)*

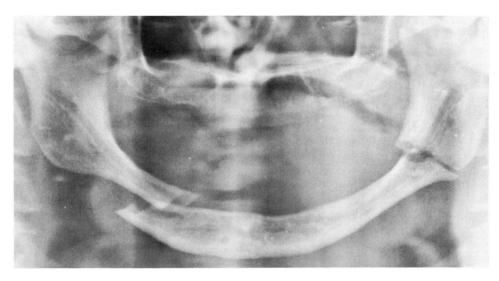

Figure 7-15 Mandibular fracture. Panorex examination in edentulous (without teeth) patient shows fractures of left angle and right body of mandible. *(From Rogers LF: Radiology of skeletal trauma, New York, Churchill Livingstone, 1982.)*

cause facial disfigurement if not diagnosed and properly treated.

The mandible is a prominent, exposed segment of the facial skeleton and is thus a common site for both intentional and accidental trauma. Plain radiographs with oblique views, combined with Panorex tomography, can demonstrate most mandibular

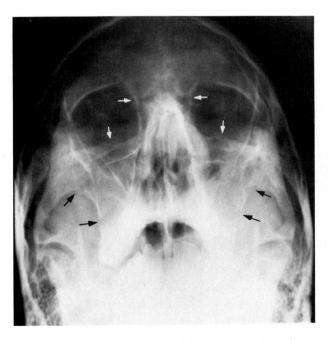

Figure 7-16 LeFort II fracture. Waters' projection shows large separated fragment produced by multiple fractures *(arrows). (From Dolan K, Jacoby C, and Smoker W: The radiology of facial features, RadioGraphics 4:576-663, 1984.)*

fractures (Figure 7-15). The angle of the mandible is the most frequent site of fracture, although fractures can involve any portion of the body and the condylar and coronoid processes. Because the mandible functions essentially as a bony ring, bilateral fractures are common.

LeFort fractures refer to severe injuries in which separation at the fracture site results in the formation of a large, complex detached fragment that is unstable and may have its position altered relative to its site of origin. LeFort fractures involve bilateral and horizontal fractures of the maxillae and are classified as types I, II, or III, depending on the extent of injury (Figure 7-16).

TUMORS OF THE CENTRAL NERVOUS SYSTEM

Intracranial neoplasms present clinically with seizure disorders or gradual neurologic deficits (difficulty thinking, slow comprehension, weakness, headache). The specific clinical presentation and radiographic appearance depend on the location of the tumor and the site of the subsequent mass effect. MRI is generally considered to be the most sensitive technique for detecting most suspected brain tumors. In general, both the tumor and its surrounding edema have high signal intensity on T2-weighted images. In addition to its exquisite sensitivity in detecting pathologic alteration of normal tissue constituents, MRI provides excellent delineation of tumor extent and can show associated abnormalities such as hydrocephalus. This modality is of special value in imaging neoplasms of the brain-stem and posterior fossa, which may be poorly seen on CT.

CT with contrast enhancement is an excellent examination for evaluating a patient with suspected brain tumor. It is of special value for detecting punctate or larger calcification that cannot be shown by MRI. Although skull radiographs were used in the past to demonstrate tumoral calcification, bone erosion, and displacement of the calcified pineal gland, plain films are no longer indicated, since this information can be more effectively obtained on CT scans.

Before the advent of CT, cerebral arteriography was used to show such evidence of brain tumors as mass effect, contralateral displacement of midline arteries and veins, abnormal vessels with tumor staining, and early venous filling. At present, the major use of arteriography is to precisely delineate the arterial and venous anatomy before surgical therapy and to evaluate those cases in which a vascular anomaly is a strong consideration in the differential diagnosis of a tumor. Radionuclide brain scans have a relatively high rate of detection of cerebral tumors but are far less specific than CT or MRI.

Glioma

Gliomas are the most common primary brain tumors. They spread by direct extension and can cross from one cerebral hemisphere to the other through connecting white matter tracts such as the corpus callosum. Gliomas have a peak incidence in middle adult life and are infrequent in persons less than 30 years of age.

Glioblastomas are highly malignant lesions that are predominantly cerebral, although similar tumors may occur in the brainstem, cerebellum, or spinal cord. Astrocytomas are slowly growing tumors that have an infiltrative character and can form large cavities or pseudocysts. Favored sites are the cerebrum, cerebellum, thalamus, optic chiasm, and pons.

Less frequent types of gliomas are ependymoma, medulloblastoma, and oligodendrocytoma. Ependymomas most commonly arise from the walls of the fourth ventricle, especially in children, and from the lateral ventricles in adults. Medulloblastomas are rapidly growing tumors that develop in the posterior part of the vermis in children and, rarely, in the cerebellar hemisphere in adults. The tumor tends to spread through the subarachnoid space, with metastatic deposits occurring anywhere within the brain or spinal column. Oligodendrocytomas are slow-growing lesions that usually arise in the cerebrum and have a tendency to calcify.

On MRI scans (Figure 7-17), gliomas typically appear as masses of high signal intensity on T2-weighted images. They may be of low intensity or isointense on T1-weighted sequences.

On noncontrast CT scans, gliomas most commonly are seen as single, nonhomogeneous masses. Low-grade astrocytomas tend to be low-density lesions (Figure 7-18); glioblastomas most frequently

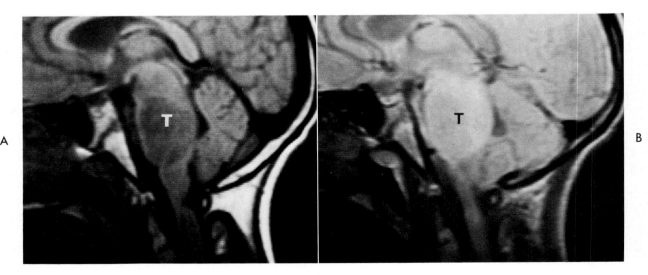

Figure 7-17 Brainstem glioma. Sagittal MRI scans show enlargement of brain stem involving pons and midbrain. Note that various imaging techniques can alter characteristics of tumor (T). On T1-weighted, image, **A,** tumor is gray (low-intensity signal); on T2-weighted, image, **B,** tumor now appears white (high-intensity signal).

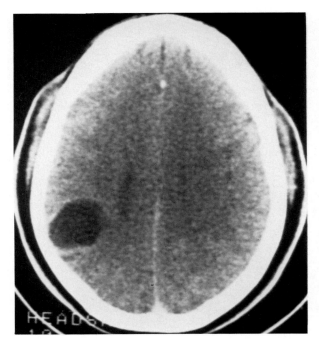

Figure 7-18 Cystic astrocytoma. CT scan shows hypodense mass with thin rim of contrast enhancement.

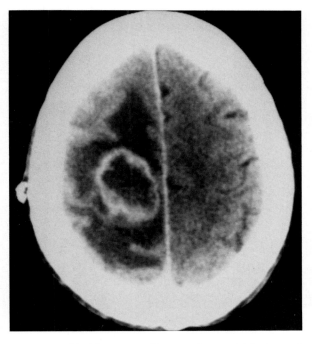

Figure 7-19 Glioblastoma. CT scan shows thick, irregular ring-enhancing lesion associated with large amount of surrounding low-attenuation edema.

contain areas of both increased and decreased density, although a broad spectrum of CT appearances can occur. Edema is often seen in the adjacent subcortical white matter. After the intravenous injection of contrast material, virtually all gliomas enhance, with the most malignant lesions tending to enhance to the greatest degree (Figure 7-19). The most common pattern is an irregular ring of contrast enhancement, representing solid vascularized tumor, surrounding a central low-density area of necrosis. Contrast enhancement also can appear as patches of increased density distributed irregularly throughout a low-density lesion or as rounded nodules of increased density within the mass.

Meningioma

Meningioma is a benign tumor that arises from arachnoid lining cells and is attached to the dura. The most common sites of meningioma are the convexity of the calvarium, olfactory groove, tuberculum sellae, parasagittal region, Sylvian fissure, cerebellopontine angle, and spinal canal.

Because meningiomas tend to be isointense with brain on both T1- and T2-weighted images, anatomic distortion is the key to the MRI diagnosis (Figure 7-20). A thin rim of low intensity may separate the tumor from adjacent brain. Calcification within a meningioma may produce nonuniform signal or fo-

cal signal void. Surrounding edema may make the lesion easier to identify. Just as the detection of meningiomas by CT is facilitated by the use of iodinated contrast material, paramagnetic contrast agents can enhance the detection of meningiomas on MRI.

CT typically shows a meningioma as a rounded, sharply delineated, isodense or hyperdense tumor abutting a dural surface. Calcification often is seen within the mass on noncontrast scans. After the intravenous injection of contrast material, there is intense homogeneous enhancement, which reflects the highly vascular nature of the tumor (Figure 7-21).

Pronounced dilation of meningeal and diploic vessels, which provide part of the blood supply to the tumor, may produce prominent grooves in the calvarium on plain films of the skull. Calvarial hyperostosis (increased density) may develop because of invasion of the bone by tumor cells that stimulate osteoblastic activity. Dense calcification or granular psammomatous deposits may be seen within the tumor (Figure 7-22).

Arteriography can demonstrate the feeding arteries, which most commonly arise from both the internal and external carotid artery circulation. Preoperative embolization of the external carotid artery supply can decrease the amount of blood loss at surgery.

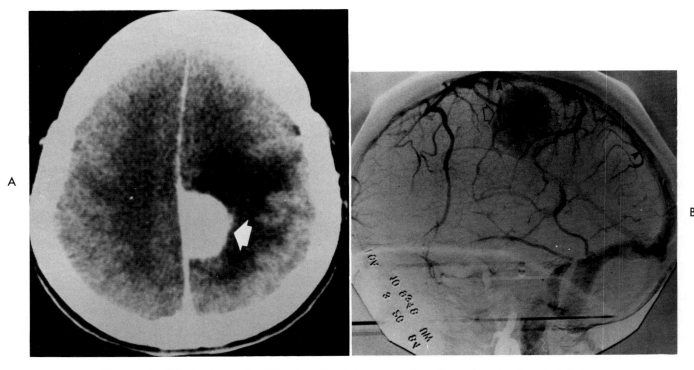

Figure 7-20 Meningioma. Huge mass *(arrowheads)* that appears hypointense on T1-weighted coronal MRI scan, **A,** and hyperintense on T2-weighted image, **B.** Note dramatic shift of ventricle *(v)* caused by mass effect of tumor. Arrows point to areas of hemorrhage within neoplasm (arrowheads).

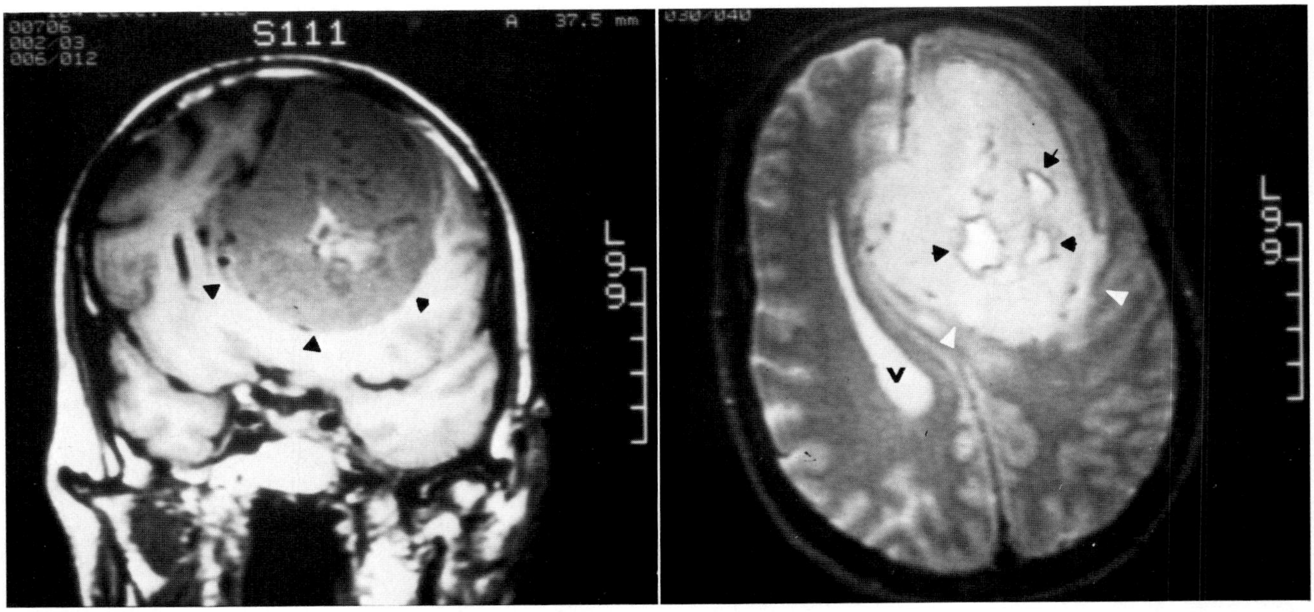

Figure 7-21 Meningioma. **A,** CT scan after intravenous injection of contrast material shows uniformly enhancing mass *(arrow)* with surrounding low-density edema attached to falx. **B,** Venous phase of carotid arteriogram shows characteristic prominent vascular blush *(arrow)* of meningioma. Note that superior sagittal sinus *(arrowheads)* is patent.

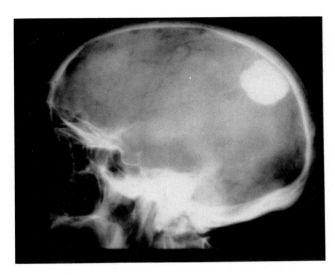

Figure 7-22 Parietal meningioma. Plain skull film shows dense calcification in tumor.

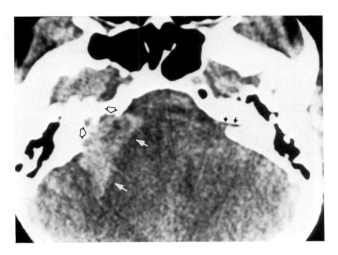

Figure 7-23 Acoustic neuroma. CT scan shows widening and erosion of right internal auditory canal *(open arrows)* associated with large extra-axial mass *(white arrows)* in right cerebellopontine angle. Solid black arrows point to normal internal auditory canal on left. *(From Williams AL and Haughton VM: Cranial computed tomography, St. Louis, The CV Mosby Co, 1985.)*

Acoustic neuroma

Acoustic neuroma is a slowly growing benign tumor that may occur as a solitary lesion or as part of the syndrome of neurofibromatosis. The tumor arises from Schwann cells in the vestibular portion of the auditory (eighth cranial) nerve. It usually originates in the internal auditory canal and extends into the cerebellopontine angle cistern.

MRI scans (T1-weighted) exquisitely show the tumor as a focal or generalized enlargement of the eighth cranial nerve. This technique can even demonstrate small intracanalicular tumors confined to the internal auditory canal, which may be impossible to show on CT unless contrast material (metrizamide or air) is administered into the ventricular system. CT scans demonstrate enlargement and erosion of the internal auditory canal and a uniformly enhancing mass in the cerebellopontine angle (Figure 7-23). Very large tumors may compress the fourth ventricle and lead to the development of hydrocephalus.

Pituitary adenoma

Pituitary adenomas, almost all of which arise in the anterior lobe, constitute more than 10% of all intracranial tumors. Most are nonsecreting **chromophobe adenomas.** As chromophobe tumors enlarge, the adjoining secreting cells within the sella turcica are compressed, leading to diminished secretion and decreased levels of growth hormone, gonadotropins, thyrotropic hormone, and adrenocorticotrophic hormone (ACTH). Large chromophobe adenomas can extend upward to distort the region of the optic chiasm, whereas lateral expansion of tumor can

compress the cranial nerves passing within the cavernous sinus.

Hormone-secreting pituitary tumors can cause clinical symptoms even if too small to produce mechanical mass effect. Hypersecretion of growth hormone results in gigantism in adolescents (before the epiphyses have closed) and acromegaly in adults (after the epiphyses have closed). Excess secretion of ACTH by a pituitary tumor results in the hypersecretion of steroid hormones from the adrenal cortical cortex and symptoms of Cushing's disease. Hypersecretion of thyroid-stimulating hormone (TSH) leads to hyperthyroidism; excess secretion of prolactin by a pituitary tumor in women causes the amenorrhea/galactorrhea syndrome.

Thin-section CT and MRI are the examinations of choice in evaluating a patient with a suspected pituitary tumor. After the intravenous administration of contrast material, large pituitary tumors are typically homogeneous and hyperdense with respect to surrounding brain tissue. Most pituitary microadenomas are of lower density than the normal pituitary gland. CT can also demonstrate adjacent bone erosion, tumor extension beyond the confines of the sella, and impression on nearby structures such as the third ventricle, optic nerves, or optic chiasm (Figure 7-24).

Coronal T1-weighted MRI scans show a microadenoma as a low-intensity focal lesion associated with contralateral deviation of the pituitary stalk and

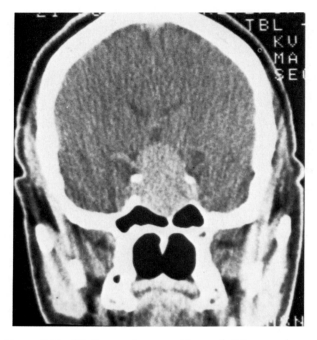

Figure 7-24 Pituitary adenoma. Coronal CT scan shows enhancing mass filling and extending out from pituitary fossa. Note erosion of base of sella.

an upwardly convex contour of the gland (Figure 7-25). After the injection of a paramagnetic contrast agent, the pituitary tumor can be clearly demonstrated as a high-intensity area on T1-weighted images.

Although plain skull radiographs can show enlargement of the sella turcica, erosion of the dorsum sellae, and a double floor resulting from the unequal downward growth of the mass, this imaging modality now is of value only in the incidental detection of sellar enlargement on films taken for other purposes.

Craniopharyngioma

Craniopharyngioma is a benign tumor that contains both cystic and solid components. The lesion usually originates above the sella turcica, depressing the optic chiasm and extending up into the third ventricle. Less commonly, a craniopharyngioma lies within the sella, where it compresses the pituitary gland and may erode adjacent bony walls.

Most craniopharyngiomas have calcification that can be detected on plain skull films or CT scans (Figure 7-26). In cystic lesions the shell-like calcification lies along the periphery of the tumor; in mixed or solid lesions, the calcification is nodular, amorphous, or cloudlike. CT clearly demonstrates the cystic and solid components of the mass. After the intravenous administration of contrast material, there is variable enhancement, depending on the

A 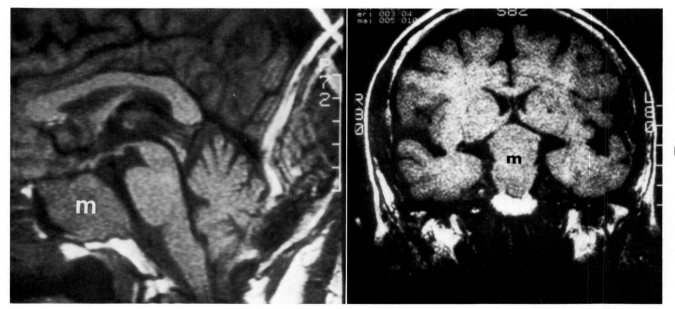 B

Figure 7-25 Pituitary adenoma. **A,** Sagittal and, **B,** coronal MRI scans demonstrate large mass (*m*) that arises from sella turcica and extends upward to fill suprasellar cistern.

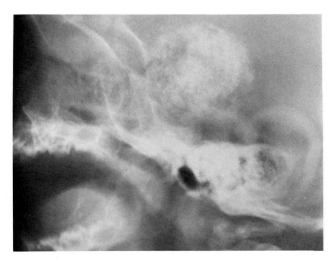

Figure 7-26 Craniopharyngioma. Plain skull radiograph shows large suprasellar calcified mass in child.

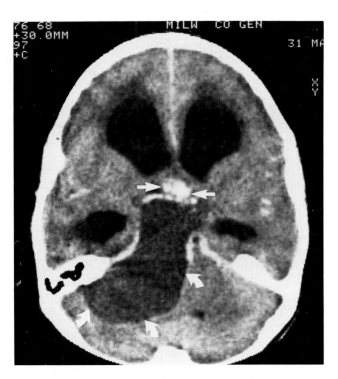

Figure 7-27 Craniopharyngioma. CT scan shows rim-enhancing tumor that contains dense calcification *(straight arrows)* and large cystic component *(curved arrows)* that extends into posterior fossa. Note associated hydrocephalus. *(From Williams AL and Haughton VM: Cranial computed tomography, St. Louis, The CV Mosby Co, 1985.)*

type of calcification and the amount of cystic components within the tumor (Figure 7-27). CT can also demonstrate hydrocephalus if the tumor has expanded to obstruct one or both of the foramina of Monro.

The MRI appearance of craniopharyngioma depends on the tissue components of the tumor. Cystic areas have low signal intensity on T1-weighted scans and high signal intensity on T2-weighted scans; fat-containing regions have high signal intensity on T1-weighted images and are of moderate intensity on T2-weighted scans (Figure 7-28). Large areas of calcification appear dark on all imaging sequences.

Pineal tumors

The most common tumors of the pineal gland are germinomas and teratomas, both of which occur predominantly in males less than 25 years of age and may be associated with precocious puberty.

On CT, germinomas appear as hyperdense or isodense masses that tend to deform or displace the posterior aspect of the third ventricle and often obliterate the quadrigeminal cistern. Punctate calcification can often be detected within the mass (Figure 7-29). Intense enhancement of the tumor occurs after the injection of contrast material. Teratomas in the pineal region typically appear as hypodense masses with internal calcification. Occasionally, other formed elements (e.g., teeth) can occur. Contrast enhancement is usually much less pronounced than with germinomas. Large pineal tumors may cause obstructive hydrocephalus with ventricular dilation.

A small number of tumors with the histologic

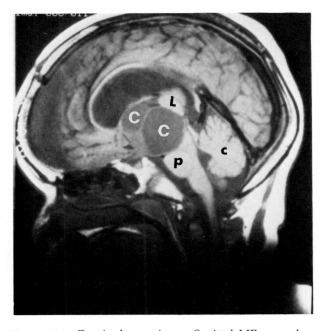

Figure 7-28 Craniopharyngioma. Sagittal MR scan demonstrates large multiloculated suprasellar mass with cystic *(C)* and lipid *(L)* components. *p,* Pons; *c,* cerebellum.

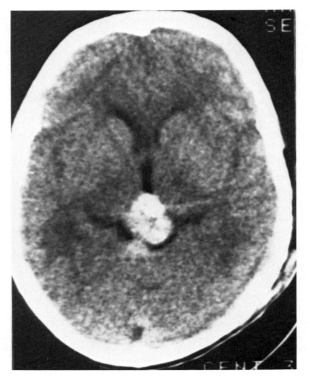

Figure 7-29 Pineal teratoma. Nonenhanced CT scan shows inhomogeneous mass containing large amount of calcification.

appearance of pinealomas appear elsewhere in the brain at some distance from the normal pineal gland. These "ectopic pinealomas" generally occur in the anterior aspect of the third ventricle or within the suprasellar cistern. They may produce a clinical triad of bitemporal hemianopsia, hypopituitarism, and diabetes insipidus that simulates a craniopharyngioma.

Chordoma

Chordomas are tumors that arise from remnants of the notochord (the embryonic neural tube). Although any part of the vertebral column and base of the skull can be involved, the most common sites are the clivus and the lower lumbosacral region. The tumors are locally invasive but do not metastasize. Chordomas arising at the base of the skull produce the striking clinical picture of multiple cranial nerve palsies on one or both sides combined with a retropharyngeal mass and erosion of the clivus.

On plain radiographs, a chordoma tends to be a bulky mass causing ill-defined bone destruction or cortical expansion. Flocculent (fluffy or cloudlike) calcification may develop within a large soft-tissue mass (Figure 7-30, *A*). On CT scans, chordomas at the base of the skull tend to appear as lesions that are slightly denser than brain tissue and often dem-

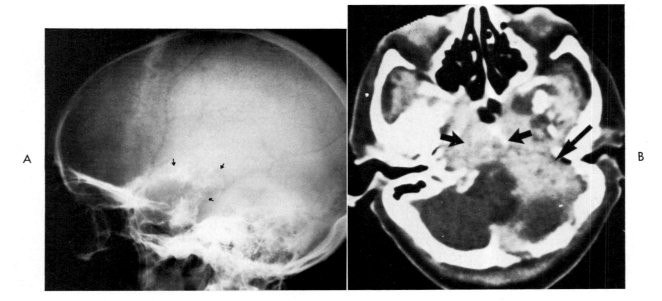

Figure 7-30 Chordoma. **A,** Plain skull radiograph shows dense calcification (*arrows*) within large soft-tissue mass that has eroded dorsum sellae and upper portion of clivus. **B,** In another patient, CT scan shows enlarging mass with destruction of entire clivus (*short arrows*) and only small bone fragments remaining. Left petrous pyramid is also destroyed (*long arrow*). (*B from Levine HL, Kleefield J, and Rao KCVG: In Lee SH and Rao KCVG, editors: Cranial computed tomography. New York, McGraw-Hill Book Co, 1983.*)

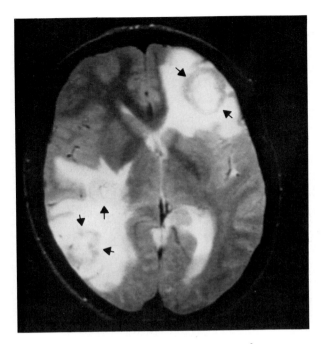

Figure 7-31 Metastases. Axial MRI scan demonstrates three large masses *(arrows)* surrounded by extensive high signal intensity edema.

onstrate moderate contrast enhancement (Figure 7-30, *B*).

Metastatic carcinoma

Carcinomas usually reach the brain by hematogenous spread. Infrequently, epithelial malignancies of the nasopharynx can spread into the cranial cavity through neural foramina or by direct invasion through bone. The most common neoplasms that metastasize to the brain arise in the lung and breast. Melanomas, colon carcinomas, and testicular and kidney tumors also cause brain metastases.

On T2-weighted MRI scans, metastases appear as single or multiple masses of high signal intensity that most commonly are situated at the gray matter–white matter junction (Figure 7-31). Additional lesions can often be demonstrated after the injection of a paramagnetic contrast agent. On CT, brain metastases typically appear as multiple enhancing lesions of various sizes with surrounding sizes of low-density edema (Figures 7-32 and 7-33). On noncontrast scans, metastatic deposits may be hypodense, hyperdense, or similar in density to normal brain tissue, depending on such factors as cellular density, tumor neovascularity, and degree of necrosis. In general, metastases from lung, breast, kidney, and colon tend to be hypodense or isodense; hyperdense metastases often reflect hemorrhage or calcification within or adjacent to the tumor.

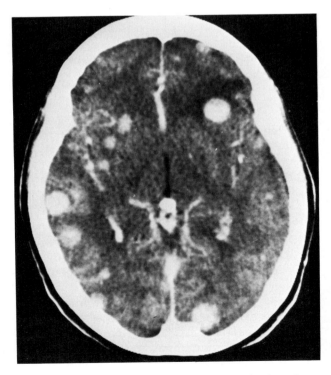

Figure 7-32 Metastases. CT scan shows multiple enhancing masses of various shapes and sizes representing hematogenous metastases from carcinoma of breast.

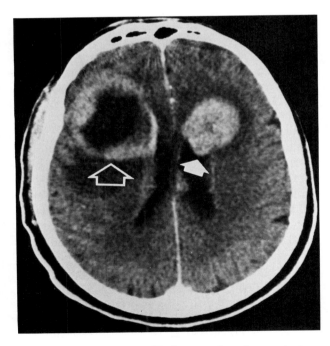

Figure 7-33 Metastases. CT shows enhancing metastases from squamous cell carcinoma of lung that are both ring-enhancing *(open arrow)* and solid *(solid arrow).*

Single metastatic deposits in the brain may be indistinguishable from primary tumors. However, since primary brain neoplasms are unusual in older patients, single lesions in this population should suggest metastatic disease.

INFECTIONS OF THE CENTRAL NERVOUS SYSTEM

With the widespread availability of antibiotics, infectious disease of the CNS is now much less common than previously. Nevertheless, bacterial, fungal, viral, or protozoal organisms can infect the brain parenchyma, meningeal linings, and bones of the skull.

Meningitis

Meningitis is an acute inflammation of the pia mater and arachnoid, the membranes covering the brain and spinal cord. Infecting organisms can reach the meninges from a middle ear, upper respiratory tract, or frontal sinus infection, or they can be spread through the bloodstream from an infection in the lungs or other site. Bacterial meningitis is most commonly due to *Haemophilus influenzae* in neonates and young children and to meningococci and pneumococci in adolescents and adults. Viral meningitis may be caused by mumps, poliovirus, and occasionally by herpes simplex. A chronic form of meningitis can be due to tuberculous infection.

Although the meninges initially demonstrate vascular congestion, edema, and minute hemorrhages, the underlying brain remains intact. CT scans are normal during most acute episodes of meningitis and remain normal if appropriate therapy is promptly instituted. If the infection extends to involve the cortex of the brain and the ependymal lining of the ventricles, noncontrast scans demonstrate increased density in the basal cisterns, interhemispheric fissure, and choroid plexus. This appearance, which frequently simulates contrast enhancement, probably reflects a fibrinous or hemorrhagic exudate with a high protein level in the subarachnoid space of the interhemispheric fissure and basal cisterns. Diffuse brain swelling may symmetrically compress the lateral and third ventricles. Focal edema may produce localized areas of low density. CT is also of value in the early detection of such complications of acute meningitis as arterial or venous vasculitis or thrombosis with infarction (Figure 7-34), hydrocephalus caused by adhesions or thickening of the arachnoid at the base of the brain, subdural effusion or empyema, and brain abscess.

Although acute bacterial meningitis is best evaluated by CT with bone-window settings, plain films

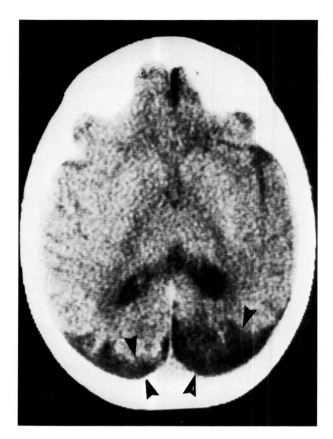

Figure 7-34 Brain infarctions resulting from childhood meningitis. In this 12-year-old girl with cortical blindness as a result of previous meningitis at age 2, CT scan shows bilateral occipital lobe infarctions (*arrowheads*) as low-density lesions. Spasm of cerebral vessels caused by meningitis led to subsequent infarction.

of the sinuses and skull can demonstrate cranial osteomyelitis, paranasal sinusitis, or a skull fracture as the underlying cause of meningitis. Chest radiographs may show a silent area of pneumonia or a lung abscess.

Encephalitis

Encephalitis is a viral inflammation of the brain and meninges that produces symptoms ranging from mild headache and fever to severe cerebral dysfunction, seizures, and coma. Encephalitis caused by herpes simplex is an often fatal, fulminant process. The earliest and predominant CT finding in herpetic encephalitis is poorly marginated, hypodense areas in the temporal and frontal lobes, which are the characteristic sites of involvement in gross pathologic specimens. The low density probably represents a combination of tissue necrosis and focal brain edema. A mass effect is common and may

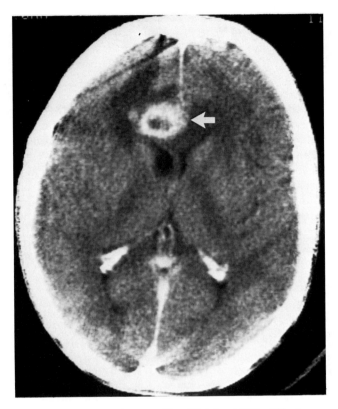

Figure 7-35 Brain abscess *(Candida)* in AIDS. CT shows cystic lesion with thick zone of enhancement *(arrow)* near genu of corpus callosum. *(From Kelly WM and Brant-Zawadzki MB: Acquired immunodeficiency syndrome: neurologic findings, Radiology 149:485-491, 1983.)*

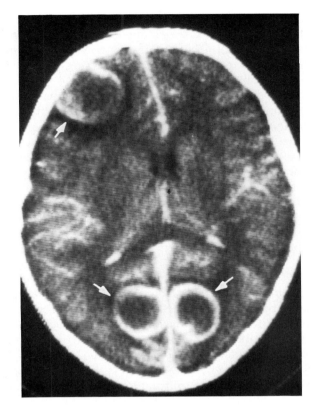

Figure 7-36 Pyogenic brain abscesses. CT scan shows one frontal and two occipital lesions *(arrows)* with relatively thin, uniform rings of enhancement.

be seen as a midline shift or as a focal mass compressing the ventricles or the Sylvian cisterns. Compromise of the blood-brain barrier in areas of rapid, more progressive hemorrhagic necrosis results in a nonhomogeneous pattern of contrast enhancement. Follow-up scans typically demonstrate widespread low-density encephalomalacia involving the temporal and frontal lobes.

In addition to confirming the clinical diagnosis and excluding the presence of an abscess or tumor, CT is important in the evaluation of herpes simplex encephalitis to indicate the best site for biopsy. A definitive diagnosis of herpes infection is essential before beginning treatment with adenine arabinoside, a chemotherapeutic agent that may be neurotoxic, mutagenic, and carcinogenic.

Brain abscess

Brain abscesses usually are a result of chronic infections of the middle ear, paranasal sinuses, or mastoid air cells or to systemic infections (pneumonia, bacterial endocarditis, osteomyelitis). The most common organisms causing brain abscesses are streptococci. In patients with AIDS, brain abscesses are often caused by unusual organisms such as toxoplasmosis and cryptococcosis.

The earliest CT sign of brain abscess is an area of low density with poorly defined borders and a mass effect reflecting vascular congestion and edema. Further progression of the inflammatory process leads to cerebral softening that may undergo necrosis and liquefaction and result in a true abscess. Noncontrast scans continue to demonstrate an ill-defined, low-density area with a mass effect on the ventricular system or midline structures. After the intravenous administration of contrast material, an oval or circular peripheral ring of contrast enhancement outlines the abscess capsule (Figure 7-35). Although the wall is usually thin and of uniform thickness, an irregularly thick wall may be seen that mimics the wall of a malignant glioma. Multiple abscesses suggest the possibility of septic emboli from a systemic infection (Figure 7-36).

CT can be used to assess the results of therapy

of a brain abscess and to document complications. This modality can demonstrate the often fatal intraventricular rupture of an abscess and the development of increased intracranial pressure that may lead to brain herniation.

Plain skull radiographs may show evidence of underlying sinusitis, mastoiditis, or osteomyelitis, although this is better evaluated by CT scanning with bone-window settings. Infection by gas-forming organisms occasionally produces an air-fluid level within the abscess cavity.

Because CT is far better than other modalities (radionuclide studies, arteriography) in assessing brain abscesses, if a CT scanner is unavailable the patient should probably be transferred to another facility where CT can be performed.

Subdural empyema

Subdural empyema is a suppurative process in the space between the inner surface of the dura and the outer surface of the arachnoid. The most common cause of subdural empyema is the spread of infection from the frontal or ethmoid sinuses. Less frequently, subdural empyema may be a result of mastoiditis, middle ear infection, purulent meningitis, penetrating wounds to the skull, craniectomy, or osteomyelitis of the skull. Subdural empyema is often bilateral and is associated with a high mortality rate even if properly treated. The most common location of a

subdural empyema is over the cerebral convexity; the base of the skull is usually spared.

CT is the procedure of choice in evaluating the patient with suspected subdural empyema. Noncontrast scans demonstrate a crescentic or lentiform (lenslike), extra-axial hypodense collection (representing pus) adjacent to the inner border of the skull. There is compression and displacement of the ipsilateral ventricular structures. After the intravenous administration of contrast material, a narrow zone of enhancement of relatively uniform thickness separates the hypodense extracerebral collection from the brain surface (Figure 7-37). CT can also demonstrate involvement of the adjacent parenchyma by means of retrograde thrombophlebitis with resultant infarction or abscess formation, signs associated with a poor prognosis.

Extradural abscess

Extradural abscess (Figure 7-38) is almost invariably associated with osteomyelitis in a cranial bone originating from an infection in the ear or paranasal sinuses. The infectious process is localized outside the dural membrane and beneath the inner table of the skull. The frontal region is most frequently affected because of its close relation to the frontal sinuses and the ease with which the dura can be stripped from the bone.

Noncontrast CT scans demonstrate the epidural

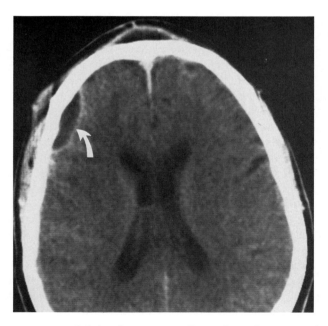

Figure 7-37 Subdural empyema. Lens-shaped extra-axial hypodense collection *(arrow)* that complicated severe sinus infection. Note thin rim of peripheral contrast enhancement.

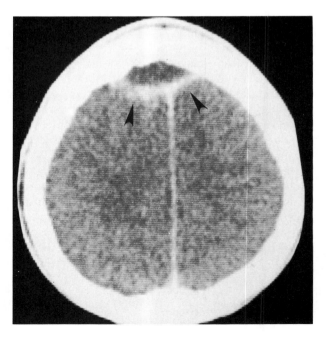

Figure 7-38 Extradural abscess. (From Lee SH and Rao KVCG, editors: Cranial computed tomography, New York 1983, McGraw-Hill Book Co.)

infection as a poorly defined area of low density adjacent to the inner table of the skull. An adjacent area of bone destruction or evidence of paranasal sinus or mastoid infection (fluid, soft-tissue thickening) often can be demonstrated on CT or plain skull radiographs. After the intravenous administration of contrast material, the inflamed dural membrane appears as a thickened zone of enhancement on the convex inner side of the lesion. If the collection lies in the midline, the attachment of the falx is displaced inward and separated from the adjacent skull, thus identifying its extradural location.

Osteomyelitis of the skull

Osteomyelitis of the skull is most commonly due to direct extension of a suppurative process from the paranasal sinuses, mastoid air cells, or scalp. As with osteomyelitis elsewhere in the skeleton, the radiographic changes often develop 1 to 2 weeks after the onset of clinical symptoms and signs.

Acute osteomyelitis first appears radiographically as multiple small, poorly defined areas of lucency (Figure 7-39). Over the next several weeks, the lucencies enlarge and coalesce centrally with an expanding perimeter of small satellite foci. As the infection becomes more chronic (especially with syphilis, tuberculosis, or fungal infections), attempts at bone regeneration produce multiple areas of poorly defined reactive sclerosis.

VASCULAR DISEASE OF THE CENTRAL NERVOUS SYSTEM

The term **cerebrovascular disease** refers to any process that is caused by an abnormality of the blood vessels or blood supply to the brain. Pathologic processes causing cerebrovascular disease include abnormalities of the vessel wall, occlusion by thrombus or emboli, rupture of blood vessels with subsequent hemorrhage, and decreased cerebral blood flow caused by lowered blood pressure or narrowed lumen caliber. Cerebrovascular diseases include arteriosclerosis, hypertensive hemorrhage, arteritis, aneurysms, and arteriovenous malformations.

The radiographic evaluation of cerebrovascular disease depends on the presenting symptoms and the most likely diagnosis. For ease of classification, patients with cerebrovascular disease can be divided into three categories: completed stroke, transient ischemic attacks (TIAS), and intracranial hemorrhage.

Stroke syndrome

The term **stroke** denotes the sudden and dramatic development of a focal neurologic deficit, which may vary from dense hemiplegia (paralysis on one side of the body) and coma to only a trivial neurologic disorder. The specific neurologic defect depends on the arteries involved. Strokes most commonly involve the circulation of the internal carotid arteries

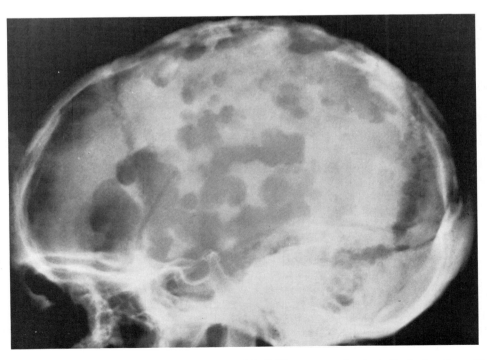

Figure 7-39 Osteomyelitis of skull (blastomycosis). Diffuse areas of osteolytic destruction affect most of calvarium.

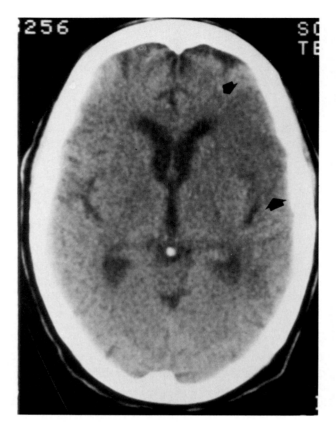

Figure 7-40   Acute left middle cerebral artery infarct. CT scan obtained 20 hours after onset of acute hemiparesis and aphasia shows obliteration of normal sulci *(arrows)* in involved hemisphere. There is low density of gray and white matter in distribution of left middle cerebral artery.

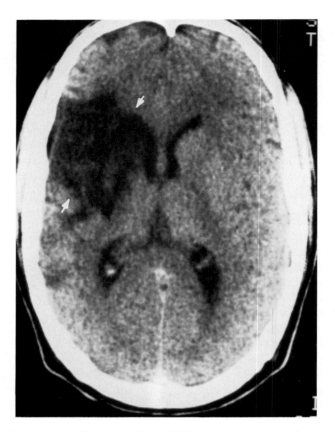

Figure 7-41   Chronic right middle cerebral artery infarct. Low-attenuation region with sharply defined borders *(arrows)*, and some dilation of adjacent ventricle.

and are seen with symptoms that include acute hemiparesis (weakness of one side of the body) and dysarthria (difficulty speaking).

The purpose of radiographic evaluation in the acute stroke patient is not to confirm the diagnosis of a stroke but to exclude other processes that can simulate the clinical findings (parenchymal hemorrhage, subdural hematoma). Although the abrupt onset of a stroke may permit differentiation from other conditions that have a more gradual onset of symptoms, patients with focal neurologic deficits of various causes may initially be found comatose, so that the history of gradual onset is not elicited. Obviously, it is essential to exclude an intracranial hemorrhage before considering the possibility of treating the stroke patient with anticoagulant therapy.

Noncontrast CT (or MRI, if available) is the examination of choice for the evaluation of the stroke patient. Intravenous contrast material is contraindicated because it is a toxic substance that can cross the disrupted blood-brain barrier in the region of a

cerebral infarct and lead to increased edema and a slower recovery for the patient. CT and MRI scans are normal in patients with small infarctions and in the early hours of large infarctions. The initial appearance (8 to 24 hours) of a cerebral infarction is a triangular or wedge-shaped area of hypodensity on CT (Figure 7-40) and high signal on T2-weighted MRI sequences involving both the cortex and the underlying white matter down to the ventricular surface. The abnormality is confined to the vascular territory of the involved artery. Although little or no mass effect is evident during the first day, progressive edema produces a mass effect that is maximal 7 to 10 days after the acute event. As an infarct ages, brain tissue atrophies, and the adjacent sulci and ventricular system enlarge (Figure 7-41). In patients with classic stroke symptoms, follow-up CT or MRI scans are not indicated.

Transient ischemic attacks

Transient ischemic attacks (TIAs) present as focal neurologic deficits that completely resolve within 24 hours. They may result from emboli originating from

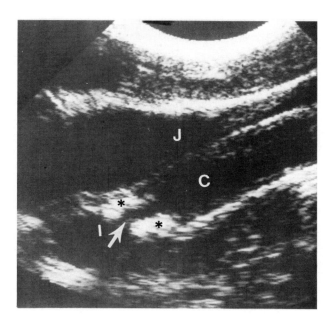

Figure 7-42 Ultrasound of cervical arteriosclerotic occlusive disease. There is severe narrowing *(arrow)* of origin of internal carotid artery *(I)* by densely echogenic arteriosclerotic plaque *(asterisks)*. C, common carotid artery; J, jugular vein.

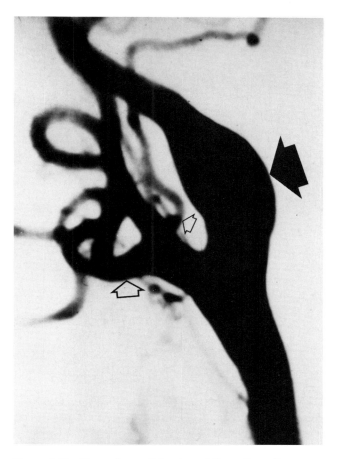

Figure 7-43 Normal carotid artery bifurcation. Common carotid arteriogram shows bulbous origin of internal carotid artery *(solid arrow)* and multiple branches of external carotid artery *(open arrows)*.

the surface of an arteriosclerotic ulcerated plaque, which causes temporary occlusion of cerebral vessels, or from stenosis of an extracerebral artery, which leads to a reduction in critical blood perfusion. Because almost two thirds of arteriosclerotic strokes are preceded by TIAs and the 5-year cumulative risk of stroke in patients with TIAs may be as high as 50%, accurate diagnosis and appropriate treatment (antiplatelet therapy, anticoagulation therapy, or carotid endarterectomy) are essential.

The most common location of surgically treatable arteriosclerotic disease causing TIAs is the region of the carotid bifurcation in the neck. In patients with an asymptomatic bruit (rumbling noise heard by a stethoscope) or an unclear history of a TIA, carotid duplex scanning is often the initial screening study (Figure 7-42). This technique combines high-resolution ultrasound imaging and Doppler ultrasound with spectral analysis into a "duplex" unit that avoids many of the problems associated with each of these modalities when used alone. In most cases, carotid duplex scanning can reliably determine whether there is significant disease to warrant more invasive procedures (angiography). Patients with a normal or near-normal carotid duplex scan do not need to undergo more invasive diagnostic procedures to assess the carotid bifurcation. Limitations of the usefulness of carotid duplex scanning include

its extreme operator dependence and the fact that 10% of patients cannot be successfully imaged with carotid duplex scanning because of anatomic factors (patients with extreme high carotid bifurcations and those with short, thick necks). Using ultrasound techniques, it may be impossible to differentiate patients with a total occlusion of the internal carotid artery from those with a tiny residual lumen. This is an important clinical distinction because patients with even a small remaining lumen can undergo a successful carotid endarterectomy (surgical removal of atherosclerotic plaque).

Patients with a clear-cut episode of a TIA or a neurologic deficit usually are subjected to an angiographic study for evaluating the carotid arteries. Either intravenous or intra-arterial digital subtraction angiography (DSA) or selective intra-arterial carotid arteriography can be used to demonstrate TIA-producing stenotic or ulcerative lesions that may be amenable to surgical therapy (Figures 7-43 to 7-45).

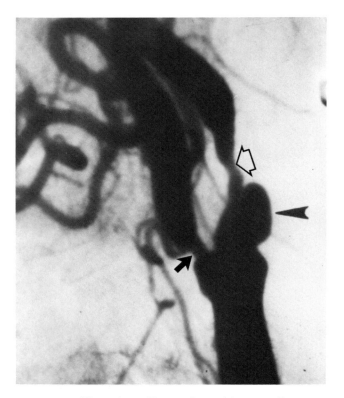

Figure 7-44 Ulceration of internal carotid artery. Common carotid arteriogram shows ulcerated lesion *(arrowhead)* at origin of internal carotid artery with severe stenosis of internal carotid *(open arrow)* and external carotid *(black arrow)* arteries.

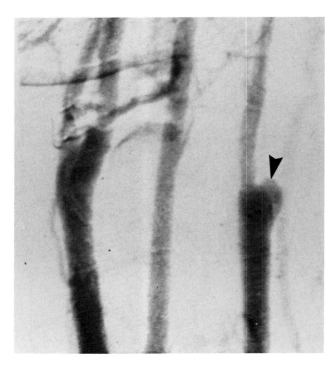

Figure 7-45 Occluded internal carotid artery. Intravenous digital subtraction angiogram shows occlusion of left internal carotid artery at its origin *(arrowhead).*

Angiographic evaluation of the aortic arch and vertebral arteries is infrequently indicated in evaluating patients with TIAs, both because surgery on the origins of the great vessels and posterior circulation is difficult and not established and also because of the higher morbidity from arch and vertebral angiograms reported in some studies.

Intraparenchymal hemorrhage

Aside from head trauma, the principle cause of intraparenchymal hemorrhage is hypertensive vascular disease. Less frequent causes are rupture of a congenital berry aneurysm or an arteriovenous malformation. Hypertensive hemorrhages result in oval or circular collections that displace the surrounding brain and can cause a significant mass effect. Although they can occur at any location within the brain, hypertensive hemorrhages are most frequent in the basal ganglia, white matter, thalamus, cerebellar hemispheres, and pons. A frequent complication is rupture of the hemorrhage into the ventricular system or subarachnoid space. Intraparenchymal hemorrhages resulting from congenital

"berry" aneurysms usually are associated with subarachnoid hemorrhage and tend to develop in regions where these congenital vascular anomalies most commonly occur. These include the sylvian fissure (middle cerebral artery) and the midline subfrontal area (anterior communicating artery). Arteriovenous malformations occur throughout the brain and tend to bleed into the white matter.

Patients with a suspected intraparenchymal hemorrhage should be evaluated with MRI or a noncontrast CT scan. A fresh hematoma appears on CT as a homogeneously dense, well-defined lesion with a round to oval configuration (Figure 7-46). Hematomas produce ventricular compression and, when large, considerable midline shift and brain herniation. Steroid therapy, especially in nontraumatic hematomas, usually controls the edema that produces much of the mass effect. A hematoma that is not homogeneously dense suggests hemorrhage occurring within a tumor, an inflammatory process, or an infarction. As the hematoma ages, its density changes. On CT, after passing through an isodense stage the hematoma becomes hypodense; by 6

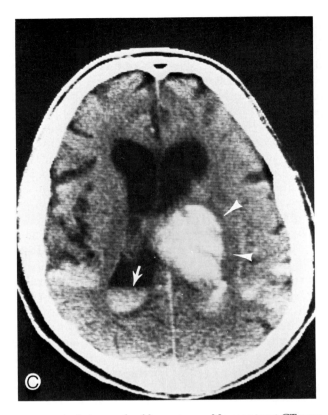

Figure 7-46 Intracerebral hematoma. Noncontrast CT scan shows homogeneous, high-density area in left thalamus. Low-density area *(arrowheads)* adjacent to hematoma represents associated ischemia and edema. Hematoma has entered ventricular system, and prominent CSF-blood level is seen in dependent lateral ventricle *(arrow)*. Such extension of blood into ventricular system is extremely poor prognostic sign. Mass effect caused by hematoma has compressed third ventricle and foramen of Monro and resulted in obstructive enlargement of lateral ventricles. *(From Drayer BP: In Rosenberg RN and Heinz ER, editors: The clinical neurosciences. IV. Neuroradiology. New York, Churchill Livingstone, 1984.)*

months it appears as a well-defined, low-density region that is often considerably smaller than the original lesion. Contrast enhancement usually develops about the periphery of a hematoma after 7 to 10 days. On MRI, the high signal intensity within a hematoma (caused by the conversion of normal hemoglobin to methemoglobin) arises after a few days and continues for several months (Figure 7-47). Once the methemoglobin is completely converted to paramagnetic hemosiderin, the hematoma has very low signal intensity on T2-weighted sequences.

Arteriography is not indicated in patients with classic hypertensive hematomas. However, arteriography is of value in those patients in whom an aneurysm or arteriovenous malformation is suspected as the underlying cause of the hematoma. In

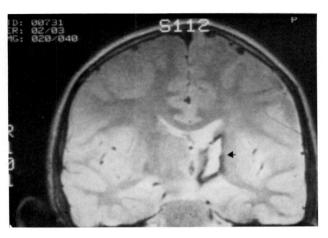

Figure 7-47 Intracerebral hematoma. Coronal T2-weighted MRI scan shows large hematoma in left thalamic region *(arrow)*. Hematoma consists of two portions: central area of increased signal intensity representing methemoglobin, and surrounding area of low signal intensity representing hemosiderin.

patients with a suspected aneurysm, it is important to determine the number of aneurysms, the aneurysm that has ruptured, the location of the neck of the aneurysm, and the patency of the circle of Willis. Statistically, the largest of multiple aneurysms is the one that has ruptured; it is rare for an aneurysm less than 5 mm in diameter to rupture. Because an aneurysm generally ruptures at its apex, an irregular, multiloculated dome suggests a prior rupture. Spasm in adjacent vessels and adjacent hematomas also assist in identifying which of several aneurysms has bled.

In patients less than 20 years of age, arteriovenous malformation is the most common cause of nontraumatic intraparenchymal hemorrhage. On MRI (Figure 7-48) a cerebrovascular malformation appears as a mass of vascular structures of varying intensity, depending on whether there is rapid flow (black) or slow flow (white). On CT the malformation consists of an irregular tangle of vessels (best seen after the intravenous injection of contrast material) and markedly dilated veins draining from the central tangle (Figure 7-49, *A*). Arteriography demonstrates an irregular, racemose tangle of abnormal vessels that are fed by dilated cerebral or cerebellar arteries (Figure 7-49, *B*). There is rapid shunting of blood into dilated, tortuous draining veins. Because of the often multiple sources of blood flow to an arteriovenous malformation, the arteriographic evaluation should include selective injections of contrast material into both internal and external carotid arteries.

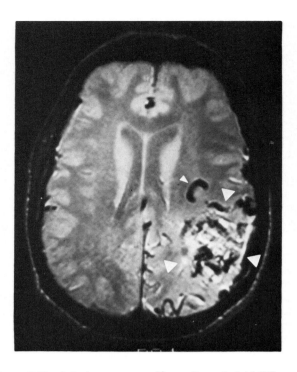

Figure 7-48 Arteriovenous malformation. Axial MRI scan shows large left parietal mass *(large arrowheads)* consisting of vascular structures of varying intensity, depending on whether there is rapid flow *(black)* or slow flow *(white)*. Note markedly dilated vessel *(small arrowhead)* that feeds malformation.

Subarachnoid hemorrhage

A major cause of subarachnoid hemorrhage is rupture of a berry aneurysm (Figure 7-50). Patients with this condition usually have a generalized excruciating headache followed by unconsciousness. The radiographic procedure of choice is a noncontrast CT scan, which can demonstrate high-density blood in the subarachnoid spaces of the basal cisterns in more than 95% of cases. Bleeding may extend into the brain parenchyma adjacent to the aneurysm. Contrast-enhanced CT scans are not indicated in subarachnoid hemorrhage, since the surgeon will not operate for a suspected aneurysm without an angiogram and the patient would thus be exposed to the risk of an excessive load of contrast material.

The timing of angiography in subarachnoid hemorrhage depends on the philosophy of the surgeon. Blood in the subarachnoid space is an irritant that causes vasospasm of the vessels of the circle of Willis and middle cerebral artery. This vasospasm, which can lead to cerebral ischemia and frank infarction, is greatest 3 to 14 days after the acute episode. If emergency surgery within the first 72 hours after the hemorrhage is planned, emergency selective angiography is indicated. If surgical intervention is to be delayed, angiography should be postponed until just before surgery. The most common locations for berry aneurysms are the origins of the posterior cerebral and anterior communicating arteries and the trifurcation of the middle cerebral artery. Because of the 20% incidence of multiple aneurysms, the angiographic procedure should include evaluation of the internal carotid and vertebral arteries bilaterally.

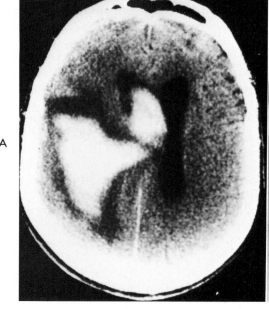

A

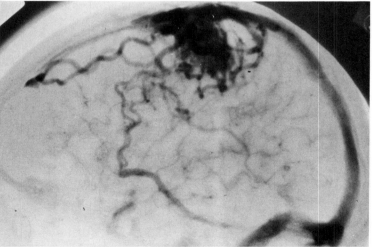

B

Figure 7-49 Arteriovenous malformation with hemorrhage. **A,** CT scan in 34-year-old comatose man shows high-density hemorrhage in right parietal lobe that extends into ventricular system. **B,** Carotid arteriogram shows dilated blood vessels constituting arteriovenous malformation.

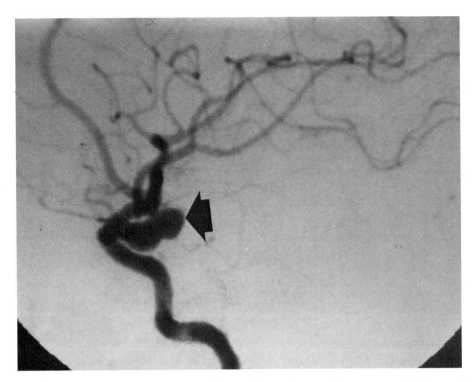

Figure 7-50 Ruptured berry aneurysm. Left carotid arteriogram demonstrates left supraclinoid aneurysm of internal carotid artery. Posterior bulge of aneurysm *(arrow)* represents site of rupture.

MULTIPLE SCLEROSIS

Multiple sclerosis is a demyelinating disorder that presents as recurrent attacks of focal neurologic deficits that primarily involve the spinal cord, optic nerves, and central white matter of the brain. The disease has a peak incidence between 20 and 40 years of age, a strong predominance in women, and a clinical course characterized by multiple relapses and remissions. Impairment of nerve conduction caused by the degeneration of myelin sheaths leads to such symptoms as double vision, nystagmus (involuntary, rapid movement of the eyeball in all directions), loss of balance and poor coordination, shaking tremor and muscular weakness, difficulty in speaking clearly, and bladder dysfunction.

MRI is the modality of choice for demonstrating the plaques of demyelinization that are characteristic of multiple sclerosis. The plaques appear as multiple areas of increased signal intensity that primarily involve the periventricular white matter, cerebellum, brainstem, and spinal cord (Figure 7-51). CT shows old inactive disease as well-defined areas of decreased attenuation in the deep white matter and periventricular regions. In the acute phase, CT after the intravenous demonstration of contrast material

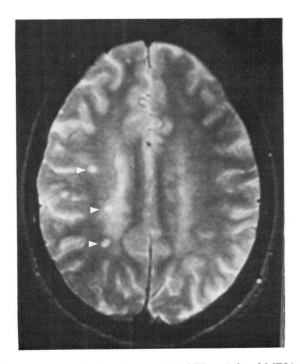

Figure 7-51 Multiple sclerosis. Axial T2-weighted MRI image in 35-year-old woman shows characteristic areas of increased signal intensity *(arrowheads)* in deep white matter.

demonstrates a mixture of nonenhancing focal areas of decreased density (representing old areas of demyelinization) and enhancing regions that represent active foci.

EPILEPSY AND CONVULSIVE DISORDERS

Epilepsy is a condition in which brain impulses are temporarily disturbed, resulting in a spectrum of symptoms ranging from loss of consciousness for a few seconds to violent seizures (shaking and thrashing movements of all extremities). Although most cases of epilepsy are idiopathic, the disorder can be a result of injury (penetrating or nonpenetrating trauma, depressed skull fracture), birth trauma, or infection.

The mildest type of epilepsy, which primarily occurs in children, is called **petit mal.** This results in brief episodes of loss of consciousness that may be associated with mild muscular twitching. Petit mal epilepsy usually disappears in young adulthood.

Grand mal epilepsy refers to generalized convulsions associated with the patient falling to the floor, hypersalivating (foaming at the mouth), and losing control of urine and sometimes feces. In many cases an approaching seizure is heralded by an aura, such as a ringing in the ears, a tingling sensation in the fingers, or spots before the eyes. After a seizure, the patient tends to be groggy and unaware of what has happened (postictal state).

In the patient who has an acute seizure, the initial effort should be directed toward stabilizing the patient (securing adequate ventilation and perfusion) and stopping the seizure. Subsequently, a careful history, physical examination, and appropriate laboratory studies should be performed to exclude reversible chemical causes of seizures such as hypoglycemia, hyponatremia or hypernatremia, and hypocalcemia or hypercalcemia. If the patient does not respond to routine anticonvulsive treatment, CT may be indicated to search for possible surgical causes of an acute seizure disorder (e.g., subdural hematoma, intracerebral hematoma). These conditions can be adequately assessed with a noncontrast CT scan (see page 238); plain skull radiographs are not required.

Whenever possible, the radiographic evaluation of a patient with a seizure disorder should be done when the patient is clinically stable. The appropriate procedure is a contrast-enhanced CT scan or an MRI scan to search for an unsuspected brain tumor or arteriovenous malformation (Figure 7-52). Since most seizure disorders are due to small areas of cortical brain injury resulting from trauma or infarction, CT or MRI scans are usually normal. If the scan is

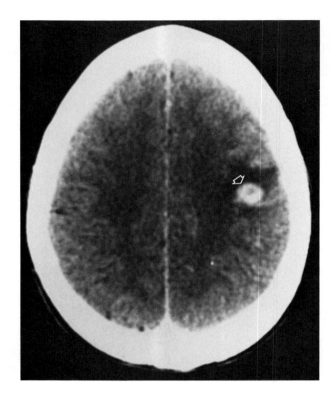

Figure 7-52 Seizure disorder caused by astrocytoma. CT scan after intravenous injection of contrast material in 27-year-old woman with focal right arm seizures shows enhancing left cerebral tumor (*arrow*) surrounded by low-density edema. As in this patient, most seizure disorders can be evaluated with contrast-enhanced CT scan (or MRI scan).

normal, no further radiographic examination is indicated.

DEGENERATIVE DISEASES

Normal aging

During normal aging, a gradual loss of neurons results in enlargement of the ventricular system and sulci (Figure 7-53). Demyelination, which is also a part of normal aging, leads to the development of low density in the periventricular regions on CT and high signal intensity on T2-weighted MR images (Figure 7-54).

Alzheimer's disease

Alzheimer's disease (presenile dementia) is a diffuse form of progressive cerebral atrophy that develops at an earlier age than the senile period. CT and MRI demonstrate nonspecific findings of cerebral atrophy, including symmetrically enlarged ventricles with prominence of the cortical sulci (Figure 7-55).

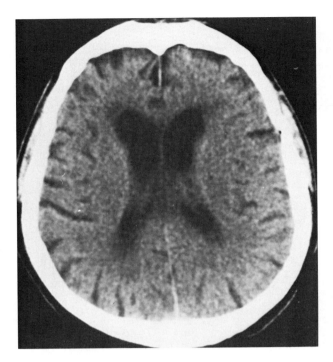

Figure 7-53 Normal aging. CT scan of 70-year-old man shows generalized ventricular dilation with prominence of sulci over surfaces of cerebral hemisphere.

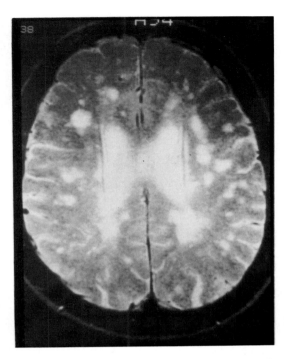

Figure 7-54 Degenerative changes of aging. Axial MRI scan demonstrates multiple areas of increased signal intensity around ventricles and in deep white matter, consistent with cerebral ischemia or infarction.

Huntington's disease

Huntington's disease is an inherited condition (autosomal dominant) that predominantly involves men and presents in the early to middle adult years with dementia and typical choreiform movements (involuntary movements that are rapid, jerky, and without stop). The pathologic hallmark of Huntington's disease is atrophy of the caudate nucleus and putamen, which produces the typical CT appearance of focal dilation of the frontal horns and a loss of their normal concave shape (Figure 7-56). Generalized enlargement of the ventricles and dilation of the cortical sulci can also occur.

Parkinson's disease

Parkinson's disease (shaking palsy) is a progressive degenerative disease characterized by stooped posture, stiffness and slowness of movement, fixed facial expression, and involuntary rhythmic tremor of the limbs that disappears with voluntary movement. A disorder of middle or later life, Parkinson's disease is very gradually progressive and exhibits a prolonged course.

The major degenerative changes in nerve cells in Parkinson's disease occur in the basal ganglia, especially the globus pallidus, substantia nigra, and

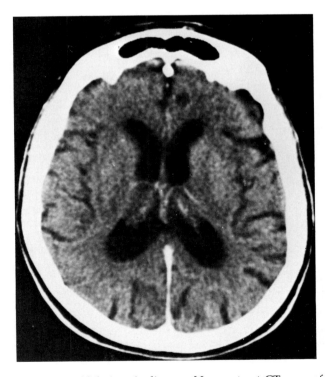

Figure 7-55 Alzheimer's disease. Noncontrast CT scan of 56-year-old woman with progressive dementia shows generalized enlargement of ventricular system and sulci.

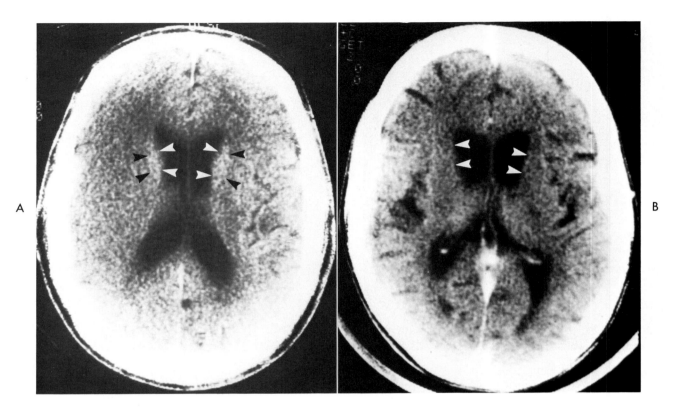

Figure 7-56 Huntington's disease. **A,** CT scan in normal patient shows heads of caudate nucleus *(black arrowheads)* producing normal concavity of frontal horns *(white arrowheads).* **B,** In patient with Huntington's disease, atrophy of caudate nucleus causes characteristic loss of normal concavity *(white arrowheads)* of frontal horns.

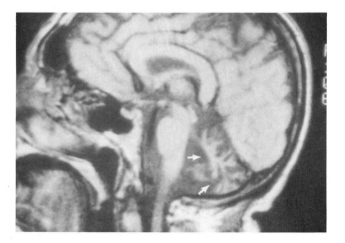

Figure 7-57 Cerebellar atrophy. Sagittal MRI scan shows dramatic loss of substance of vermis of cerebellum *(arrows)* in patient with severe alcoholism.

the fibers of the corpus striatum. The essence of the condition seems to be an enzyme defect that results in an inadequate production of the neuronal transmitter substance, dopamine. The most recent method of treatment is the administration of L-dopa, a substance that is converted to dopamine in the brain. Although this drug therapy does not stop the neuronal degeneration, it dramatically improves both the appearance and behavior of the patient.

CT scans in patients with Parkinson's disease often demonstrate cortical atrophy. However, because this condition is usually seen in older individuals, the ventricular enlargement and prominent cortical sulci found on CT scans may be indistinguishable from that caused by the normal aging process.

Cerebellar atrophy

Isolated atrophy of the cerebellum may represent an inherited disorder, a degenerative disease, or the toxic effect of the prolonged use of such drugs as alcohol and dilantin (Figure 7-57).

Amyotrophic lateral sclerosis (Lou Gehrig's disease)

In this relentlessly progressive condition of unknown cause, there is widespread selective atrophy and loss of motor nerve cells leading to extensive paralysis and death from respiratory weakness or aspiration pneumonia. Although this disease cannot be diagnosed radiographically, CT, MRI, or myelography is often performed to exclude a spinal malignancy that could produce a similar clinical appearance.

HYDROCEPHALUS

Hydrocephalus refers to dilation of the ventricular system that is usually associated with increased intracranial pressure. In **noncommunicating** (obstructive) hydrocephalus, there is an obstruction to the flow of CSF somewhere along the ventricular pathways from the lateral ventricles to the outlets of the fourth ventricle. Enlargement of the lateral ventricles with normal-sized third and fourth ventricles indicates an obstruction at the level of the foramina of Monro. This is most commonly due to a colloid cyst (Figure 7-58) or suprasellar tumor, especially craniopharyngioma. Enlargement of the lateral and third ventricles with a normal-sized fourth ventricle indicates an obstruction at the level of the aqueduct of Sylvius (Figure 7-59). The most common causes of this appearance are congenital aqueduct stenosis or occlusion and neoplasm (pinealoma, teratoma). Enlargement of the entire ventricular system (with the fourth ventricle often dilated out of proportion) indicates an obstruction at the level of the outlet of the fourth ventricle (Figure 7-60), a condition that may reflect congenital atresia, infection, neoplasm, or downward herniation of the cerebellar tonsils through the foramen magnum.

In the much more common **communicating** hydrocephalus, the ventricular fluid passes freely into the extraventricular subarachnoid space. There is generalized ventricular enlargement with normal or absent sulci. Obstruction of the normal CSF pathway distal to the fourth ventricle usually involves the subarachnoid space at the basal cisterns, cerebral convexity, or foramen magnum. Causes include in-

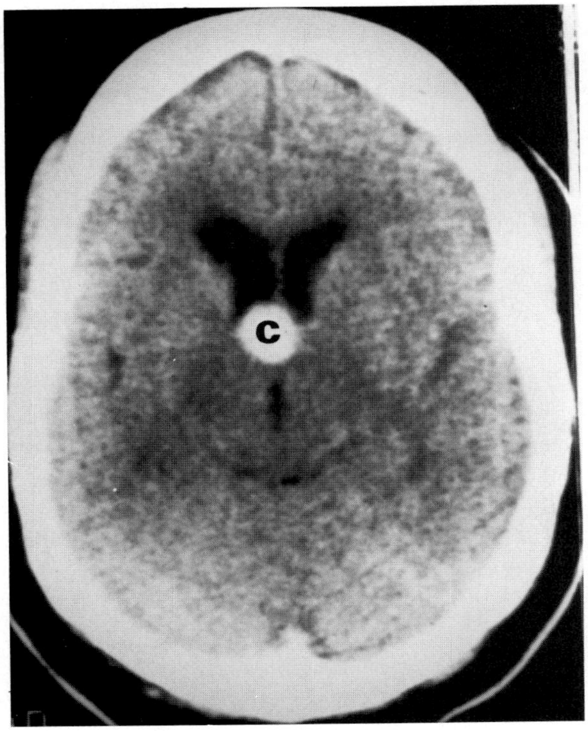

Figure 7-58 Hydrocephalus with obstruction at level of foramen of Monro. Bilateral enlargement of frontal horns with normal-sized third ventricle in patient with hyperdense colloid cyst *(c)*.

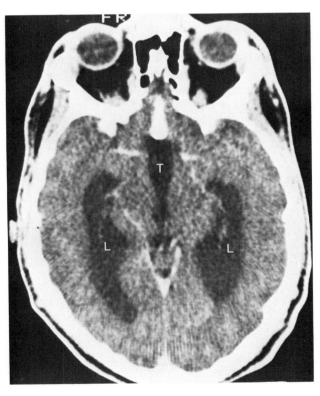

Figure 7-59 Hydrocephalus caused by obstruction at level of aqueduct. Dilation of lateral *(L)* and third *(T)* ventricles in patient with congenital hydrocephalus. Symptoms of headache and papilledema resolved after ventricular shunting.

fection (meningitis, empyema), subarachnoid or subdural hemorrhage, congenital anomalies, neoplasm, and dural venous thrombosis. A similar radiographic pattern is seen in **"normal-pressure"** hydrocephalus, a syndrome of gait ataxia, urinary incontinence, and dementia associated with ventricular dilation and relatively normal CSF pressure.

The diagnosis of dilated ventricles can be easily made by CT or MRI (Figure 7-61). Ultrasound can show the ventricular dilation either in utero or after birth as long as the sound waves can traverse the open fontanels.

Generalized enlargement of the ventricular system can also be due to the overproduction of CSF by a papilloma (Figure 7-62) or carcinoma arising in the choroid plexus (CSF-secreting vascular tissue in the ventricles). These rare tumors usually occur in the fourth ventricle in adults and the lateral ventricles in children.

Hydrocephalus can often be treated by the placement of a shunt between the dilated ventricles and the heart or the peritoneal cavity. Successful shunting causes a decrease in the intracranial pressure and ventricular size; the latter can be monitored by CT or MRI.

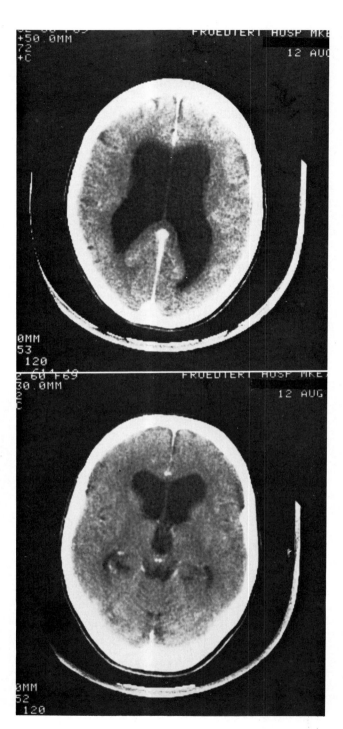

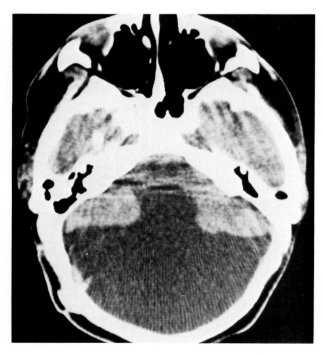

Figure 7-60 Hydrocephalus caused by obstruction at level of outlet of fourth ventricle. Huge low-density cyst (Dandy-Walker cyst) occupies most of enlarged posterior fossa and represents extension of dilated fourth ventricle.

Figure 7-61 Communicating hydrocephalus. Generalized ventricular enlargement in 69-year-old patient with classic clinical triad of ataxia, dementia, and incontinence. Note absence of dilated sulci seen in obstructive hydrocephalus. *(From Williams AL and Haughton VM: Cranial computed tomography, St. Louis, CV Mosby Co, 1985.)*

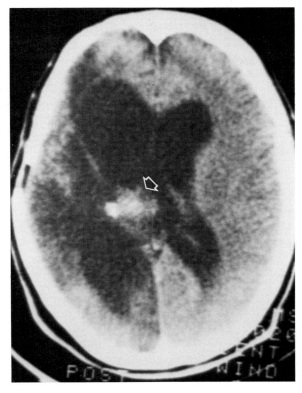

Figure 7-62 Choroid plexus papilloma. Enhancing ventricular mass *(arrow)* causing pronounced generalized enlargement of ventricular system.

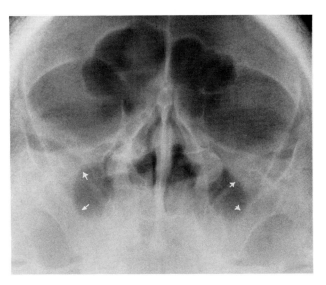

Figure 7-63 Chronic sinusitis. Mucosal thickening appears as soft-tissue density *(arrows)* lining walls of maxillary antra.

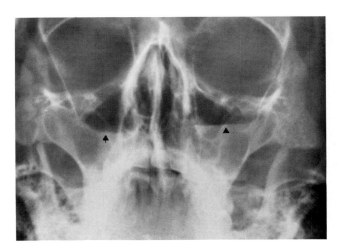

Figure 7-64 Acute sinusitis. There is mucosal thickening involving most of paranasal sinuses and air-fluid levels *(arrows)* in both maxillary antra.

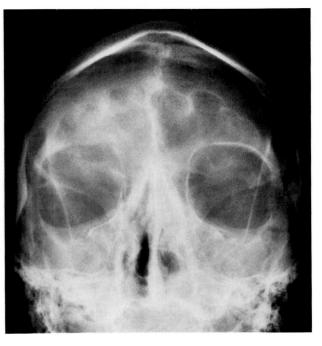

Figure 7-65 Mucormycosis causing pansinusitis with osteomyelitis. Destruction of roof of right orbit and outer margins of right frontal sinus are present.

SINUSITIS

The paranasal sinuses (maxillary, ethmoid, frontal, and sphenoid) are paired air-filled cavities that are lined with a mucous membrane that is directly continuous with the nasal mucosa. The size and shape of the sinuses vary in different age periods, in different individuals, and on the two sides of the same individual. At birth, the maxillary sinus is only a slitlike space that later expands to fill the maxilla and is thus responsible for the growth of the face. The ethmoid sinuses can be seen radiographically by age 6, whereas the frontal sinuses usually are not well demonstrated until about age 10. The sphenoid sinuses begin to develop around age 2 or 3 and are fully developed by late adolescence.

Viral infection of the upper respiratory tract may lead to obstruction of drainage of the paranasal sinuses and the development of localized pain, tenderness, and fever. Radiographically, acute or chronic sinusitis causes mucosal thickening that appears as a soft-tissue density lining the walls of the involved sinuses (Figure 7-63). The maxillary antra are most commonly affected and are best visualized on the Waters' projection. An air-fluid level in a sinus is usually considered a manifestation of acute inflammatory disease (Figure 7-64). To demonstrate this finding, it is essential that all sinus films be obtained with the patient erect and with the use of a horizontal beam. The destruction of the bony wall of a sinus is an ominous sign indicating secondary osteomyelitis (Figure 7-65).

QUESTIONS

1. The imaging modality of choice to evaluate patients with suspected neurologic dysfunction caused from head trauma is _____ .
   A. Ultrasound   C. CT
   B. MRI   D. Skull radiographs

2. Arterial bleeding sometimes associated with head trauma can cause _____ hematomas.
   A. Intracranial   C. Epidural
   B. Subdural   D. Acute

3. Venous bleeding sometimes associated with head trauma can cause _____ hematomas.
   A. Intracranial   C. Epidural
   B. Subdural   D. Acute

4. Movement of the brain within the calavarium following blunt trauma to the skull sometimes results in a cerebral _____ .
   A. Subdural hema-   C. Acute hematoma
      toma   D. Contusion
   B. Epidural hematoma

5. Bleeding into the ventricular system due to injury to surface veins, cerebral parenchyma, or cortical arteries can cause _____ hemorrhage.
   A. Epidural   C. Epiarachnoid
   B. Subdural   D. Subarachnoid

6. Plain radiographs of the facial bones should always be made with the patient in the _____ position if possible.
   A. Supine   C. Lateral decubitus
   B. Erect   D. Anterior

7. The most common primary brain tumor is a _____ .
   A. Glioma   C. Meningioma
   B. Glioblastoma   D. Neurinoma

8. A benign tumor that arises from arachnoid lining cells and is attached the dura is named _____ .
   A. Glioma   C. Meningioma
   B. Glioblastoma   D. Neurinoma

9. The most common neoplasms that metastasize to the brain arise in the _____ and _____ .
   A. Lung, stomach C. Stomach, breast
   B. Lung, breast   D. Breast, prostate

10. A viral inflammation of the brain and meninges is called _____ .
    A. Meningitis   C. Encephalitis
    B. Hydrocephalus D. Encephalomalacia

11. The best imaging modality to evaluate brain abscesses is _____ .

12. The two imaging procedures of choice to evaluate the extent of a stroke in the brain are _____ and _____ .

13. The initials *TIA* mean _____ .

14. The imaging modality of choice to demonstrate the plaques of demyelinization that are characteristic of multiple sclerosis is _____ .

15. A condition in which brain impulses are temporarily disturbed, the results of which range from loss of consciousness to violent seizures, is termed _____ .

16. A diffuse form of progressive cerebral atrophy that develops at an earlier age than the senile period is called _____ .

17. A progressive degenerative disease characterized by involuntary tremors of the extremities that disappear with voluntary movement is named _____ .

18. Sinus radiographs should be taken using a _____ beam and with the patient in the _____ position.

19. The pathologic condition that refers to dilation of the ventricular system and is usually associated with increased intracranial pressure is _____ .

20. If a patient needing facial or sinus radiographs is unable to stand or sit erect, a _____ using a _____ beam may be performed to demonstrate any air or fluid levels that may be present.

_____ 21. Convolutions on the surface of the cerebrum

_____ 22. The basic unit of the nervous system

_____ 23. Combination of 12 pairs of cranial nerves, 31 pairs of spinal nerves, autonomic nerves, and ganglia

_____ 24. Impulse conduction to and from the central nervous system

_____ 25. Entity consisting of the brain and spinal cord

_____ 26. Fatty covering that insulates axons

_____ 27. Junction where impulses are passed from one neuron to another

_____ 28. Part of nervous system that supplies the striated skeletal muscles

_____ 29. Projection leading from the nerve cell body

_____ 30. Part of the nervous system that supplies smooth muscle, cardiac muscle, and glandular epithelial tissue

_____ 31. Shallow grooves on the surface of the cerebrum

_____ 32. Projection leading to a nerve cell body

A. Dendrites

B. Dura mater

C. Axon

D. Gyri

E. Monro

F. Pia mater

G. Reflex arc

H. Corpus callosum

I. Synapse

J. Neuron

K. Hydrocephalus

L. Arachnoid

M. Somatic

N. Peripheral nervous system

O. Sulci

P. Myelin sheath

Q. Fourth ventricle

R. Autonomic

S. Falx cerebri

T. CNS

U. Meningitis

V. Mesencephalon

W. Third ventricle

X. Tentorium cerebelli

Y. Aqueduct of Sylvius

_____ 33. White matter connecting the two cerebral hemispheres

_____ 34. Midbrain

_____ 35. Transparent covering of the brain and spinal cord

_____ 36. Projects down into the longitudinal fissure to separate the cerebral hemispheres

_____ 37. Slitlike space between the right and left thalami

_____ 38. Inflammation of the protective layers of the brain

_____ 39. Covering over the cerebellum that separates it from the occipital lobe of the cerebrum

_____ 40. Cobweb-like covering of the brain

_____ 41. Diamond-shaped space in front of the cerebellum and behind the medulla and pons

_____ 42. Outermost covering of the brain

_____ 43. Canal connecting the third and fourth ventricles

_____ 44. Result of an obstruction of cerebrospinal spinal fluid

_____ 45. Foramen connecting the third and lateral ventricles

BIBLIOGRAPHY

Brant-Zawadzki M and Norman D: Magnetic resonance imaging of the central nervous system, New York, Raven Press, 1987.

Lee SH and Rao KCVG: Cranial computed tomography and MRI, New York, McGraw-Hill Book Co, 1987.

Ramsey RG: Neuroradiology with computed tomography, Philadelphia, WB Saunders Co, 1987.

CHAPTER 8

Hematopoietic System

PREREQUISITE KNOWLEDGE

The student should have a basic knowledge of the physiology of the hematopoietic system.

GOALS

To acquaint the student radiographer with the pathophysiology and radiographic manifestations of all of the common and some of the unusual disorders of the hematopoietic system

OBJECTIVES

1. Describe the physiology of the hematopoietic system
2. Identify blood structures on diagrams
3. Be able to define terminology relating to the hematopoietic system
4. Be able to describe the various pathologic conditions affecting the hematopoietic system and their radiographic manifestations

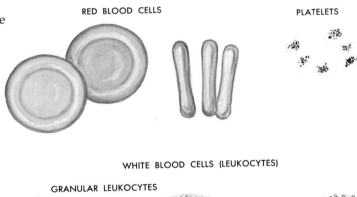

RED BLOOD CELLS PLATELETS

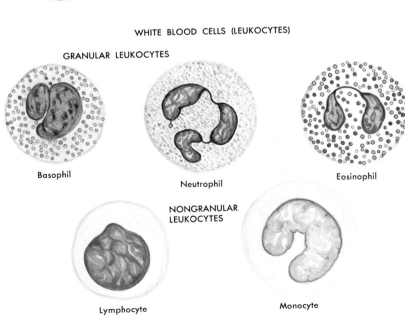

WHITE BLOOD CELLS (LEUKOCYTES)

GRANULAR LEUKOCYTES

Basophil

Neutrophil

Eosinophil

NONGRANULAR LEUKOCYTES

Lymphocyte

Monocyte

Although the hematopoietic system cannot be directly imaged, many blood disorders result in abnormalities that can be demonstrated radiogaphically. Technical factors may have to be increased or decreased in patients who manifest advanced stages of these diseases (see Table 1-1). The radiographer must be aware of the severe pain experienced by patients undergoing a sickle cell crisis. Patients with advanced leukemia or lymphoma who have an altered immune status may require protective isolation. Because many hematopoietic system diseases cause significant demineralization of bone, the radiographer must be alert to the possibility of pathologic fracture and thus exercise caution when moving and positioning these patients.

DISEASES OF THE BLOOD

Blood and the cells within it are vital to life. An adequate blood supply to all body tissues is necessary to bring oxygen, nutrients, salts, and hormones to the cells and to carry away the waste products of cellular metabolism. The components of blood are also a major defense against infection, toxic substances, and foreign antigens.

Red bone marrow (found in vertebrae and flat bones such as the sternum, ribs, skull, and proximal femurs) and lymph nodes are the blood-forming tissues of the body. Red blood cells (erythrocytes) and platelets (thrombocytes) are made in red bone marrow, whereas white blood cells (leukocytes) are produced in both red marrow and lymphoid tissue.

Erythrocytes are biconcave disks without a nucleus that contain **hemoglobin,** an iron-based protein that carries oxygen from the respiratory tract to the body's tissues. In a normal person, there are 4.5 to 6 million red blood cells in each cubic millimeter of blood. The amount of hemoglobin per deciliter is approximately 14 g in women and 15 g in men.

Leukocytes, or white blood cells, normally number from 5000 to 10,000/mm^3 of blood. Unlike erythrocytes, there are several types of white blood cells. **Neutrophils (polymorphonuclear leukocytes),** which make up 55% to 75% of white blood cells, defend the body against bacteria by ingesting these foreign organisms and destroying them (phagocytosis). The number of polymorphonuclear leukocytes in the blood is enormously increased in acute infections because the bone marrow rapidly releases into the bloodstream the large numbers of these cells kept in reserve. **Eosinophils** (1% to 4%) are red-staining cells whose number markedly increases in allergic and parasitic conditions. The third type of leukocyte is the **basophil** (0% to 1%), which contains granules that stain blue. These three types of cells are formed in the sinusoids of the bone marrow and, as with red blood cells, go through immature stages before the adult form is reached.

Lymphocytes represent about 25% to 40% of white blood cells. They play a major role in the immune system and are involved in the synthesis of antibodies and the production of immunoglobulins.

The final type of white blood cell is the monocyte, which is actively phagocytic and plays an important part in the inflammatory process. **Monocytes** are formed in the bone marrow and represent about 2% to 8% of white blood cells.

Platelets are the smallest blood cells and are essential for blood clotting. Normally, there are about 150,000 to 400,000 platelets in every cubic millimeter of blood.

DISEASES OF RED BLOOD CELLS

Anemia

Anemia refers to a decrease in the amount of oxygen-carrying hemoglobin in the blood. This reduction can be due to improper formation of new red blood cells, an increased rate of red blood cell destruction, or a loss of red blood cells as a result of prolonged bleeding. Regardless of the cause, a hemoglobin deficiency makes the anemic person appear pale. This is best appreciated in the mucous membranes of the mouth and conjunctiva and in the nail beds. A decrease in the oxygen-carrying hemoglobin impairs the delivery of an adequate oxygen supply to the cells and tissues, leading to fatigue and muscular weakness and often to shortness of breath on exertion (dyspnea). To meet the body's need for more oxygen, the respiratory rate is increased and the heart beats more rapidly.

Iron deficiency anemia

Iron deficiency is the most common cause of anemia. It most frequently results from chronic blood loss, as from an ulcer, a malignant tumor, or excessive bleeding during menstruation (menorrhagia). Other causes of iron deficiency anemia include inadequate dietary intake of iron and increased iron loss caused by intestinal parasites. Iron deficiency anemia also may develop during pregnancy because the mother's iron supply is depleted by red blood cell development in the fetus.

Hemolytic anemia

The underlying abnormality in hemolytic anemia is a shortened life span of the red blood cells with resulting hemolysis and the release of hemoglobin into the plasma. Most hemolytic anemias are caused by a hereditary defect that may produce abnormal red cells or abnormal hemoglobin. Less commonly, hemolytic anemia is acquired and related to circulating antibodies from autoimmune or allergic reactions (e.g., drugs such as sulfonamide) or the malaria parasite.

Spherocytosis, sickle cell anemia, and thalassemia are the major hereditary hemolytic anemias. In spherocytosis the erythrocytes have a circular rather than a biconcave shape, making them fragile and susceptible to rupture. In sickle cell anemia, which is generally confined to blacks, the hemoglobin molecule is abnormal and the red cells are crescent- or sickle-shaped and tend to rupture. A defect in hemoglobin formation is also responsible for thalassemia, which predominantly occurs in persons living about the Mediterranean, especially those of Italian, Greek, or Sicilian descent.

The breakdown of hemoglobin produces bilirubin, a pigmented substance that is normally detoxified by the liver and converted into bile. The accumulation of large amounts of this orange pigment in the plasma causes the tissues to have a yellow appearance (jaundice).

The hemolytic anemias produce a variety of radiographic abnormalities. Although the radiographic findings are similar in the various types of hemolytic anemia, they tend to be most severe in thalassemia and least prominent in spherocytosis. Extensive marrow hyperplasia, the result of ineffective erythropoiesis and rapid destruction of newly formed red blood cells, causes generalized osteoporosis with pronounced widening of the medullary spaces and thinning of the cortices in long and tubular bones (Figrue 8-1). As the fine secondary trabeculae are resorbed, new bone is laid down on the surviving trabeculae, thickening them and producing a coarsened pattern. Normal modeling of long bones does not occur because the expanding marrow flattens or even bulges the normally concave surfaces of the shafts.

In the skull there is widening of the diploic space and thinning or complete obliteration of the outer table. When the hyperplastic marrow perforates or destroys the outer table, it proliferates under the invisible periosteum, and new bone spicules are laid down perpendicular to the inner table. This produces the characteristic hair-on-end appearance of vertical striations in a radial pattern (Figure 8-2).

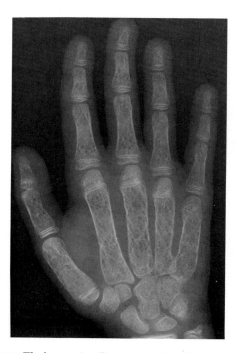

Figure 8-1 Thalassemia. Pronounced widening of medullary spaces with thinning of cortical margins. Note absence of normal modeling caused by pressure of expanding marrow space. Localized radiolucencies simulating multiple osteolytic lesions represent tumerous collections of hypoplastic marrow.

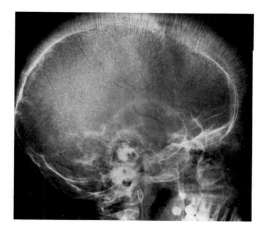

Figure 8-2 Thalassemia. Lateral projection of skull demonstrates hair-on-end appearance. Note normal appearance of calvarium inferior to internal occipital protuberance, an area in which there is no red marrow, and poor pneumatization of visualized paranasal sinuses.

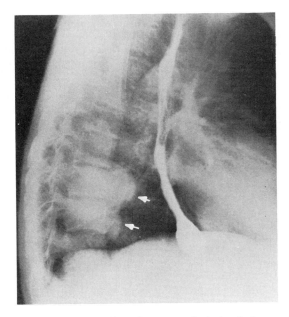

Figure 8-3 Extramedullary hematopoiesis in thalassemia. A lateral projection of chest demonstrates lobulated posterior mediastinal masses of hematopoietic tissue *(arrows)* in lower thoracic region. *(From Leigh TF: Radiol Clin North Am 1:377-393, 1963.)*

Extramedullary hematopoiesis is a compensatory mechanism of the reticuloendothelial system (liver, spleen, lymph nodes) in patients with prolonged erythrocyte deficiency resulting from the destruction of red blood cells or the inability of normal blood-forming organs to produce them. Paravertebral collections of hematopoietic tissue may appear on chest radiographs as single or multiple, smooth or lobulated, posterior mediastinal masses that are usually located at the lower thoracic levels (Figure 8-3).

In sickle cell anemia expansile pressure of the adjacent intervertebral disks produces characteristic biconcave indentations on both the superior and inferior margins of the softened vertebral bodies ("fish vertebra") (Figure 8-4, *A*). Another typical appearance is the development of localized steplike central depressions of multiple vertebral endplates (Figure 8-4, *B*). This is probably caused by circulatory stasis and ischemia, which retard growth in the central portion of the vertebral cartilaginous growth plate. The periphery of the growth plate, which has a different blood supply, continues to grow at a more normal rate. Bulging of the abnormally shaped red blood cells in sickle cell anemia typically causes focal ischemia and infarction in multiple tissues. Bone infarcts commonly occur in infants and children.

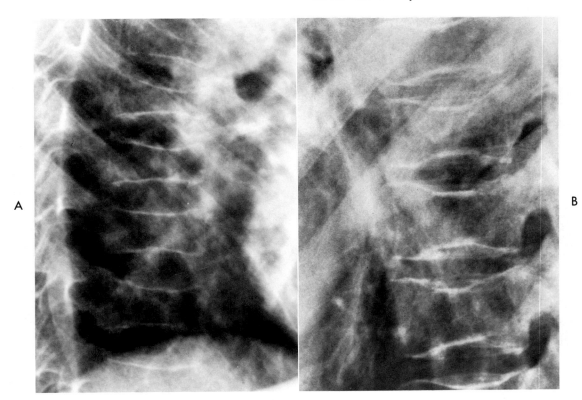

Figure 8-4 Sickle cell anemia. **A,** Biconcave indentations on both superior and inferior margins of soft vertebral bodies produce characteristic fish vertebrae. **B,** Localized steplike central depressions of multiple vertebral endplates.

These most frequently involve the small bones of the hands and feet, producing an irregular area of bone destruction with overlying periosteal calcification that may be indistinguishable from osteomyelitis. In older children and adults bone infarction may initially appear as an ill-defined lucent area that then becomes irregularly calcified. Acute osteomyelitis, often caused by *Salmonella* infection, is a common complication in sickle cell disease. The resulting lytic destruction and periosteal reaction may be extensive, often involving the entire shaft and multiple bones (Figure 8-5). Radiographically, it may be impossible to distinguish between osteomyelitis and bone infarction without infection. (Figure 8-6).

Throughout their lives, patients with sickle cell anemia are plagued by recurrent painful crises. These episodes are due to recurrent vaso-occlusive phenomena and may appear with explosive suddenness and attack various parts of the body, especially the abdomen, chest, and joints. It is often difficult to distinguish between a painful sickle crisis and some other type of acute process such as biliary colic, appendicitis, or a perforated viscus. In the extremities a sickle crisis may mimic osteomyelitis or acute arthritis such as gout or rheumatoid arthritis.

The most common extraskeletal abnormality in the hemolytic anemias is cardiomegaly caused by severe anemia and increased cardiac output. The heart has a globular configuration reflecting enlargement of all chambers. Increased pulmonary blood flow produces engorgement of the pulmonary vessels, giving a hypervascular appearance to the lungs. Pulmonary infarction, pulmonary edema and congestive failure, and pneumonia are frequent complications.

Renal abnormalities can be demonstrated by excretory urography in about two thirds of patients with sickle cell disease. A serious complication is renal papillary necrosis, which is probably related to vessel obstruction within the papillae and may produce sinuses or cavity formation within one or more papillae.

Hemolytic anemia of the newborn (erythroblastosis fetalis), can result when the mother is Rh negative and the fetus has Rh positive blood inherited

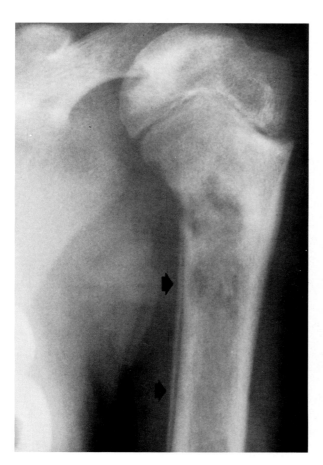

Figure 8-5 Acute osteomyelitis in sickle cell anemia. There is diffuse lytic destruction of proximal humerus along with extensive periosteal reaction *(arrows).*

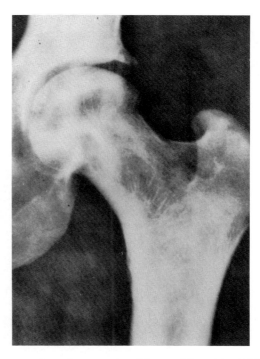

Figure 8-6 Aseptic necrosis of femoral head in sickle cell anemia. Mottled areas of increased and decreased density reflecting osteonecrosis without collapse. Trabeculae in neck and intertrochanteric region are thickened by apposition of new bone. Solid layer of new bone along inner aspect of cortex of femoral shaft causes narrowing of medullary canal. *(From Moseley JE: Semin Roentgenol 9:169-184, 1984.)*

from the father. Although the fetal and maternal circulations are separate, fetal blood can enter the mother's blood through ruptures in the placenta occurring at delivery. The mother thus becomes sensitized to the Rh factor of the fetus and makes antibodies against it. Any antibodies reaching the fetal blood through the placenta in future pregnancies cause hemolysis of the fetal red blood cells. The severity of the disease ranges from mild anemia with jaundice to fetal death.

Blood testing to determine whether Rh incompatibility exists is now an essential part of prenatal care. If an Rh negative mother delivers or aborts an Rh positive infant, she is given a vaccine of Rh immunoglobin within 24 hours to prevent the production of antibodies against the Rh factor.

Megaloblastic anemia

A deficiency of vitamin B_{12} or folic acid leads to defective DNA synthesis and an anemia in which there is a decreased number of red blood cells, although each cell contains the normal amount of hemoglobin. The most common cause of vitamin B_{12} deficiency is pernicious anemia, in which there is inadequate intrinsic factor secretion related to atrophy of the gastric mucosa. Intrinsic factor acts as a carrier in the small bowel absorption of vitamin B_{12}, which is essential for erythrocyte development. Gastric atrophy is seen radiographically as a tubular

stomach with a bald appearance that reflects a decrease or absence of the usually prominent rugal folds (Figure 8-7). It must be emphasized, however, that radiographic findings of atrophic gastritis are often seen in older persons with no evidence of pernicious anemia.

A deficiency of folic acid (and vitamin B_{12}) may also be related to intestinal malabsorption. This may be related to intestinal parasites or bacterial overproduction, especially in patients with stasis of bowel contents as in blind loop syndrome and multiple jejunal diverticula. Other causes of megaloblastic anemia include a poor diet, such as strict vegetarianism, in which there are no sources of vitamin B_{12}, or long-term alcoholism, in which no folic acid is available.

Aplastic anemia

A generalized failure of the bone marrow to function (aplastic anemia) results in decreased levels of erythrocytes, leukocytes, and platelets. In addition to anemia the patient cannot fight infection (a white blood cell function) and has a bleeding tendency (platelet depletion). Causes of aplastic anemia include exposure to chemical agents, drugs, or infections or invasion of the bone marrow by cancer. Regular blood transfusions are generally necessary for survival. Bone marrow transplantation is a new technique for treating these patients.

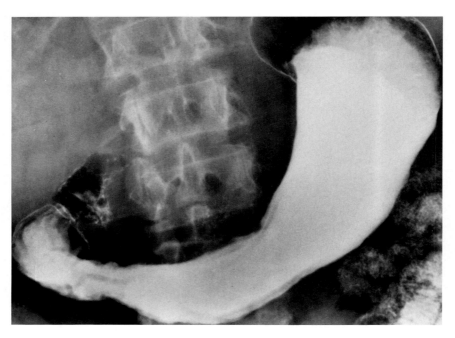

Figure 8-7 Megaloblastic anemia in patient with chronic atrophic gastritis, which presents as tubular stomach with striking decrease in usually prominent rugal folds.

Myelophthisic anemia

Infiltration of bone marrow with tumor cells, or encroachment on marrow cavities caused by cortical thickening, can result in severe anemia and pancytopenia (decreased red and white blood cells and platelets). Tumors may arise from cells that are normally found in the bone marrow (leukemia, lymphoma, myeloma), or the marrow may be invaded by extensive metastases to bone (carcinomas of the breast, prostate, lung, thyroid). Less common causes of marrow replacement include lipid storage disorders (Gaucher's disease), osteopetrosis (marble bones), and myelofibrosis.

Polycythemia

Primary polycythemia (polycythemia vera)

Polycythemia vera is a hematologic disorder characterized by hyperplasia of the bone marrow that results in increased production of erythrocytes, granulocytes, and platelets. The disease is slowly progressive and produces symptoms associated with increased blood volume and viscosity. Cerebrovascular and peripheral vascular insufficiency are common, and many patients give a history of some thrombotic or hemorrhagic event during the course of their disease. There is an increased incidence of peptic ulcer disease, and the excessive cellular proliferation often results in increased levels of uric acid with secondary gout and the formation of urate stones. The spleen is often massively enlarged and may be seen as a left upper quadrant mass.

Increased blood volume in polycythemia vera can lead to prominence of the pulmonary vascular shadows, usually without the cardiomegaly associated with the increased pulmonary vascularity that occurs in patients with congenital heart disease (Figure 8-8). Intravascular thrombosis may cause pulmonary infarctions that appear as focal areas of consolidation or as bands of fibrosis.

Secondary polycythemia

Secondary polycythemia may be the result of long-term inadequate oxygen supply in patients with severe chronic pulmonary disease or congenital cyanotic heart disease, or it may develop in persons living at high altitudes. An elevated hemoglobin concentration may also be caused by certain neoplasms (renal cell carcinoma, hepatoma, cerebellar hemangioblastoma) that result in an increased production of erythropoietin that stimulates red blood cell formation.

Because secondary polycythemia is a compensatory phenomenon, the pulmonary vasculature is normal in appearance and there is no evidence of

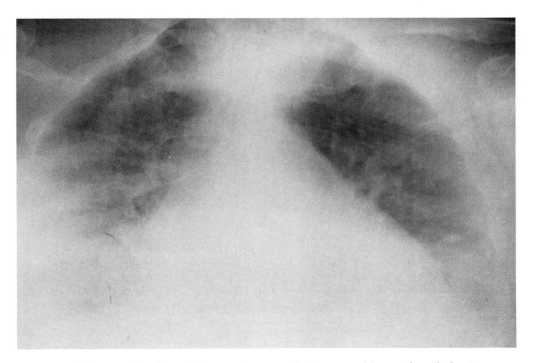

Figure 8-8 Primary polycythemia. Severe hypoventilation caused by profound obesity causes engorgement of pulmonary vessels. Although cardiomegaly is uncommon in polycythemia, in this case it reflects pronounced elevation of diaphragm as result of huge abdominal girth and some underlying cardiac decompensation.

the disease on chest radiographs. In children with severe secondary polycythemia caused by cyanotic heart disease, the skull may show thickened tables and a hair-on-end appearance similar to the findings in congenital hemolytic anemias.

DISEASES OF WHITE BLOOD CELLS

Leukemia

Leukemia is a neoplastic proliferation of white blood cells. The two major types of leukemia are named for the site of malignancy. **Myelocytic** leukemia is a cancer of the bone marrow, in which the primitive white blood cells are called myelocytes. In this condition there is a huge increase in the number of circulating granulocytes with a decreased production of red blood cells and platelets. **Lymphatic** leukemia is a malignancy of the lymph nodes. In this condition the only white blood cells that are dramatically increased are lymphocytes.

Leukemia may be chronic or acute. Acute lymphocytic leukemia, which has an abrupt onset and progresses rapidly, is the most common form in children. Acute myelocytic leukemia is more common in adults. Chronic leukemias run a more prolonged course and may involve either cell type.

Because of the exuberant white cell production, there is generally a decrease in the number of circulating red blood cells and platelets. This results in a typical clinical appearance of weakness, shortness of breath, and cardiac palpitations. A decrease in the number of platelets interferes with the blood-clotting mechanism and results in a bleeding tendency. Even though there are more circulating white blood cells than normal, most are immature and thus the patient becomes highly susceptible to infection. Diffuse

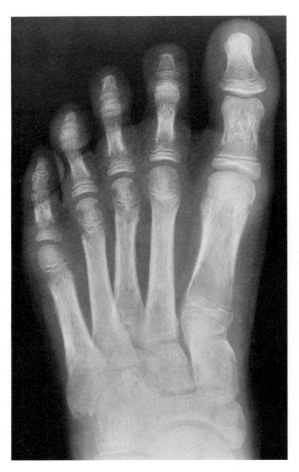

Figure 8-9 Acute leukemia. In addition to radiolucent metaphyseal bands, there is frank bone destruction with cortical erosion involving many metatarsals and proximal phalanges.

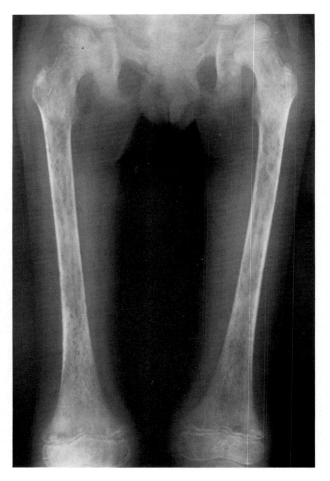

Figure 8-10 Acute leukemia. Proliferation of neoplastic cells in marrow has caused extensive destruction of bone in both femurs.

infiltration of white cells in the spleen and liver may cause massive enlargement of these organs (hepatosplenomegaly).

In childhood leukemia radiographically detectable skeletal involvement is extremely common as a result of the infiltration of leukemic cells in the marrow. The earliest radiographic sign of disease is usually a transverse radiolucent band at the metaphyseal ends of the long bones, most commonly about the knees, ankles, and wrists (Figure 8-9). Although in infancy this appearance is nonspecific and also occurs with malnutrition or systemic disease, the presence of these transverse lucent metaphyseal bands after the age of 2 strongly suggests acute leukemia.

As the proliferation of neoplastic cells in the marrow becomes more extensive, actual destruction of bone may occur. This may cause patchy lytic lesions, a permeative moth-eaten appearance, or diffuse destruction with cortical erosion (Figure 8-10). A reactive response to proliferating leukemic cells can cause patchy or uniform osteosclerosis; subperiosteal proliferation incites the formation of periosteal new bone. Diffuse skeletal demineralization may result in vertebral compression fractures.

Enlargement of mediastinal and hilar lymph nodes is the most common abnormality on chest radiographs. Diffuse bilateral reticular changes may simulate lymphangitic spread of carcinoma. The nonspecific pulmonary infiltrates seen in patients with acute leukemia are usually due to hemorrhage or secondary infection.

The radiographic abnormalities in chronic leukemia are often similar to those in the acute disease, although their frequency and degree may vary. Skeletal changes are much less common and are usually limited to generalized demineralization in the flat bones, where active marrow persists in adulthood. The demonstration of focal areas of destruction, or periosteal new bone formation, suggests transformation into an acute phase of the disease.

Hilar and mediastinal adenopathy are common, especially in chronic lymphocytic leukemia. Congestive heart failure commonly results from the associated severe anemia.

Marked splenomegaly is an almost constant finding in patients with chronic leukemia (Figure 8-11). Leukemic infiltration of the gastrointestinal tract can produce single or multiple intraluminal filling defects or appear as an infiltrative process that may be indistinguishable from carcinoma. Renal infiltration can cause bilateral enlargement of the kidneys. In chronic lymphocytic leukemia, enlargement of retroperitoneal or mesenteric lymph nodes can cause

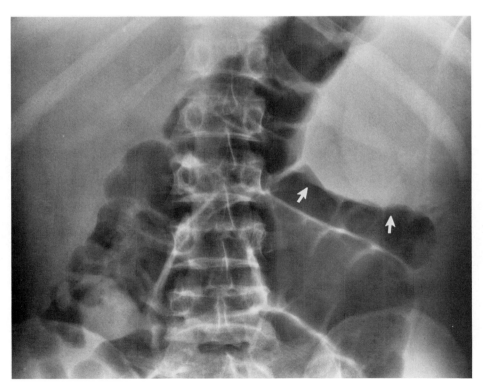

Figure 8-11 Chronic leukemia. Massive splenomegaly causes downward displacement of splenic flexure of colon. Arrow points to inferior margin of spleen.

displacement or obstruction of structures in the genitourinary or gastrointestinal tracts.

Lymphoma

Lymphomas are neoplasms of the lymphoreticular system, which includes the lymph nodes, spleen, and the lymphoid tissues of parenchymal organs such as the gastrointestinal tract, lung, or skin. They are usually divided into two major types: Hodgkin's and non-Hodgkin's lymphomas. Ninety percent of cases of Hodgkin's disease originate in the lymph nodes; 10% are of extranodal origin. In contrast, parenchymal organs are more often involved in non-Hodgkin's lymphomas, about 40% of which are of extranodal origin. Mediastinal lymph node enlargement is the most common radiographic finding in lymphoma (Figure 8-12). It is seen on initial chest radiographs of about half the patients with Hodgkin's disease and about one third of those with non-Hodgkin's lymphoma. Mediastinal lymph node enlargement is usually asymmetric but bilateral. Involvement of anterior mediastinal and retrosternal nodes is common, a major factor in the differential diagnosis from sarcoidosis, which rarely produces radiographically visible enlargement of nodes in the anterior compartment. Calcification may develop in intrathoracic lymph nodes after mediastinal irradiation.

Involvement of the pulmonary parenchyma and pleura usually occurs by direct extension from mediastinal nodes along the lymphatic vessels of the bronchovascular sheaths. Radiographically, this may appear as a coarse interstitial pattern (Figure 8-13), as solitary or multiple ill-defined nodules, or as patchy areas of parenchymal infiltrate that may

coalesce to form a large homogeneous mass. At times, it may be difficult to distinguish a superimposed infection after radiation therapy or chemotherapy from the continued spread of lymphomatous tissue. Pleural effusion occurs in up to one third of patients with thoracic lymphoma; extension of the tumor to the pericardium can cause pericardial effusion.

About 5% to 10% of patients with lymphoma have involvement of the gastrointestinal tract, primarily of the stomach and small bowel. Gastric lymphoma often is seen as a large, bulky polypoid mass, usually irregular and ulcerated, that may be indistinguishable from a carcinoma (Figure 8-14). A multiplicity of malignant ulcers or an aneurysmal appearance of a single huge ulcer (the diameter of which exceeds that of the adjacent gastric lumen) is characteristic of lymphoma. Additional findings suggestive of lymphoma include relative flexibility of the gastric wall, enlargement of the spleen, and associated prominence of retrogastric and other regional lymph nodes that cause extrinsic impressions on the barium-filled stomach. Other manifestations of gastric lymphoma include thickening, distortion, and nodularity of rugal folds (Figure 8-15) and generalized gastric narrowing caused by a severe fibrotic reaction.

Lymphoma can produce virtually any pattern of abnormality in the small bowel. The disease may be localized to a single intestinal segment, be multifocal, or cause diffuse involvement. The major radiographic appearances include irregular thickening of mucosal folds, large ulcerating masses, and multiple intraluminal or intramural filling defects simulating metastatic disease.

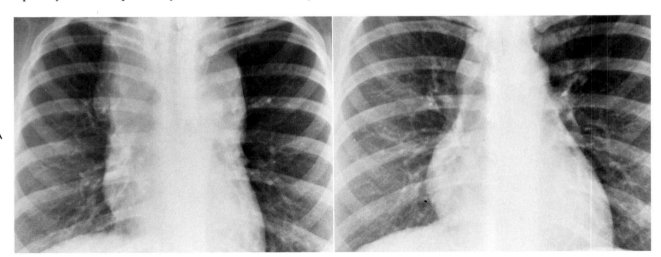

A B

Figure 8-12 Lymphoma. **A,** Initial chest film demonstrates marked widening of upper half of mediastinum caused by pronounced lymphadenopathy. **B,** After chemotherapy, there is dramatic decrease in width of upper mediastinum.

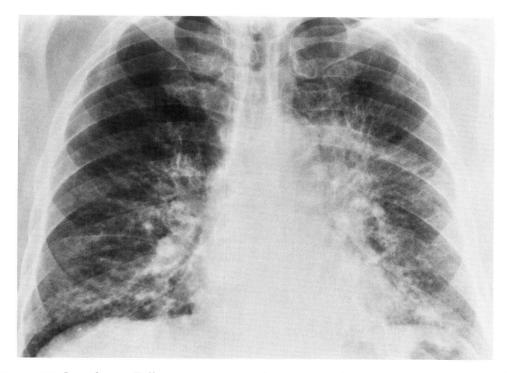

Figure 8-13 Lymphoma. Diffuse reticular and reticulonodular changes causing prominence of interstitial lung markings. Note enlargement of left hilar region.

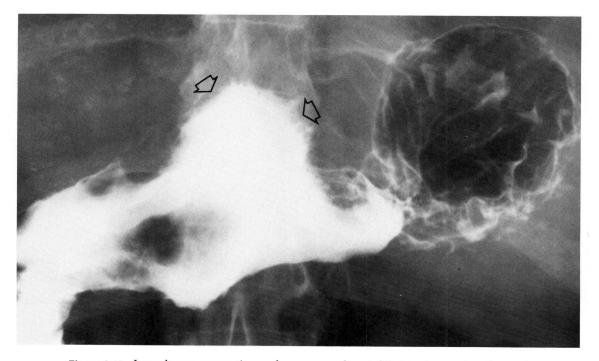

Figure 8-14 Lymphoma presenting as large mass almost filled by huge ulcer *(arrows)*.

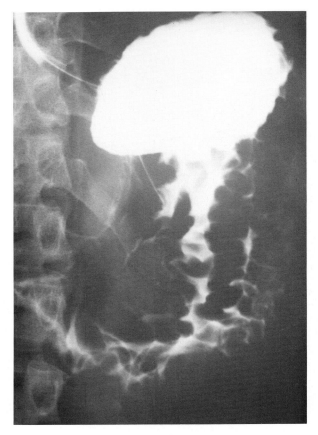

Figure 8-15 Lymphoma of stomach. Note diffuse thickening, distortion, and nodularity of gastric folds.

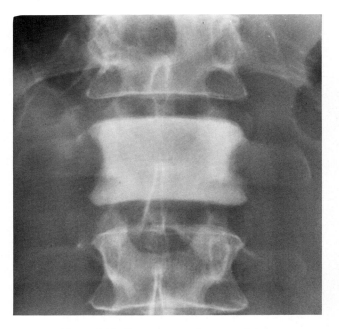

Figure 8-16 Lymphoma. Ivory vertebra.

Skeletal involvement can be demonstrated in about 15% of patients with lymphoma. Direct extension from adjacent lymph nodes causes bone erosion, especially of the anterior surface of the upper lumbar and lower thoracic spine. Paravertebral soft-tissue masses may occur. The hematogenous spread of lymphoma produces a mottled pattern of destruction and sclerosis that may simulate metastatic disease. Dense vertebral sclerosis (ivory vertebra) may develop in Hodgkin's disease (Figure 8-16).

Diffuse lymphomatous infiltration may cause renal enlargement with distortion, elongation, and compression of the calyces (Figure 8-17). Single or multiple renal nodules or perirenal masses may displace or distort the kidney. Diffuse retroperitoneal lymphoma can displace the kidneys or ureters and obliterate one or both psoas margins.

Once the diagnosis of lymphoma is made, it is essential to determine the status of the abdominal and pelvic lymph nodes. This is necessary for both the initial staging and treatment planning and for assessing the efficacy of treatment and detecting tumor recurrence.

There is controversy about the best radiographic approach for the staging of a patient with known lymphoma. Although lymphography has long been a most accurate examination for demonstrating lymphomatous involvement of abdominal and pelvic nodes, noninvasive cross-sectional imaging techniques (CT and ultrasound) are now considered by many to be the diagnostic methods of choice. Unlike CT and ultrasound, which rely primarily on an increase in node size as a criterion for determining tumor involvement, lymphography can detect mi-

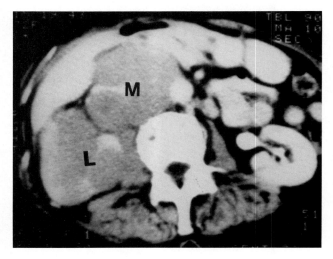

Figure 8-17 Lymphoma. Right kidney is completely replaced by lymphomatous mass (L). Note extensive involvement of lymph nodes (M).

croscopic tumor foci and alterations in architecture within normal-sized nodes. It can also distinguish large nodes that contain tumor from similarly enlarged nodes that demonstrate only benign reactive changes. After formal staging procedures, abdominal radiographs can demonstrate retained contrast material within lymph nodes and thus provide an inexpensive and accurate mean for assessing the effect of therapy and detecting relapse. However, lymph nodes in the upper para-aortic, retrocrural, renal hilus, or splenic hilus, porta hepatis, and mesenteric areas cannot be adequately examined by lymphography and require CT or ultrasound (Figure 8-18). CT can also be used to check on the response to treatment, especially since there may be insufficient residual contrast on postlymphography abdominal films to make a diagnosis.

In practice, CT is generally the first procedure used in staging lymphoma patients, especially those with non-Hodgkin's lymphoma which tends to produce bulky masses in the mesenteric and high retrocrural areas where the contrast material used in lymphography does not reach. An abnormal CT scan eliminates the need for the more invasive lymphography; a normal CT scan obtained at 2 cm intervals can exclude retroperitoneal adenopathy with high confidence. Lymphography is of value primarily in Hodgkin's disease, which infrequently involves the mesenteric nodes, often does not produce bulky masses, and may cause alterations of internal architecture only (which cannot be detected with CT) in normal-sized nodes. Lymphography is also indicated when CT is equivocal because of either a lack of fat or gross motion artifacts.

Infectious mononucleosis

Mononucleosis is a self-limited viral disease of the lymphoreticular system characterized by vague symptoms of mild fever, fatigue, sore throat, and swollen lymph nodes. It primarily infects young adults and, although often termed the "kissing disease," is not particularly contagious. Blood tests show an elevated white cell count with an abnormally high percentage of atypical lymphocytes that resemble monocytes. The diagnosis is based on the presence of antibodies to the virus in the blood.

Generalized lymphadenopathy and splenomegaly are characteristic clinical and radiographic findings in infectious mononucleosis. Hilar lymph node enlargement, usually bilateral, can be demonstrated in about 15% of cases (Figure 8-19). Pneumonia is a

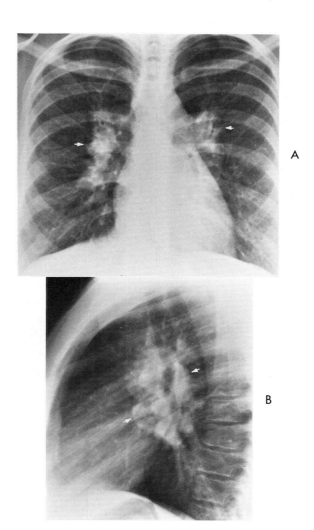

Figure 8-19 Infectious mononucleosis. **A,** Frontal and, **B,** lateral projections of chest demonstrate marked enlargement of hilar lymph nodes bilaterally *(arrows)*.

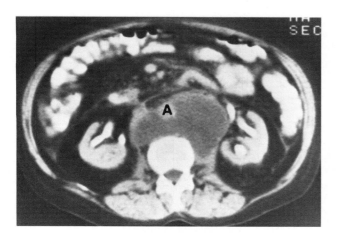

Figure 8-18 Lymphoma. CT scan demonstrates anterior displacement of abdominal aorta *(A)* away from spine caused by lymphomatous involvement of retro-aortic and para-aortic nodes.

rare complication that can appear as a diffuse reticular pattern indicating interstitial disease or as a patchy, nonspecific air space consolidation.

DISEASES OF PLATELETS (BLEEDING DISORDERS)

Blood coagulation (clotting) is a complicated mechanism requiring platelets, calcium, and 12 coenzymes and proteins called **coagulation factors.** A deficiency in quantity or activity of any of these materials may lead to an inability to control hemorrhage or even to spontaneous bleeding.

Hemophilia

Hemophilia is an inherited (sex-linked recessive gene) anomaly of blood coagulation that appears clinically only in males. Patients with this disease have a decreased or absent serum concentration of antihemophilic globulin (factor VIII) and suffer a lifelong tendency to spontaneous hemorrhage or severe bleeding from even minor cuts or injuries.

The major radiographic changes in hemophilia are complications of recurrent bleeding into the joints, which most commonly involve the knees, elbows, and ankles. Initially, the hemorrhage produces a generalized nonspecific soft-tissue prominence of the distended joint. Deposition of iron pigment may produce areas of cloudy increased density in the periarticular soft tissues. Although complete resorption of intra-articular blood may leave no residual change, subsequent episodes of bleeding result in synovial hypertrophy. In chronic disease the hyperplastic synovium causes cartilage destruction and joint space narrowing and often leads to the development of multiple subchondral cysts of vary-

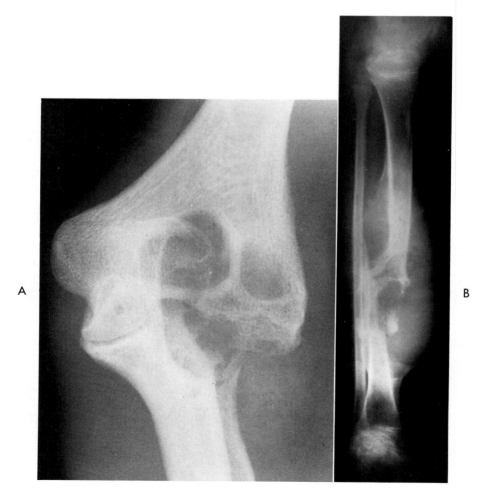

Figure 8-20 Hemophilia. **A,** Large subchondral cysts about elbow. **B,** Destructive, expansile lesion of lower tibial shaft. *(From Stoker DJ and Murray RO: Semin Roentgenol 9:185-193, 1974.)*

ing sizes in the immediate juxta-articular bone (Figure 8-20, *A*). Destruction of articular cartilage and continued use of the damaged joint lead to subchondral sclerosis and collapse, extensive and bizarre spur formation, and often marked soft-tissue calcification. Hemorrhage extending into the adjacent bony structures may cause extensive destruction (pseudotumor of hemophilia), which can mimic a malignant tumor (Figure 8-20, *B*).

Repeated joint hemorrhages lead to increased blood flow in the region of the epiphysis and growth plate. These structures may ossify prematurely, become abnormally large, or fuse prematurely with the metaphysis. Increased blood flow and atrophy of bone and muscle that may follow an episode of joint bleeding result in severe osteoporosis. Common signs suggestive, although not pathognomonic, of hemophilia include widening and deepening of the intercondylar notch of the femur (Figure 8-21) and "squaring" of the inferior border of the patella. Asymmetric growth of the distal tibial epiphysis may result in "slanting" of the tibiotalar joint. Hemarthrosis can cause occlusion of epiphyseal vessels and result in avascular necrosis. This most com-

monly involves the femoral and radial heads, both of which have a totally intracapsular epiphysis and are therefore especially vulnerable to deprivation of their vascular supply from compression by a tense joint effusion.

As in the other bleeding disorders, submucosal bleeding into the wall of the gastrointestinal tract may develop in patients with hemophilia. This most commonly involves the small bowel and produces a short or long segment with regular thickening of folds. In the colon bleeding may produce the thumbprinting pattern of sharply defined, fingerlike marginal indentations along the contours of the colon wall.

Purpura (thrombocytopenia)

Purpura refers to a deficiency in the number of platelets causing spontaneous hemorrhages in the skin, mucous membranes of the mouth, and internal organs. In the skin, purpura leads to the development of small, flat red spots (petechiae) or larger hemorrhagic areas (ecchymoses).

Acute idiopathic thrombocytopenic purpura typically has the sudden onset of severe purpura 1 to 2 weeks after a sore throat or upper respiratory infection in an otherwise healthy child. In most patients the disorder is self-limited and clears spon-

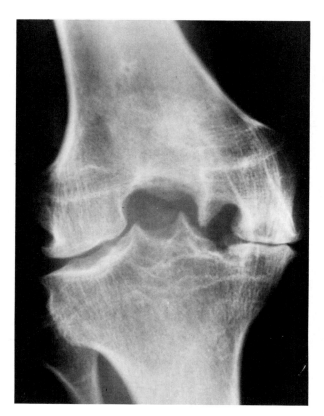

Figure 8-21 Hemophilia. Intercondylar notch is markedly widened, and coarse trabeculae, narrowing of joint space, and hypertrophic spurring can be seen.

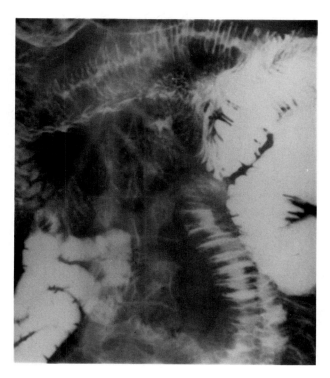

Figure 8-22 Chronic idiopathic thrombocytopenic purpura. Hemorrhage into wall of small bowel causes regular thickening of mucosal folds.

taneously within a few weeks. Unlike the acute form, chronic idiopathic thrombocytopenic purpura occurs primarily in young women and has an insidious onset with a relatively long history of easy bruising and menorrhagia. This condition is generally considered to be an autoimmune disorder, since most patients have a circulating platelet autoantibody that develops without underlying disease or significant exposure to drugs.

Purpura can also be a complication of conditions that suppress the bone marrow (aplastic anemia) or infiltrate the bone marrow with tumor cells (leukemia, lymphoma, myeloma, metastases).

The radiographic changes caused by either acute or chronic idiopathic thrombocytopenic purpura primarily involve the gastrointestinal tract. Hemorrhage into the small bowel produces characteristic uniform, regular thickening of mucosal folds in the affected intestinal segment (Figure 8-22). Splenomegaly is commonly present; splenectomy is often required to remove this important site of platelet destruction and major source of synthesis of platelet antibodies.

QUESTIONS

1. When diseases of the hematopoietic system result in demineralization of bone, the radiographer must be alert to the possibility of _____.
   A. Patient infection
   B. Self infection
   C. Pathologic fracture
   D. Syncope

2. Red blood cells are called _____.
   A. Erythrocytes
   B. Leukocytes
   C. Thrombocytes
   D. Hemoglobin

3. Platelets are called _____.
   A. Erythrocytes
   B. Leukocytes
   C. Thrombocytes
   D. Lymphocytes

4. White blood cells are called _____.
   A. Erythrocytes
   B. Leukocytes
   C. Thrombocytes
   D. Paracytes

5. The smallest blood cells, platelets, are essential for what process?
   A. Immunity
   B. Clotting
   C. Carrying oxygen
   D. Fighting infection

6. Lymphocytes play a major role in the _____ system.
   A. Endocrine
   B. Hematopoietic
   C. Immune
   D. Metabolic

7. The term _____ refers to a decrease in the amount of oxygen-carrying hemoglobin in the blood.
   A. Spherocytosis
   B. Thalassemia
   C. Anemia
   D. Hematopoiesis

8. What type of anemia can cause painful bone infarcts and is generally confined to the black race?
   A. Spherocytosis
   B. Thalassemia
   C. Sickle cell
   D. Salmonella

9. A hematologic disorder characterized by an increase in the production of erythrocytes, granulocytes, and platelets is _____.
   A. Polycythemia vera
   B. Erythrocytosis
   C. Sickle cell anemia
   D. Hemolytic anemia

10. A cancerous disease of the hematopoietic system characterized by an increase in white blood cells is _____.
    A. Anemia
    B. Thrombocytopenia
    C. Leukemia
    D. Hemophilia

11. What is the name of an inherited anomaly of blood coagulation?
    A. Sickle cell anemia
    B. Hemophilia
    C. Leukemia
    D. Leukocytosis

12. What pathologic condition refers to a deficiency in the number of platelets resulting in spontaneous hemorrhages in the skin, internal organs, and mucous membranes of the mouth?
    A. Hemophilia
    B. Purpura
    C. Leukemia
    D. Sickle cell anemia

BIBLIOGRAPHY

Reynolds J: Radiologic manifestations of sickle cell hemoglobulinopathy, JAMA 238:247-250, 1977.

Korsten J et al: Extramedullary hematopoiesis in patients with thalassemia anemia, Radiology 95:257-264, 1970.

Stoker DJ and Murray RO: Skeletal changes in hemophilia and other bleeding disorders, Semin Roentgenol 9:185-193, 1974.

Pear BL: Skeletal manifestations of the lymphomas and leukemias, Semin Roentgenol 9:229-240, 1974.

CHAPTER 9

Endocrine System

PREREQUISITE KNOWLEDGE

The student should have a basic knowledge of the anatomy and physiology of the endocrine system. In addition, proper learning and understanding of the material will be facilitated if the student has some clinical experience in general radiography and film evaluation, including a concept of the newer imaging modalities (ultrasound, CT, MRI) used to study the various body systems affected by endocrine abnormalities.

GOALS

To acquaint the student radiographer with the pathophysiology and radiographic manifestations of all of the common and some of the unusal disorders of the endocrine system

OBJECTIVES

1. Describe the physiology of the endocrine system
2. Identify anatomic structures on both diagrams and images of the endocrine system
3. Be able to define terminology relating to the endocrine system
4. Be able to describe the various pathologic conditions affecting the endocrine system and their radiographic manifestations

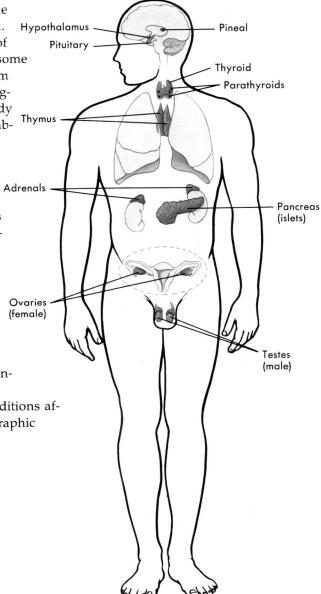

Hypothalamus
Pituitary
Pineal
Thyroid
Parathyroids
Thymus
Adrenals
Pancreas (islets)
Ovaries (female)
Testes (male)

Imaging modalities are used to diagnose both the underlying endocrine disorder and the secondary changes that may occur in various areas of the body. Disorders of the endocrine glands themselves are usually evaluated by ultrasound, CT, MRI, and radionuclide scanning. Secondary pathologic manifestations elsewhere in the body are generally evaluated on plain radiographs, for which the routine exposure techniques may have to be altered (see Table 1-1). For example, Cushing's syndrome causes extensive osteoporosis that requires a decrease in kVp to adequately visualize the demineralized bones. It should also be noted that patients with this condition can easily sustain pathologic fractures and thus should always be handled with caution.

DISEASES OF THE ENDOCRINE SYSTEM

The endocrine system is a biochemical communication network through which several small glands control a broad range of vital body activities. The endocrine glands secrete chemical messengers called hormones, which circulate in the blood and may affect a single target organ or the entire body. Hormones may be proteins (growth hormone), steroids (cortisone), peptides (antidiuretic hormone), amino acids (thyroxine), or amines (epinephrine). They range from large to small molecules and have chemical structures of varying complexity.

The major endocrine glands are the pituitary, adrenal, thyroid, and parathyroid glands. Inadequate **(hypoactive)** or excess **(hyperactive)** production of hormones from these endocrine glands can give rise to a wide variety of clinical symptoms and radiographic abnormalities.

Because hormones are powerful chemicals, it is essential that their circulating levels be carefully controlled. One type of control is called the "negative feedback mechanism." In this system, an adequate level of a hormone in the blood automatically stops the release of additional hormone (somewhat like a thermostat). As the blood level of the hormone decreases, the gland is stimulated to secrete more of it. Another control mechanism is the production of two different hormones whose actions are opposite to each other. For example, insulin is secreted by the pancreas when the blood sugar level rises. When the blood sugar level falls below normal, a second hormone, glucagon, is secreted by the pancreas to raise the blood sugar. Thus these two hormones are balanced so that a proper blood sugar level is continually maintained.

ADRENAL GLANDS

Physiology of the adrenal glands

The adrenal glands are situated at the top of each kidney and consist of an outer cortex and an inner medulla. The adrenal cortex secretes several different types of steroid hormones, which can be divided into three general groups. The **mineralocorticoids** (primarily aldosterone) regulate salt and water balance by causing sodium retention and potassium excretion by the kidneys. The production of aldosterone is primarily regulated by the secretion of renin from specialized cells (juxtaglomerular apparatus) in the kidney. Reduced blood volume (as in hemorrhage) causes low blood pressure that is detected by the juxtaglomerular apparatus and eventually results in increased aldosterone secretion from the adrenal cortex. **Glucocorticoids** (especially cortisone) regulate carbohydrate metabolism and are under the regulation of ACTH from the anterior pituitary gland. Cortisone also depresses the inflammatory response to almost all forms of injury, thus leading to its use in the treatment of trauma, rheumatoid arthritis, bursitis, and asthma, and as an immunosuppressive agent to help limit rejection after organ transplantation. **Androgens** are sex hormones that tend to masculinize the body, to retain amino acids, and to enhance protein synthesis. It is these hormones that are used both illegally and unwisely by athletes to attempt to increase their body strength.

The adrenal medulla secretes epinephrine (adrenaline) and norepinephrine. These "fight or flight" hormones are secreted in stress situations when additional energy and strength are needed. Epinephrine stimulates heart activity, raises blood pressure, and increases the level of blood glucose. By constricting some blood vessels and dilating others, epinephrine shunts blood to active muscles where oxygen and nutrients are urgently needed.

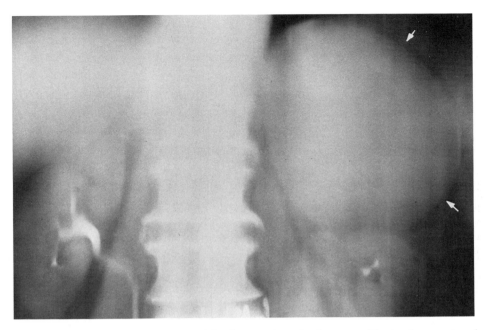

Figure 9-1 Cushing's syndrome caused by large adrenal adenoma. Nephrotomogram demonstrates huge suprarenal mass *(arrows)* causing indentation and downward displacement of left kidney.

Diseases of the adrenal cortex

Cushing's syndrome

The excess production of glucocorticoid hormones in Cushing's syndrome may be due to generalized bilateral hyperplasia of the adrenal cortex or may be a result of a functioning adrenal or even nonadrenal tumor. It can also be the result of the exogenous administration of cortisone. Excess secretion of glucocorticoid hormones mobilizes lipids and increases their level in the blood. This produces a characteristic obesity that is confined to the trunk of the body and is associated with a round, moon-shaped face and a pathognomonic fat pad that forms behind the shoulders (buffalo hump). Retention of salt and water results in hypertension.

Generalized enlargement of the adrenal glands is best demonstrated by CT, which shows thickening of the wings of the adrenal gland that appear to have a stellate or Y-shaped configuration in cross section. Ultrasound can also show diffuse adrenal gland enlargement.

Benign and malignant tumors of the adrenal cortex are less common causes of Cushing's syndrome than is nontumorous adrenal hyperfunction. As a general rule, the larger an adrenal cortical tumor and the more abrupt the onset of clinical symptoms and signs, the more likely the tumor is to be malignant. However, the differentiation between adenoma and carcinoma may be impossible at the time of histo-

logic examination, and only the clinical course may define the nature of the tumor. On extretory urography with nephrotomography, a left-sided adrenal mass tends to rotate the upper pole of the kidney laterally so that the axis of the kidney no longer parallels the psoas margin. Larger left-sided masses may displace the kidney downward or indent the posterior aspect of the stomach (Figure 9-1). On the right, a mass commonly indents the superior aspect of the right kidney and displaces it downward. CT and ultrasound can demonstrate an adrenal tumor (Figure 9-2). CT is often of more value because the abundance of retroperitoneal fat may prevent an optimal ultrasound examination. Adrenal venography has been widely used to demonstrate adrenal masses and also permits the aspiration of blood samples for assessing the level of adrenal hormones.

Cushing's syndrome produces radiographic changes in multiple systems. Diffuse osteoporosis causes generalized skeletal demineralization that may lead to the collapse of vertebral bodies, spontaneous fractures, and aseptic necrosis of the head of the femur or humerus. Widening of the mediastinum as a result of excessive fat deposition sometimes develops in Cushing's syndrome and can be confirmed by CT. Hypercalciuria caused by the elevated steroid levels can lead to renal calculi and nephrocalcinosis.

Imaging of the sella turcica by conventional to-

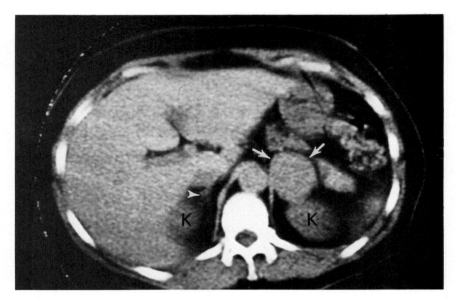

Figure 9-2 Cushing's syndrome caused by functioning cortical adenoma; 4-cm mass in left adrenal gland *(arrows)* is seen posterior to tail of pancreas and anterior to kidney *(K)*. Arrowhead points to normal right adrenal gland. *(From Lee JKT, Sagel SS, and Stanley RJ, editors: Computed body tomography, New York, Raven Press, 1983.)*

mography or CT is important in the routine assessment of the patient with Cushing's syndrome. Most patients with nontumorous adrenal hyperfunction are found at surgery to have an intrasellar lesion. It is important to emphasize, however, that small pituitary microadenomas may be present in asymptomatic patients. After adrenal surgery, a pituitary adenoma develops in up to one third of the patients and produces progressive sellar enlargement. For this reason, yearly follow-up sellar tomograms may be indicated after adrenalectomy.

Nonpituitary tumors producing ACTH may cause adrenal hyperfunction and Cushing's syndrome. The most common sites of origin are the lung, thymus, and pancreas; about half of these tumors can be demonstrated on chest radiographs.

Aldosteronism

An overproduction of mineralocorticoid hormones produced by the most superficial layer of the cortex causes retention of sodium and water and abnormal loss of potassium in the urine. This results in hypertension, muscular weakness or paralysis, and excessive thirst (polydypsia). Aldosteronism may be due to an adrenal cortical adenoma (Conn's syndrome) or to bilateral hyperplasia of the superficial cortical layer. The clinical manifestations of aldosteronism can be cured by the resection of an adenoma but are little affected by the removal of both adrenal glands in the patient with bilateral hyper-

plasia. Therefore the role of radiographic imaging is to demonstrate the location of adenomas that may be otherwise difficult to detect during exploratory surgery.

Because aldosteronomas are often very small (unlike the large cortical adenomas in patients with Cushing's syndrome), excretory urography with tomography has little usefulness. CT is the major imaging modality and demonstrates the small adrenal cortical adenoma as a contour abnormality of the gland (Figure 9-3). Adrenal venography with biochemical assay of a sample of adrenal blood is another important technique for localizing aldosteronomas.

Aldosteronism may also be the result of renin-secreting tumors, renal artery stenosis, malignant hypertension, and bilateral chronic renal disease.

Adrenogenital syndrome

The adrenogenital syndrome (adrenal virilism) is caused by the excessive secretion of androgenically active substances by the adrenal gland. In the congenital form, a specific enzyme deficiency that prevents the formation of androgenic hormones causes continuous ACTH stimulation and bilateral hyperplasia. The elevated levels of androgens result in accelerated skeletal maturation along with premature epiphyseal fusion that may lead to dwarfism.

Most cases of acquired adrenogenital syndrome are due to adrenal cortical tumors that can be de-

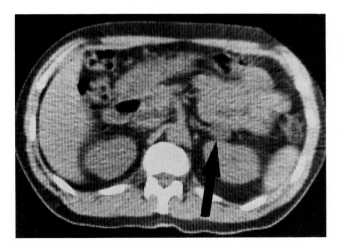

Figure 9-3 Aldosteronoma. Small mass *(arrow)* anterior to left kidney.

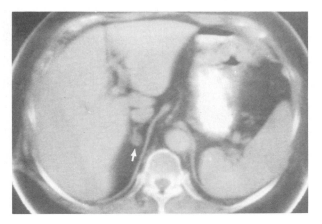

Figure 9-4 Adrenogenital syndrome caused by functioning adrenal carcinoma. Large mass in left upper quadrant *(arrow)* displacing spleen *(S)* anteriorly. Multiple round metastases are present in liver. *(From Karstaedt N et al: Computed tomography of the adrenal gland, Radiology 129:723-730, 1978.)*

tected by CT (Figure 9-4), ultrasound, or adrenal venography. In women the tumor causes masculinization with the development of hair on the face (hirsutism). The breasts diminish, the clitoris enlarges, and ovulation and menstruation cease.

Hypoadrenalism

The clinical manifestations of adrenal insufficiency vary from those of a chronic insidious disorder (easy fatigability, anorexia, weakness, weight loss, increased melanin pigmentation) to an acute collapse with hypotension, rapid pulse, vomiting, and diarrhea.

The most common cause of adrenal insufficiency is the excessive administration of steroids. Primary adrenal cortical insufficiency (Addison's disease) results from progressive cortical destruction, which must involve more than 90% of the glands before clinical signs of adrenal insufficiency appear. In the past, Addison's disease was usually attributed to tuberculosis; at present most cases reflect idiopathic atrophy, probably on an autoimmune basis. In areas where the disease is endemic, histoplasmosis is an occasional cause of adrenal insufficiency (Figure 9-5). Acute inflammatory disease causes generalized enlargement of the adrenal glands, which can be demonstrated by a variety of imaging techniques. Other radiographic findings occasionally seen in patients with adrenal insufficiency include a small heart and calcification of the cartilage of the ear.

Adrenal carcinoma

About half of adrenal carcinomas are functioning tumors that cause Cushing's syndrome, virilization, feminization, or aldosteronism. The tumors grow

rapidly and are usually large masses at the time of clinical presentation.

Excretory urography demonstrates an adrenal carcinoma as a nonspecific suprarenal mass that is often lobulated and tends to displace the kidney without evidence of invasion. Ultrasound shows the tumor as a complex mass that may be difficult to separate from an upper pole renal tumor. CT demonstrates an adrenal carcinoma as a large mass that often contains low-density areas resulting from necrosis or prior hemorrhage (Figure 9-6). Because lymphatic and hepatic metastases are common at the time of clinical presentation, CT scans at multiple

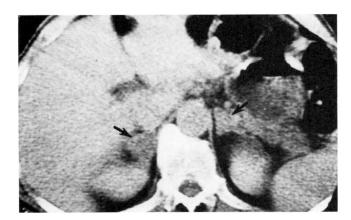

Figure 9-5 Adrenocortical insufficiency caused by disseminated histoplasmosis. CT scan demonstrates bilateral adrenal enlargement *(arrows)*. *(From Karstaedt N et al: Computed tomography of the adrenal gland, Radiology 129:723-730, 1978.)*

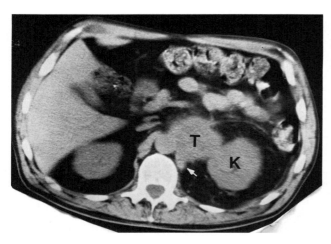

Figure 9-6 Large soft-tissue tumor *(T)* invading antero-medial aspect of left kidney *(K)* and left crus of diaphragm *(arrow)*. *(Courtesy of Nolan Krastaedt, M.D., and Neil Wolf-man, M.D.)*

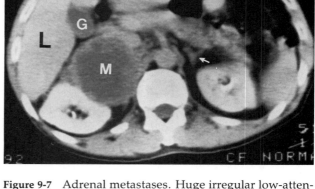

Figure 9-7 Adrenal metastases. Huge irregular low-attenuation mass *(M)* representing adrenal metastasis from oat cell carcinoma of lung. Left adrenal gland *(arrow)* is normal. *L,* Liver; *G,* gallbladder.

abdominal levels are necessary to define the extent of the primary tumor and to detect metastases before attempted surgical resection. Extension of the tumor into the renal vein and vena cava can also be detected by CT, especially after the injection of intravenous contrast material.

Metastases to the adrenal glands

The adrenal gland is one of the most common sites of metastatic disease. The primary tumors that most frequently metastasize to the adrenal gland are carcinomas of the lung and breast; carcinomas of the kidney, ovary, and gastrointestinal tract; and melanomas. Metastatic enlargement of an adrenal gland can cause downward displacement of the kidney with flattening of the upper pole. Ultrasound and CT demonstrate adrenal metastases as solid, soft-tissue masses that vary considerably in size and are frequently bilateral (Figure 9-7). However, the ultrasound and CT patterns are indistinguishable from those of primary malignancies of the gland. Therefore when a known primary tumor exists elsewhere, it is usually assumed that an adrenal mass is metastatic. If necessary, a needle biopsy using ultrasound guidance may be of value to determine whether the adrenal lesion is primary or metastatic.

Diseases of the adrenal medulla

Pheochromocytoma

A pheochromocytoma is a tumor that most commonly arises in the adrenal medulla and produces an excess of vasopressor substances (epinephrine and norepinephrine) that can cause an uncommon

but curable form of hypertension. About 10% of pheochromocytomas are extra-adrenal in origin. About 10% of patients have bilateral tumors, and a similar percentage of pheochromocytomas are malignant.

Because in almost all patients the diagnosis of a pheochromocytoma can be made with biochemical tests, radiographic imaging serves as a confirmatory study and as a means of localizing the tumor. Excretory urography, even with nephrotomography, may be of limited value because the kidney is often not displaced even when an adrenal pheochromocytoma is large.

CT and ultrasound are very useful in the localization of pheochromocytomas. The cross-sectional images not only detail the extent of the adrenal lesion but also define the status of adjacent structures and can demonstrate bilateral or multiple pheochromocytomas, extra-adrenal tumors, and metastases. Pheochromocytomas generally appear as round, oval, or pear-shaped masses that are slightly less echogenic than liver and kidney parenchyma on ultrasound and have an attenuation value less than these organs on CT (Figure 9-8).

Most extra-adrenal pheochromocytomas arise in the abdomen (Figure 9-9); a few are found in the chest or neck. The tumor may be located anywhere along the sympathetic nervous system, in the organ of Zuckerkandl, and in chemoreceptor tissues such as the carotid body or the glomus jugulare, in the wall of the urinary bladder, or even in the kidney or ureter. Masses may displace the ureter or kidney or may appear as filling defects in the bladder.

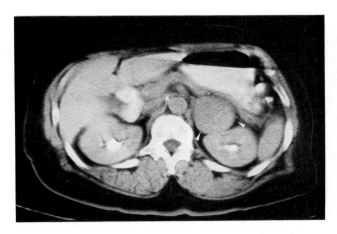

Figure 9-8 Pheochromocytoma. Large pear-shaped mass (*arrows*) anterior to left kidney.

In patients with pheochromocytomas, the arterial injection of contrast material causes a marked elevation in blood pressure that must be controlled by α-adrenergic blocking agents. Therefore arteriography is hazardous in these patients.

Neuroblastoma

Neuroblastoma, a tumor of adrenal medullary origin, is the second most common malignancy in children. About 10% of these tumors arise outside the adrenal gland, primarily in sympathetic ganglia in the neck, chest, abdomen, or pelvis. The tumor is highly malignant and tends to attain great size before detection.

Calcification is common in neuroblastoma (occurring in about 50% of cases) in contrast to the relatively infrequent calcification in Wilms' tumor, from which neuroblastoma must be differentiated. Calcification in a neuroblastoma has a fine granular or stippled appearance (Figure 9-10, *A*). Occasionally, there may be a single mass of amorphous calcification. Calcification can also develop in metastases of neuroblastoma in paravertebral lymph nodes and liver.

Excretory urography usually demonstrates downward and lateral renal displacement by the tumor mass (Figure 9-11). Neuroblastoma tends to cause the entire kidney and its collecting system to be displaced as a unit, unlike Wilms' tumor, which has an intrarenal origin and thus tends to distort and widen the pelvocalyceal system.

Because of its non-ionizing character, ultrasound is a superb modality for evaluating abdominal masses in children. A neuroblastoma appears as a solid or semisolid mass that is separate from the kidney. The tumor is often diffusely highly echogenic, probably because of necrosis and hemor-

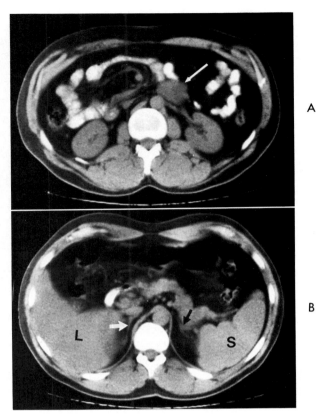

Figure 9-9 Ectopic pheochromocytoma. **A,** Soft-tissue mass (*arrows*) adjacent to aorta and in front of left renal vein. **B,** CT scan taken at higher level demonstrates that both right and left adrenal glands are normal (*arrows*). *L,* Liver; *S,* spleen. (*From Welch TJ et al: Pheochromocytoma: value of computed tomography, Radiology 148:501-503, 1983*).

rhage. CT can show evidence of tumor spread to lymph nodes and the sympathetic chain, widening of the paravertebral stripe (also seen on plain films) (Figure 9-12), and metastases to the liver and chest. This modality can also be used to assess the response to treatment.

Metastases to bone, liver, and lungs are common in neuroblastoma. Metastases to the skull typically cause spreading of cranial sutures because of plaques of tumor tissue growing along the surface of the brain. Bone destruction leads to a granular pattern of osteoporosis that is often associated with thin whiskerlike calcifications coursing outward and inward from the tables of the skull (Figure 9-10, *B*). Metastases in long tubular bones are often multiple and relatively symmetric and present a permeative destructive pattern.

Neuroblastomas arising in the chest appear as posterior mediastinal masses. Metastases to the chest most commonly cause asymmetric enlargement of mediastinal nodes; metastases to the pulmonary parenchyma are infrequent.

A 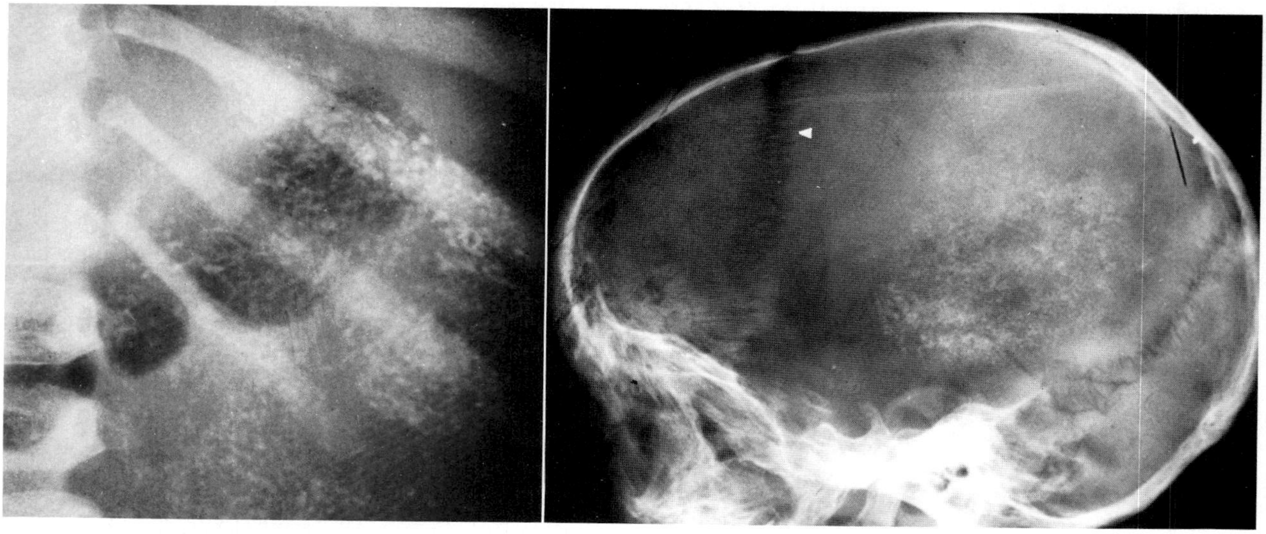   B

Figure 9-10 Neuroblastoma metastatic to bone. **A,** Plain film of upper abdomen shows diffuse granular calcification within large primary tumor. **B,** Lateral projection of skull shows similar calcifier deposits within metastastic lesion in calvarium. Note sutural widening (*arrowhead*) consistent with increased intracranial pressure. (From Eisenberg RL : Diagnostic imaging in surgery, New York, 1987, McGraw-Hill Book Co.)

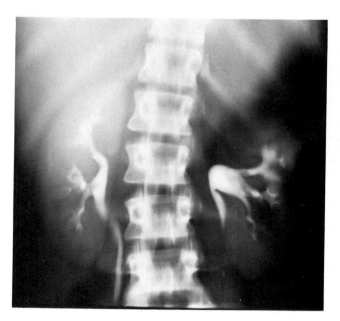

Figure 9-11 Neuroblastoma. Nephrotomogram demonstrates downward and lateral displacement of upper pole of left kidney.

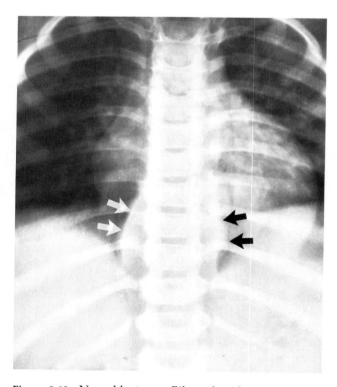

Figure 9-12 Neuroblastoma. Bilateral widening of paravertebral stripes (*arrows*) represents metastatic deposits. (*From Friedland GW et al: Uroradiology: an integrated approach. New York, Churchill Livingstone, 1983.*)

PITUITARY GLAND

The pituitary gland is often called the "master gland" because the many hormones it secretes control the level of most glandular activity throughout the body. The hormone secretion of the pituitary gland itself is controlled by the hypothalamus.

The pituitary is a tiny gland about the size of a pea that is suspended from the base of the brain by a slender stalk (infundibulum) and is situated in the bony depression of the sella turcica. It is divided into anterior and posterior portions, each of which secretes different hormones.

The anterior lobe of the pituitary gland secretes growth hormone, thyroid-stimulating hormone (TSH), adrenocorticotropic hormone (ACTH), and a group of hormones that affect the sex organs, or gonads. These gonadotropins include follicle-stimulating hormone (FSH) and luteinizing hormone (LH), which regulate the menstrual cycle and secretion of male and female sex hormones, and prolactin, which stimulates the production of milk during pregnancy and after delivery.

Growth hormone affects all parts of the body by promoting the growth and development of the tissues. Before puberty, it stimulates the growth of long bones (increasing the child's height) and the size of such organs as the liver, heart, and kidneys. After adolescence, growth hormone is secreted in lesser amounts but continues to function in promoting tissue replacement and repair. TSH controls the secretion of thyroid hormone, which regulates the body's metabolism (production and use of energy). ACTH controls the level of activity of the adrenal cortex.

The posterior lobe of the pituitary gland (neurohypophysis) produces two hormones: vasopressin (antidiuretic hormone) and oxytocin. Antidiuretic hormone (ADH) increases the rate of reabsorption of water and electrolytes by the renal tubules, thus decreasing the output of urine and protecting the individual from excessive water loss. Oxytocin causes contraction of smooth muscle, especially in the uterus, and thus strengthens contractions during labor and helps to prevent hemorrhage after delivery.

Diseases of the pituitary gland

Hyperpituitarism

Hyperpituitarism results from an excess of growth hormone produced by a tumor or generalized hyperplasia of the anterior lobe of the pituitary gland. The development of this condition before enchondral bone growth has ceased results in **gigantism;** hyperpituitarism beginning after bone growth has stopped produces **acromegaly.**

Generalized overgrowth of all the body tissues is the underlying abnormality in acromegaly. Although the long bones can no longer grow because the epiphyses are closed, the bones of the hands, feet, and face enlarge, and there is excessive growth of soft tissues. Proliferation of cartilage may cause joint space widening, especially of the metacarpophalangeal and hip joints. The slight increase in length of each of the seven articular cartilages for each digit leads to perceptible lengthening of the fingers. Overgrowth of the tips of the distal phalanges produces thick bony tufts with pointed lateral margins. The associated hypertrophy of the soft tissues produces the characteristic square, spade-shaped hand of acromegaly. Degenerative changes develop early and are associated with prominent hypertrophic spurring. Unlike typical osteoarthritis, acromegaly results in joint spaces that remain normal or are even widened.

Thickening of the heel pads (the soft tissue inferior to the plantar aspect of the calcaneus) to greater than 23 mm is highly suggestive of acromegaly (Figure 9-13). However, a similar appearance may also be seen in patients with obesity, myxedema, or generalized edema.

The bones of the skull become thickened and have increased density, often with obliteration of the diploic space. This bone thickening is especially prominent in the frontal and occipital regions, leading to characteristic frontal bossing and enlargement of the occipital protuberance. The paranasal sinuses

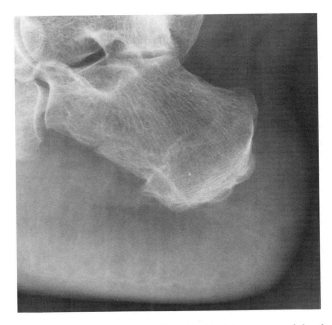

Figure 9-13 Acromegaly. Prominent thickening of heel pad, which measured 32 mm on original radiograph.

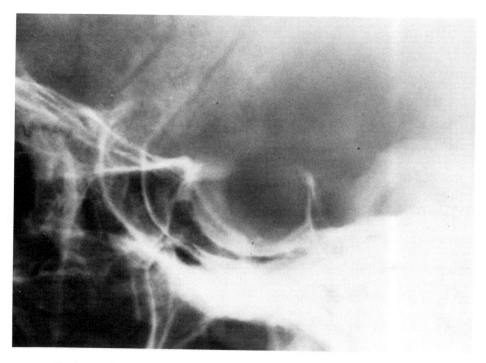

Figure 9-14 Pituitary adenoma causing acromegaly. Ballooning of sella turcica with downward displacement of floor.

(especially the frontal) become enlarged, and the mastoid processes are usually overpneumatized. Lengthening of the mandible and an increased mandibular angle produce a prognathous jaw, one of the typical clinical features of acromegaly. Thickening of the tongue may lead to slurred speech. Pituitary enlargement causes expansion and erosion of the sella turcica (Figure 9-14).

In the spine, hypertrophy of cartilage causes an increased width of the intervertebral disk spaces. An increase in the size of the vertebral bodies is best seen on lateral projections. Hypertrophy of soft tissues may produce an increased concavity of the posterior aspect of the vertebral bodies (scalloping) that is most prominent in the lumbar spine (Figure 9-15).

Extraskeletal manifestations of acromegaly include visceral enlargement, especially of the heart and kidney, enlargement of the tongue, and calcification of cartilage in the pinna of the ear.

Gigantism is manifested as an excessively large skeleton. If hypersecretion of growth hormone continues after epiphyseal closure, the soft tissue and bony changes of acromegaly are superimposed.

Hypopituitarism

Because the pituitary gland controls the level of secretion of gonadal and thyroid hormones and the

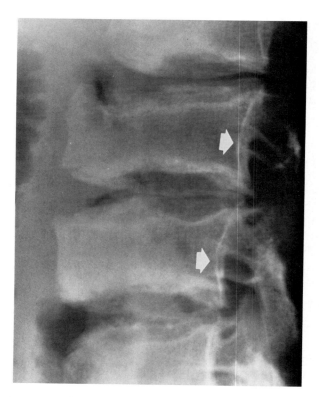

Figure 9-15 Acromegaly. Posterior scalloping *(arrows)* associated with enlargement of vertebral bodies (especially in AP dimension).

production of growth hormone, decreased function of the pituitary gland causes profound generalized disturbances in bone growth and maturation. In children, hypopituitarism typically leads to a type of dwarfism in which the delayed appearance of epiphyseal centers causes the failure of bones to grow normally in length or width. This results in a person who is small in stature and sexually immature, although well-proportioned and of normal mentality. In many patients there is a delay in the eruption of the teeth, which tend to become impacted because their size is not affected. The arrest in the growth of the skeleton occurs during childhood, when the cranial vault is proportionally greater in relation to the facial bones than in the adult. Since this discrepancy remains into adulthood in hypopituitary dwarfism, the relatively large skull may be mistakenly thought to result from hydrocephaly.

Hypopituitarism occurring after adolescence results in hypofunction of the thyroid gland, adrenal glands, and gonads but usually causes few radiologic findings. The heart and kidneys are often small, and calcification or ossification may develop in the articular cartilages.

Diabetes insipidus

The impaired ability of the kidneys to conserve water in diabetes insipidus results from low blood levels of antidiuretic hormone reflecting deficient vasopressin release by the posterior lobe of the pituitary gland in response to normal physiologic stimuli. In response to excessive water loss in the urine (polyuria), the body compensates by developing an insatiable thirst (polydypsia). Severe polyuria can lead to massive dilation of the renal pelves, calyces, and ureters. This probably represents a compensatory alteration to accommodate the huge volume of excreted urine.

It must be stressed that diabetes insipidus is completely unrelated to diabetes mellitus.

THYROID GLAND

The thyroid is a butterfly-shaped gland located in the neck at the level of the larynx. It consists of two lobes, one on each side of the trachea, and a connecting strip (isthmus) that runs anterior to the trachea and connects the lower portions of the two lobes. The thyroid lies just below the Adam's apple, the protrusion formed by the cricoid cartilage of the larynx. Microscopically, the thyroid gland consists of innumerable follicles surrounding a central core of colloid, the storage form of the active material known as thyroxine, which is the only natural iodine-containing substance in the body.

The thyroid gland picks up iodine from the bloodstream and combines it with the amino acid tyrosine to synthesize thyroid hormones, which are stored in the gland until released into the bloodstream when stimulated by TSH from the anterior lobe of the pituitary gland. The active hormone, **thyroxine,** is a small molecule that may contain either three iodine molecules (T3) or four iodine molecules (T4). These substances stimulate the rate of cellular metabolism in response to the body's need for increased energy production. The increased cellular metabolism requires additional oxygen circulated to the cells and the removal of waste materials, both of which require increased blood flow and greater cardiac output. The increased demand for oxygen stimulates the respiratory center and results in a faster rate and greater depth of breathing. Increased cellular metabolism produces heat, which is dissipated by perspiration and by increased blood flow through dilated vessels in the skin, giving the person a flushed appearance. Thyroid hormone also increases the secretion of digestive juices and the movement of ingested material through the intestinal tract.

The release of thyroid hormone is controlled by thyroid-stimulating hormone (TSH), which is secreted by the anterior lobe of the pituitary gland. This process is a negative feedback mechanism, in which a high blood level of thyroxine inhibits the anterior pituitary and TSH release, whereas a low level of thyroxine forces the anterior pituitary to release TSH again.

Diseases of the thyroid gland
Radioactive iodine scanning

Scanning after the administration of radioactive iodine is the major imaging modality for demonstrating both functioning and nonfunctioning thyroid tissue. This technique is used to localize palpable nodules, to determine the function of nodules, to detect nonpalpable lesions (especially in patients with a history of neck irradiation), and to evaluate the extent of residual tissue after surgical or radioisotopic thyroid ablation. Radionuclide scanning may be combined with uptake, stimulation, or suppression techniques to better characterize thyroid lesions.

The distribution of radioactivity is uniform throughout the normal thyroid gland (Figure 9-16). Diffuse thyroid enlargement without hyperthyroidism most frequently represents a multinodular goiter or Hashimoto's thyroiditis. In a patient with hyperthyroidism, diffuse thyroid enlargement suggests Graves' disease.

Masses within the thyroid gland appear as

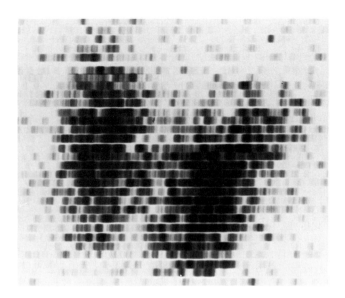

Figure 9-16 Normal radioactive iodine scan. Uniform distribution of nuclide activity throughout gland.

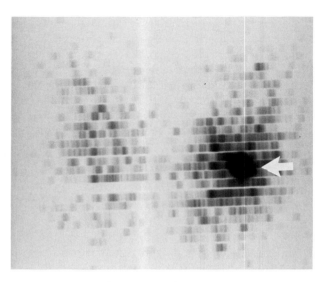

Figure 9-17 Hyperfunctioning (hot) nodule. Localized area of increased radionuclide uptake on left *(arrow)* has partially suppressed radionuclide uptake in remainder of left lobe and in entire right lobe of gland.

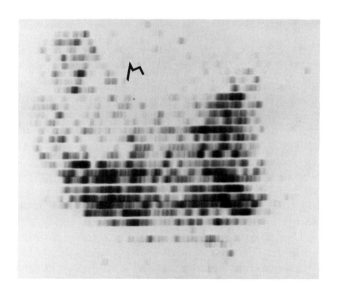

Figure 9-18 Nonfunctioning (cold) nodule *(arrow)* representing thyroid adenoma.

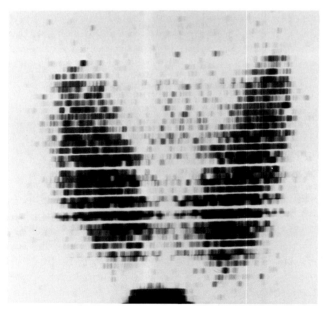

Figure 9-19 Hyperthyroidism. Radioactive iodine scan in patient with Graves' disease demonstrates diffuse enlargement of thyroid gland with prominence of pyramidal lobe and homogeneous increase in nuclide uptake.

hyperfunctioning ("hot") or poorly functioning ("cold") nodules. A hot nodule demonstrates increased radionuclide uptake compared with surrounding thyroid tissue (Figure 9-17). These hot nodules usually represent autonomously functioning thyroid tissue and are rarely malignant, although malignancy is sometimes reported elsewhere in the same gland. Large hyperfunctioning nodules may completely suppress the remaining thyroid tissue so that only the nodule itself is visualized. An autonomous nodule may eventually develop central hemorrhage or cystic change and evolve into a nonfunctioning (cold) nodule.

Cold thyroid nodules contain less nuclide per unit tissue mass than adjacent normal thyroid tissue (Figure 9-18). Most cold nodules represent poorly functioning adenomas. Thyroid cysts, carcinoma, and thyroiditis can also produce this appearance. In a young patient the absence of uptake in the region of a solitary cold thyroid nodule is associated with a 10% to 25% probability that the nodule is malignant. Although ultrasound can distinguish a thyroid cyst from the other causes of cold nodules, this modality is of little value in further characterizing noncystic thyroid masses.

Hyperthyroidism

Hyperthyroidism results from the excessive production of thyroid hormone, either from the entire gland (Graves' disease) or from one or more functioning adenomas. Graves' disease is a relatively common disorder that most often develops in the third and fourth decades and has a strong female predominance. The major clinical symptoms include nervousness, emotional lability, an inability to sleep, tremors, rapid pulse rate (tachycardia), palpitations, excessive sweating, and heat intolerance. Weight loss is frequent, usually despite an increased appetite. A characteristic physical finding is exophthalmos, outward protrusion of the eyeball caused by edema in the tissue behind the eyes.

Radioactive iodine scans in patients with Graves' disease typically demonstrate diffuse enlargement of the thyroid gland with increased radioiodine uptake (Figure 9-19). In severe disease, high-output cardiac failure may develop along with generalized cardiomegaly and pulmonary congestion. Unilateral or bilateral exophthalmos as a result of Graves' disease can be demonstrated by CT as thickening of the extraocular muscles.

Hypothyroidism

Hypothyroidism can result from any structural or functional abnormality that leads to an insufficient synthesis of thyroid hormone. Hypothyroidism dat-

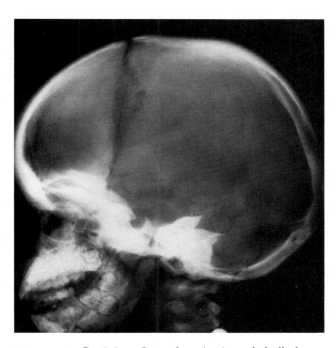

Figure 9-20 Cretinism. Lateral projection of skull shows increased density at base, small underdeveloped sinuses, and hypoplasia of teeth with delayed eruption. Retardation of facial maturation makes face appear small relative to size of calvarium.

ing from birth (cretinism) results in multiple developmental abnormalities. Children with cretinism typically have a short stature; coarse features with a protruding tongue, a broad, flattened nose, and widely set eyes; sparse hair; dry skin; and a protuberant abdomen with an umbilical hernia. The major radiographic abnormalities include a delay in the appearance and subsequent growth of ossification centers and retarded bone age. Skull changes are common and include an increase in the thickness of the cranial vault, underpneumatization of the sinuses and mastoid air cells, widened sutures with delayed closure, and a delay in the development and eruption of the teeth (Figure 9-20). Adult hypothyroidism has an insidious onset with nonspecific symptoms including lethargy, somnolence (sleeping up to 16 hours a day), constipation, cold intolerance, slowing of intellectual and motor activity, and weight gain in spite of a decreased appetite. Dry skin, stiff aching muscles, and a deepening voice with hoarseness often occur. The facial features are thickened and there is a doughy thickening of the skin (myxedema). Radiographically, the heart is typically enlarged because of pericardial effusion. Soft-tissue thickening is often seen on films of the extremities, and adynamic ileus is a common finding on abdominal radiographs.

Goiter

A goiter is an enlargement of the thyroid gland that does not result from an inflammatory or neoplastic process and is not initially associated with hyperthyroidism or myxedema. Simple (nontoxic) goiter results when one or more factors impair the capacity of the thyroid gland in the basal state to secrete the quantities of active hormones necessary to meet the needs of the body. Because the blood level of thyroid hormone is low, there is nothing to inhibit the anterior pituitary, which continues to secrete thyroid-stimulating hormone that causes the thyroid gland to enlarge. In most cases, there is a sufficient increase in both the functioning thyroid mass and the cellular activity to overcome the mild or moderate impairment of hormone synthesis, permitting the patient to remain metabolically normal though goitrous. On a radioactive iodine scan, a nontoxic goiter usually appears as symmetric or asymmetric enlargement of the thyroid gland. Plain radiographs and esophagrams often show the enlarged thyroid gland impressing or displacing the trachea and esophagus (Figure 9-21).

Although goiters were once common in endemic areas in which there was insufficient iodine in the diet, this is now a rare cause because of the commercial addition of iodine to salt and bread.

Toxic multinodular goiter may be a consequence of long-standing nontoxic goiter. In this condition, one or more areas of the gland become independent of TSH stimulation. Radioactive iodine scans most commonly show accumulation of iodine diffusely but in patchy foci throughout the gland (Figure 9-22). Another pattern consists of iodine accumulation in one or more discrete nodules within the gland, with the remainder of the gland being essentially nonfunctional.

Tumors of the thyroid gland

Benign thyroid adenomas are encapsulated tumors that vary greatly in size and usually compress adjacent tissue. They may be located within the neck, where they tend to cause deviation or compression of the trachea, or they may extend substernally and appear as masses in the superior portion of the anterior mediastinum. Calcification may develop within the mass (Figure 9-23). Thyroid adenomas can appear as hot or cold nodules, depending on their functional capacity.

The three major types of thyroid carcinomas are papillary, follicular, and medullary. Papillary carcinoma, the most common type, has peaks of incidence occurring in adolescence and young adulthood and again in later life. The tumor is usually slow-growing, and it typically spreads to regional lymph nodes, where it may remain silent for many years. Metastases to the lungs often cause only mild, nonspecific thickening of bronchovascular mark-

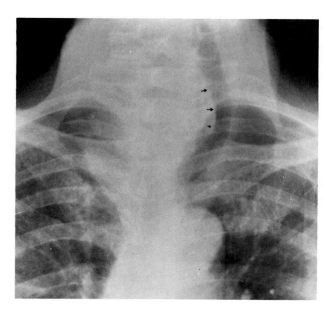

Figure 9-21 Goiter. Markedly enlarged thyroid gland appears as soft-tissue mass impressing trachea *(arrows)* and displacing it to left.

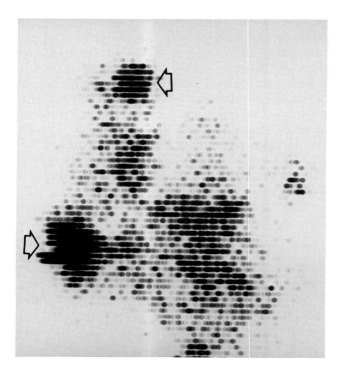

Figure 9-22 Toxic multinodular goiter. Radioactive iodine scan shows patchy uptake of nuclide and several hot nodules *(arrows)* within enlarged gland.

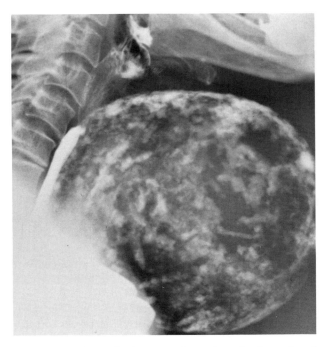

Figure 9-23 Thyroid adenoma. Lateral projection of neck shows huge calcified thyroid mass.

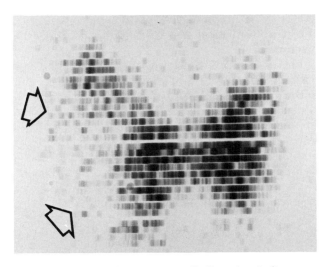

Figure 9-24 Thyroid carcinoma. Radioactive iodine scan shows solitary cold nodule (arrows) that corresponded to patient's palpable mass.

ings, although the metastases may also appear as miliary and nodular densities that predominantly involve the lower lobes.

Follicular carcinoma has a histologic appearance that closely mimics normal thyroid tissue. The tumor usually undergoes early hematogenous spread, especially to the lung and bone. Skeletal metastases, which may be the initial presentation, tend to produce entirely lytic, expansile destruction that extends into the soft tissues and is associated with little or no periosteal reaction.

Medullary carcinoma is the least common type of thyroid malignancy. At least 10% of the cases are familial, most often appearing as a component of a syndrome in which there are multiple endocrine tumors. Dense, amorphous calcifications can often be seen within the tumor.

On radioactive iodine scans, thyroid carcinoma usually appears as a solitary cold nodule that corresponds to a palpable mass (Figure 9-24). A nodule that is functioning (hot) can essentially be excluded from a diagnosis of thyroid carcinoma.

There is a substantially increased risk of thyroid cancer in persons with a history of therapeutic neck irradiation in childhood. In the past such radiation was used for benign disease such as enlargement of the tonsils, adenoids, and thymus; middle ear disease; and a variety of skin disorders, including acne.

PARATHYROID GLANDS

The parathyroids are four tiny glands, two on each side, that lie behind the upper and lower poles of the thyroid gland. They secrete **parathormone,** which is responsible for regulating the blood levels of calcium and phosphate. Parathormone raises a low serum calcium level by three mechanisms. It increases the amount of calcium absorbed from the intestinal tract by interaction with ingested vitamin D. The hormone prevents a loss of calcium through the kidneys and releases calcium from bones by stimulating osteoclastic activity. The parathyroid glands also secrete calcitonin, which decreases the serum calcium level and appears to play a role analogous to that of glucagon in the pancreas.

Diseases of the parathyroid glands
Hyperparathyroidism

Excessive secretion of parathormone leads to a generalized disorder of calcium, phosphate, and bone metabolism that results in elevated serum levels of calcium and phosphate. Primary hyperparathyroidism may be caused by a discrete adenoma or carcinoma or by generalized hyperplasia of all glands. Other causes include nonparathyroid tumors that secrete a parathormone-like substance and the familial syndrome of multiple endocrine neoplasia. Secondary hyperparathyroidism occurs more frequently than the primary form and is most often due to chronic renal failure. Tertiary hyperparathyroidism refers to the development of autonomous functioning parathyroid glands in patients who demonstrate progressive bone disease in the presence of biochemical and clinically controlled renal disease.

The radiographic findings of primary and secondary hyperparathyroidism are similar, except that in the secondary form brown tumors (focal areas of bone destruction) are rare and osteosclerosis is more common. The earliest change is subperiosteal bone resorption, which particularly involves the radial margins of the middle phalanges (Figure 9-25), the distal clavicles (Figure 9-26), and the medial aspect of the upper third of the tibias. Loss of normal cortical definition is followed by an irregularly lacy resorption, with the endosteal margin initially remaining intact. Erosions of the terminal tufts of the fingers and loss of the lamina dura of the teeth often

occur, although these are nonspecific findings that also are seen in other conditions.

Generalized loss of bone density may produce a ground-glass appearance. So-called brown tumors may become large and expansile and even simulate a malignant process (Figure 9-27). Pathologic fractures may lead to bizarre deformities. Irregular demineralization of the calvarium produces the characteristic salt-and-pepper skull (Figure 9-28).

A generalized increase in bone density (osteosclerosis) may develop in patients with hyperparathyroidism, especially when it is a result of renal failure. Thick bands of increased density adjacent to the superior and inferior margins of vertebral bodies produce the characteristic "rugger jersey" spine (Figure 9-29).

Soft-tissue calcification is common, especially in secondary hyperparathyroidism. Calcific deposits may develop in vessels, articular cartilages, menisci, joint capsules, and periarticular tissues (Figure 9-30). Elevated serum calcium and decreased excretion of calcium in the urine may result in nephrocalcinosis and urinary tract stones. An increased incidence of pancreatic calculi and pancreatitis, peptic

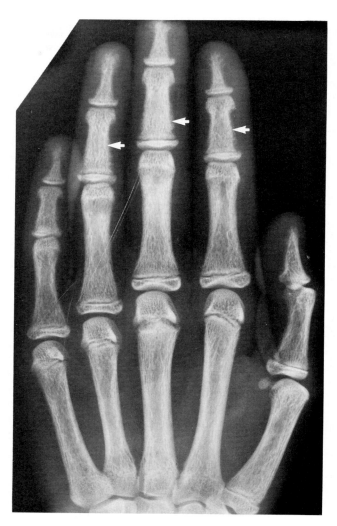

Figure 9-25 Hyperparathyroidism. Subperiosteal bone resorption that predominantly involves radial margins of middle phalanges of second, third, and fourth digits *(arrows)*. Note also resorption of terminal tufts.

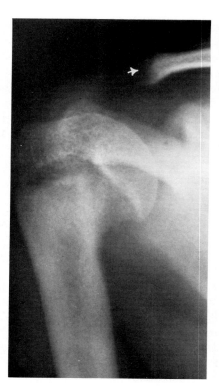

Figure 9-26 Hyperparathyroidism. Characteristic erosion of distal clavicle *(arrow)*. Metaphyseal subperiosteal resorption beneath proximal humeral head has led to pathologic fracture with slippage of humeral head.

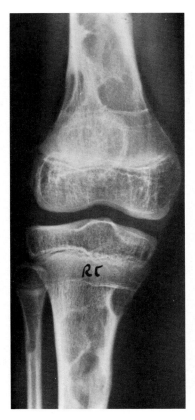

Figure 9-27 Hyperparathyroidism. Brown tumors produce multiple lytic lesions about knee.

ulcer, and gallstones also has been reported in patients with hyperparathyroidism.

The preoperative localization of a functioning parathyroid adenoma has long been a difficult radiographic problem. In many cases preoperative parathyroid localization is not required, since in patients who have not had previous neck surgery a standard bilateral neck dissection by an experienced parathyroid surgeon can be expected to have a 95% success rate in controlling hyperparathyroidism. Plain radiographs and barium studies are of virtually no value unless the tumor is huge.

The major role of sophisticated imaging modalities in the localization of functioning parathyroid adenomas is in patients who remain hypercalcemic, or in whom hypercalcemia recurs, after neck surgery for hyperparathyroidism. In these patients, normal anatomic relations are disturbed, landmarks may be absent, and scarring and adhesions distort the field and complicate the surgical technique. The illusive parathyroid tumor is also more likely to be situated in an ectopic position (Figure 9-31). Thus the success rate for parathyroid re-exploration is less than 65%.

Ultrasound, radionuclide scanning, CT, and MRI are complementary modalities for investigating the patient with hypercalcemia after parathyroid surgery. If these techniques fail to demonstrate a lesion, arteriography and venography with venous sampling may be performed for localization.

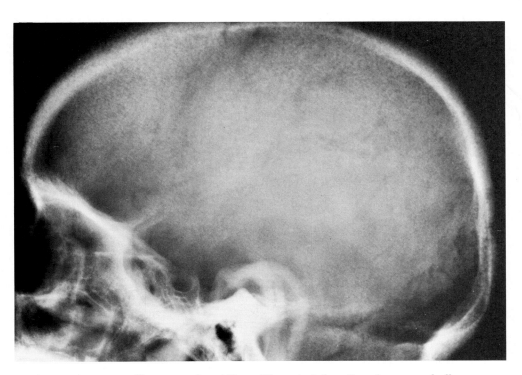

Figure 9-28 Hyperparathyroidism. Characteristic salt-and-pepper skull.

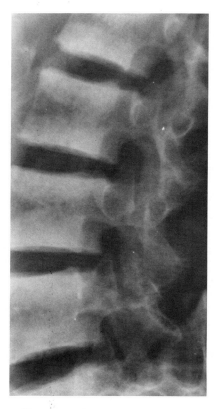

Figure 9-29 Hyperparathyroidism. Lateral projection of lumbar spine demonstrates osteosclerosis of superior and inferior margins of vertebral bodies (rugger-jersey spine).

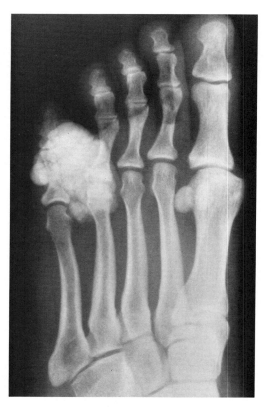

Figure 9-30 Hyperparathyroidism. Dense mass of tumoral calcification in joint capsules and periarticular soft tissues on lateral aspect of foot in patient with chronic renal disease.

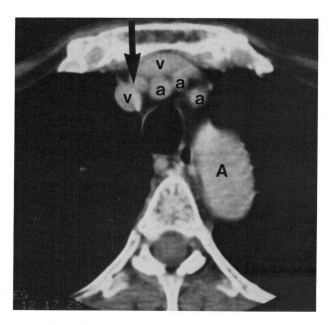

Figure 9-31 Ectopic parathyroid adenoma. CT scan shows small soft-tissue mass *(arrow)* in anterior mediastinum. *A,* Aorta; *a,* three major branches of aorta (from patient's right to left, brachiocephalic, left carotid, and left subclavian arteries); *v,* right and left brachiocephalic veins. *(From Stark DD et al: Parathyroid scanning by computed tomography, Radiology 148:297-303, 1983.)*

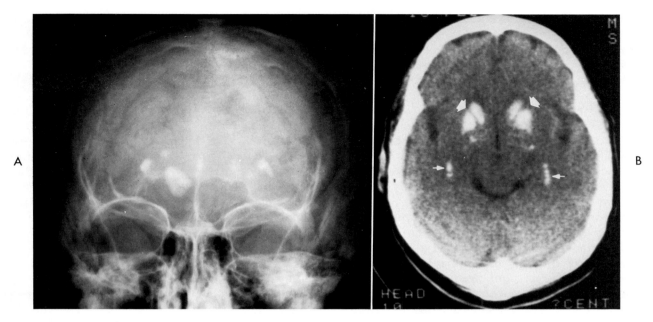

Figure 9-32 Hypoparathyroidism. **A,** Frontal projection of skull demonstrates calcification in basal ganglia bilaterally. **B,** CT scan shows characteristic bilateral calcification in basal ganglia *(broad arrows).* Note also small calcific deposits in tail of caudate nuclei *(thin arrows).*

Preoperative fine-needle aspiration biopsy using ultrasound or CT guidance can increase the specificity in localizing and confirming the exact site of a parathyroid adenoma, especially in patients who have undergone previous neck dissection. When a successful aspiration biopsy of the neck is positive for parathyroid cells, there is no doubt that abnormal parathyroid tissue is situated at this site, and this eliminates the need for extensive surgical dissection.

Hypoparathyroidism

Hypoparathyroidism usually results from injury or accidental removal of the glands during thyroidectomy and is not associated with any significant radiographic abnormalities. In the less common primary type of hypoparathyroidism, the major radiographic finding on plain skull radiographs or CT of the skull is cerebral calcification, especially involving the basal ganglia (Figure 9-32), dentate nuclei of the cerebellum, and choroid plexus. A pattern of increased density may develop in the long bones, usually localized to the metaphyseal area.

Clinically, hypoparathyroidism causes sustained muscular contraction (tetany), muscle cramps in hands and feet, and numbness and tingling of the extremities. Spasm of laryngeal muscles can cause fatal obstruction of the respiratory tract.

Pseudohypoparathyroidism and pseudopseudohypoparathyroidism

Pseudohypoparathyroidism is a hereditary disorder in which there is failure of normal end organ response to normal levels of circulating parathyroid hormone. Most patients are obese and have short stature, with round faces, opacities in the cornea or lens of the eye, short fingers, and mental retardation. The most common radiographic abnormality is shortening of the tubular bones of the hands and feet (especially the fourth and fifth metacarpals) (see Figure 1-2) and calcific or bony deposits in the skin or subcutaneous tissues. An appearance similar to rickets may develop. As in idiopathic hypoparathyroidism, calcification is often found in the brain, especially the basal ganglia.

Pseudopseudohypoparathyroidism refers to the presence of similar skeletal anomalies in other members of the patient's family in the absence of biochemical disturbances.

DIABETES MELLITUS

Diabetes mellitus is a common endocrine disorder in which beta cells in the islets of Langerhans in the pancreas fail to secrete insulin, or target cells throughout the body fail to respond to this hormone.

A lack of insulin prevents glucose from entering the cells, thus depriving the cells of their major nutrient for the production of energy. The blood glucose level increases **(hyperglycemia).**

The severity and age of onset of diabetes varies. Juvenile-onset diabetes, which develops in childhood, and insulin-dependent diabetes require the patient to undergo daily insulin injections. Non-insulin–dependent diabetes, which tends to develop later in life, is less severe and can often be controlled by diet alone. The precise cause of diabetes is unknown, although it is generally considered that heredity is an important factor.

Polyuria (excessive urination) and polydypsia (drinking large quantities of liquid) are common manifestations of diabetes. The large amount of sugar filtered through the kidneys exceeds the amount that the renal tubules can absorb. This leads to the excretion of glucose in the urine (glycosuria), which is a major sign of diabetes.

Glucose is the major fuel of the body. However, since glucose cannot enter the cells without the action of insulin, diabetic patients are forced to metabolize a large amount of fat. This produces a large number of fatty acids and ketone bodies, which can be detected in the urine. Production of fatty acids lowers the body's pH (acidosis). Severe acidosis and dehydration in a diabetic patient who fails to take enough insulin or eats a high-sugar diet can lead to diabetic coma, which may be fatal if not treated rapidly with fluids and a large dose of insulin.

A major complication of diabetes is the deposition of lipids within the walls of blood vessels (atherosclerosis). This causes arterial narrowing and even occlusion, resulting in myocardial infarction (coronary artery), stroke (carotid artery), or gangrene (peripheral artery). Excess glucose in tissues provides an excellent bacterial culture medium and leads to the frequent development of infections, which tend to heal poorly because of the generally poor circulation in diabetic patients. The kidneys are always affected by long-standing diabetes, and kidney failure is frequently the cause of death. Another complication is narrowing and rupture of minute retinal blood vessels, which may lead to blindness. Poor circulation to the nervous system may produce intractable pain, tingling sensations, loss of feeling, and paralysis.

A patient with diabetes must also be wary of developing insulin shock (hypoglycemic shock), which results from too much insulin, not enough food, or excessive exercise. The patient feels light-headed and faint, trembles, and begins to perspire. In the radiology department this may occur in diabetic patients who have not eaten or drunk before gastro-intestinal examination or other special procedures. It is essential that this condition be rapidly recognized and sugar given, usually in the form of orange juice or candy.

Diabetes mellitus produces a variety of radiographic findings that involve multiple organ systems. Atherosclerotic disease and subsequent ischemia involving the coronary, extracerebral, and peripheral circulations occur earlier and are more extensive in diabetics, especially those who smoke. Calcifications in peripheral vessels, especially those of the hands and feet, are virtually pathognomonic of the disease (Figure 9-33). Men with diabetes may demonstrate characteristic calcification of the vas deferens, which appears as bilaterally symmetric parallel tubular densities that run medially and caudally to enter the medial aspect of the seminal vesicles at the base of the prostate gland (Figure 9-34).

Diabetic persons have an increased susceptibility to infection; this especially affects the feet and may lead to severe osteomyelitis that produces bone destruction without periosteal reaction. Diabetic neuropathy with gait abnormalities and the loss of deep

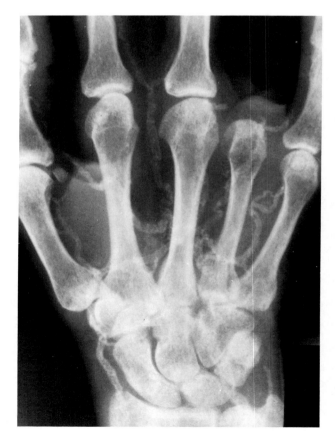

Figure 9-33 Diabetes mellitus. Typical calcification in moderate-sized vessels of hand and wrist. Note prior surgical resection of phalanges of fourth digit.

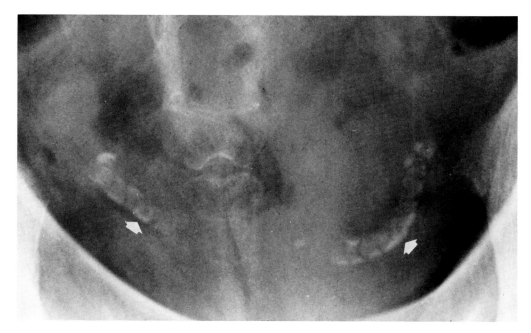

Figure 9-34 Diabetes mellitus. Bilateral calcification of vas deferens.

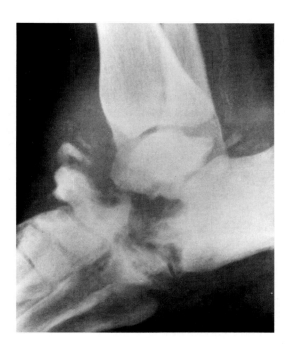

Figure 9-35 Neuropathic joint in diabetes mellitus. Severe destructive changes with calcific debris about intertarsal joints. Note characteristic vascular calcification posterior to ankle joint.

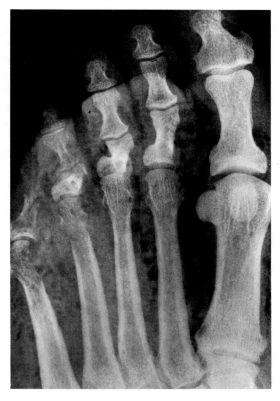

Figure 9-36 Diabetic gangrene. Diffuse destruction of phalanges and metatarsal head of fifth digit. Note large amount of gas in soft tissues of foot.

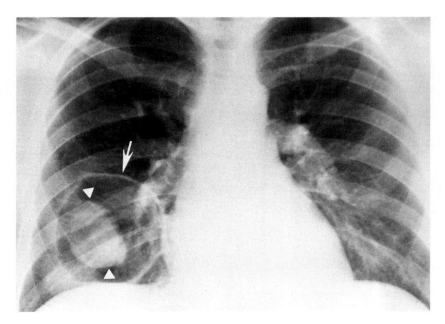

Figure 9-37 Mucormycosis in diabetic patient. Large thin-walled cavity *(arrow)* containing smooth, elliptical, homogeneous mass *(arrowheads)* representing fungus ball.

pain sensation may lead to repeated trauma on an unstable joint. Degeneration of cartilage, recurrent fracture and fragmentation of subchondral bone, soft-tissue debris, and marked proliferation of adjacent bone can lead to total disorganization of the joint (Charcot or neuropathic joint) (Figure 9-35). Vascular disease with diminished blood supply can lead to gas gangrene, in which bubbles or streaks of gas develop in the subcutaneous or deeper tissues (Figure 9-36).

Diabetic neuropathy often causes radiographically evident abnormalities in the gastrointestinal tract. Findings include decreased primary peristalsis and tertiary contractions in the esophagus, delayed gastric emptying, and dilation of the small bowel. Emphysematous cholecystitis with gas in the lumen

and wall of the gallbladder is a severe complication that occurs almost exclusively in diabetic patients.

Renal disease is a common complication and a leading cause of death in persons with diabetes. Acute and chronic pyelonephritis, renal papillary necrosis, and cystitis often occur. Diabetic neuropathy can cause dilation and atony of the bladder with incomplete emptying.

Mucormycosis infection is a devastating fungal disease that occurs virtually only in uncontrolled diabetics. It usually originates in the nose and paranasal sinuses, from which it can extend to destroy the walls of the sinus and invade the substance of the brain. Pulmonary mucormycosis is a progressive severe pneumonia that is widespread and confluent and often cavitates (Figure 9-37).

QUESTIONS

1. What organ in the body is responsible for the release of insulin?
   A. Spleen   C. Pancreas
   B. Liver   D. Small intestine

2. What organ in the body is responsible for the release of glucagon?
   A. Spleen   C. Pancreas
   B. Liver   D. Small intestine

3. The _____ glands secrete several types of steroid hormones and lie above each kidney.
   A. Adrenal   C. Pineal
   B. Pituitary   D. Thymus

4. What hormone has the ability to constrict some blood vessels while dilating others to shunt blood to active muscles where oxygen and nutrients are needed?
   A. Androgen   C. Glucocorticoids
   B. Epinephrine   D. Aldosterone

5. What hormones are known as the "fight or flight" hormones?
  A. Androgen; epinephrine
  B. Adrenaline; norepinephrine
  C. Glucocorticoid; adrenaline
  D. Androgen; glucocorticoid

6. Enlargement of the adrenal glands is best demonstrated by what diagnostic modality?
  A. Ultrasound
  B. MRI
  C. CT
  D. Plain film radiography

7. What pathologic condition is characterized by obesity of the trunk of the body, a fat pad behind the shoulders, and a moon-shaped face?
  A. Conn's syndrome
  B. Cushing's syndrome
  C. Adrenogenital syndrome
  D. Addison's syndrome

8. One complication of Cushing's syndrome that radiographers must be cautious of is _____.
  A. Buffalo hump
  B. Spontaneous fractures
  C. Hypercalciuria
  D. Sella erosion

9. Excessive administration of _____ is the most common cause of adrenal insufficiency.
  A. Adrenalin
  B. Aldosterone
  C. Steroids
  D. ACTH

10. The second most common malignancy in children is _____.
  A. Pheochromocytoma
  B. Neuroblastoma
  C. Wilms' tumor
  D. Adenoma

11. The _____ controls the hormone secretion of the pituitary gland.
  A. Cerebellum
  B. Pons
  C. Medulla oblongata
  D. Hypothalamus

12. Enlargement of the hands, feet, and face is characteristic of what pathologic condition?
  A. Adenoma
  B. Acromegaly
  C. Gigantism
  D. None of the above

13. A pea-sized gland suspended from the base of the brain, sometimes referred to as the "master gland," is called the _____.
  A. Thymus
  B. Pineal
  C. Pituitary
  D. Pinna

14. What is the name for the butterfly-shaped gland located at the level of the larynx?
  A. Thymus
  B. Thyroid
  C. Pituitary
  D. Pineal

15. Thyroid tissue is best demonstrated by what imaging modality?
  A. CT
  B. Radionuclide imaging
  C. Ultrasound
  D. Plain film radiography

16. Insufficient synthesis of thyroid hormone can lead to what pathologic condition?
  A. Hyperthyroidism
  B. Hypothyroidism
  C. Exophthalmos
  D. Graves' disease

17. What is the name for an enlargement of the thyroid gland that does not result from an inflammatory or neoplastic process?
  A. Exophthalmos
  B. Goiter
  C. Myxedema
  D. Skin thickening

18. There is a significant increased risk of thyroid cancer in people who received _____.
  A. Neck radiation in childhood
  B. Steroid therapy in childhood
  C. Chest radiographs in childhood
  D. Skull radiographs in childhood

19. If beta cells in the islets of Langerhans fail to secrete insulin, what pathologic condition results?
  A. Goiter
  B. Exophthalmos
  C. Diabetes
  D. Hypothyroidism

20. A diabetic patient who receives insulin before reporting to the radiology department for an upper gastrointestinal study should be monitored by the radiographer for any signs of developing _____.
  A. Ketoacidosis
  B. Hypoglycemic shock
  C. Acidosis
  D. Hyperglycemic shock

21. The most common complication and leading cause of death in diabetic patients is _____.
  A. Hypoglycemia
  B. Hyperglycemia
  C. Pancreatic disease
  D. Renal disease

BIBLIOGRAPHY

Beck RE: Roentgen findings in the complications of diabetes mellitus, Am J Roentgenol 82:887-896, 1959.

LeMay M: The radiologic diagnosis of pituitary disease, Radiol Clin North AM 5:303-315, 1967.

Mitty HA and Yeh HC: Radiology of the adrenals with sonography and CT, Philadelphia, WB Saunders Co., 1982.

Sandler MP, Patton JA, and Partain CL: Thyroid and parathyroid imaging, Norwalk, Appleton-Century-Crofts, 1986.

CHAPTER 10

Reproductive System

PREREQUISITE KNOWLEDGE

The student should have a basic knowledge of the anatomy and physiology of the reproductive system. In addition, proper learning and understanding of the material will be facilitated if the student has some clinical experience in reproductive system radiography and film evaluation.

GOALS

To acquaint the student radiographer with the pathophysiology and radiographic manifestations of all of the common and some of the unusual disorders of the reproductive system

OBJECTIVES

1. Describe the physiology of the reproductive system
2. Identify anatomic structures on both diagrams and radiographs of the reproductive system
3. Be able to define terminology relating to the reproductive system
4. Be able to describe the various pathologic conditions affecting the reproductive system and their radiographic manifestations
5. Be familiar with the changes in technical factors required for obtaining optimal quality radiographs

RADIOGRAPHER NOTES

Because of its nonionizing character, ultrasound has become the major modality for imaging both the male and female reproductive systems. CT and MRI are used for staging malignant tumors, and radionuclide studies are used to differentiate testicular torsion from epididymitis.

Conventional plain film radiography is virtually never indicated for disorders of the pregnant patient. The once common pelvimetry and gravid uterus examinations have been almost completely replaced by nonionizing ultrasound imaging. The two radiographic studies of the female reproductive system that are in current use are hysterosalpingography and mammography. Hysterosalpingography, which is performed using fluoroscopic guidance, evaluates the patency (openness) of the fallopian tubes. Plain radiographs are obtained only to provide a permanent record. Mammography requires dedicated equipment and a specially trained radiographer. Properly performed mammograms can detect very early breast cancer before it is symptomatic, thus decreasing the incidence of metastases and greatly improving patient survival rates. However, mammograms performed by poorly trained radiographers or on inadequate equipment may fail to demonstrate early lesions and condemn an otherwise curable woman to unnecessary suffering and even death.

It is essential that the radiographer attempt to put the patient at ease when performing an examination of the reproductive system. Although these procedures are not actually painful, they may at times be uncomfortable and are frequently embarrassing for the patient. A good professional attitude goes a long way in reassuring the patient and making these examinations as comfortable as possible.

INFLAMMATORY DISEASE

Syphilis

Syphilis is a chronic sexually transmitted systemic infection caused by the spirochete *Treponema pallidum*. The baby of an infected mother may be born with congenital syphilis. In the primary stage of infection, a chancre, or ulceration, develops on the genitals (usually the vulva of the female and the penis of the male). If untreated with antibiotics, the second phase of the disease appears as a nonitching rash that affects any part of the body. At this stage, the patient is still infectious but can be successfully treated with antibiotics. If still untreated, the disease may become dormant for many years before the development of the most serious, or tertiary, phase of the disease in which radiographic abnormalities become apparent.

Cardiovascular syphilis primarily involves the ascending aorta, which may become aneurysmally dilated and often demonstrates linear calcification of the wall (Figure 10-1). Syphilitic aortitis often involves the aortic valvular ring and produces aortic regurgitation with enlargement of the left ventricle.

Syphilitic involvement of the skeletal system most commonly produces radiographic findings of chronic osteomyelitis, which usually affects the long bones and skull. The destruction of bone incites a prominent periosteal reaction, and dense sclerosis is the most outstanding feature (Figure 10-2). Syphilis is a major cause of neuropathic joint disease (Charcot joint), in which bone resorption and total disorganization of the joint are associated with calcific and bony debris (Figure 10-3).

Syphilitic lesions developing in the cerebral cortex can cause mental disorders, deafness, and blindness. Diffuse thickening of the gastric wall can cause narrowing of the lumen indistinguishable from carcinoma.

Multiple bone abnormalities can occur in infants with congenital syphilis who are born to infected mothers (Figure 10-4). Mental retardation, deafness, and blindness are common complications.

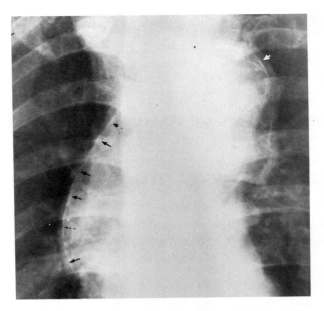

Figure 10-1 Syphilitic aortitis. Aneurysmal dilation of ascending aorta with extensive linear calcification of wall *(black arrows)*. Some calcification is also seen in distal aortic arch *(white arrow)*.

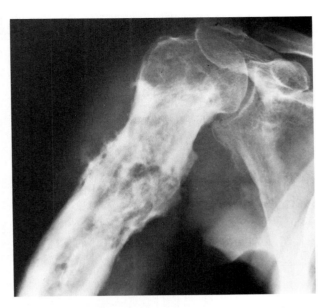

Figure 10-2 Syphilitic osteomyelitis. Diffuse lytic destruction of proximal humerus with reactive sclerosis and periosteal new bone formation.

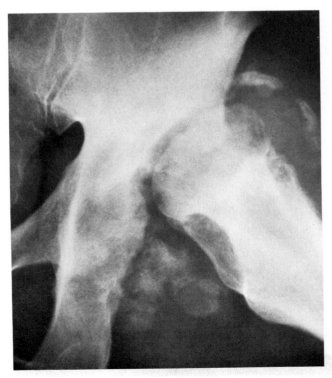

Figure 10-3 Neuropathic joint disease in syphilis. Joint fragmentation, sclerosis, and calcific debris about hip.

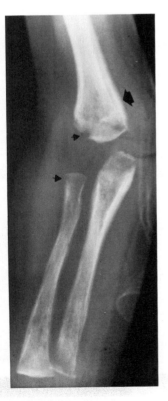

Figure 10-4 Congenital syphilis. Transverse bands of decreased density across metaphyses *(small arrows)* associated with patchy areas of bone destruction in diaphyses. There is solid periosteal new bone formation *(large arrow)*, which is best seen about distal humerus.

Gonorrhea

Gonorrhea is a bacterial infection that is one of the most common and widespread of the venereal diseases. Symptoms usually occur a few days after infection. An acute urethritis with copious discharge of pus develops in men. Women may be asymptomatic or have minimal symptoms of urethral or cervical inflammation. Gonorrhea usually responds rapidly to antibiotic therapy, but if untreated the inflammation may become chronic, spread upward, and produce fibrosis leading to urethral stricture in men (Figure 10-5) and pelvic inflammatory disease in women. A serious complication is fibrous scarring of the fallopian tubes that may result in sterility or an ectopic pregnancy.

Gonorrheal infection can cause septic arthritis leading to articular erosion and joint space narrowing.

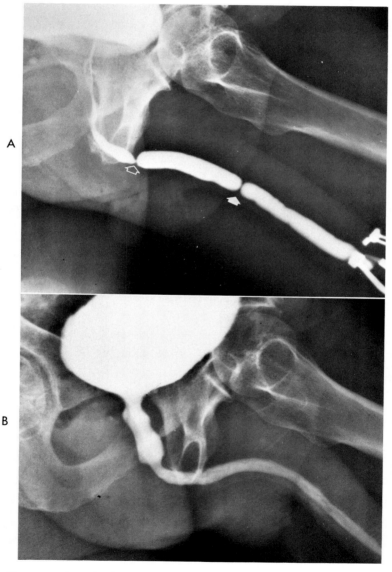

Figure 10-5   Gonococcal urethral stricture. **A,** Initial retrograde urethrogram shows diffuse stricture of bulbar urethra and high-grade stenoses in anterior *(solid arrow)* and posterior *(open arrow)* portions of urethra. **B,** After balloon dilation, voiding urethrogram shows marked improvement in appearance of urethra. *(From Russinovich NAE et al: Urol Radiol 2:33-37, 1980.)*

Male reproductive system

PHYSIOLOGY OF THE MALE REPRODUCTIVE SYSTEM

The major function of the male reproductive system is the formation of sperm **(spermatogenesis),** which begins at about age 13 and continues throughout life. Under the influence of follicle-stimulating hormone (FSH) secreted by the anterior lobe of the pituitary gland, the seminiferous tubules of the testes are stimulated to produce the male germ cells called spermatozoa. In addition to sperm cell production the testes secrete the male hormone **testosterone.** This substance stimulates the development and activity of the accessory sex organs (prostate, seminal vesicles) and is responsible for adult male sexual behavior. Testosterone causes the typically male changes that occur at puberty, including the development of facial and body hair and alterations in the larynx that result in a deepened voice. Testosterone also helps regulate metabolism by promoting growth of skeletal muscles and is thus responsible for the greater male muscular development and strength.

The final maturation of sperm occurs in the **epididymis,** a tightly coiled tube enclosed in a fibrous casing. The sperm spend about 1 to 3 weeks in this segment of the duct system, where they become motile and capable of fertilizing an ovum. The tail of the epididymis leads into the **vas deferens,** a muscular tube that passes through the inguinal canal as part of the spermatic cord and joins the duct from the **seminal vesicle** to form the ejaculatory duct. Depending on the degree of sexual activity and frequency of ejaculation, sperm may remain in the vas deferens up to 1 month with no loss of fertility. Severing of the vas deferens **(vasectomy)** is an operation performed to make a man sterile. Vasectomy interrupts the route from the epididymis to the remainder of the genital tract.

The **seminal vesicles** lie on the posterior aspect of the base of the bladder and secrete a thick liquid that is rich in fructose, a simple sugar that serves as an energy source for sperm motility after ejaculation. The seminal vesicles also secrete prostaglandin, which increases uterine contractions in the woman and helps propel the sperm toward the fallopian tubes.

The **prostate gland** lies just below the bladder and surrounds the urethra. It secretes a thin alkaline substance that constitutes the major portion of the seminal fluid volume. The alkalinity of this material is

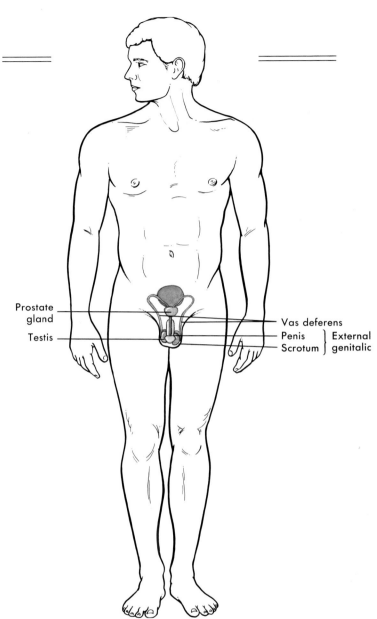

essential to sperm motility, which would otherwise be inhibited by the highly acidic vaginal secretions.

Intense sexual stimulation causes peristaltic contractions in the walls of the epididymis and vas deferens, propelling sperm into the urethra. At the same time, the seminal vesicles and prostate gland release their secretions that mix with the mucous secretion of the bulbourethral glands to form semen. The ejaculation of semen occurs when intense muscular contractions of erectile tissue cause the semen to be expressed through the urethral opening.

Male fertility is related not only to the number of sperm ejaculated but also to their size, shape, and motility. Although only one sperm fertilizes an ovum, millions of sperm seem to be necessary for fertilization to occur. Indeed, it is estimated that sterility may result when the sperm count falls below about 50 million/ml of semen.

BENIGN PROSTATIC HYPERPLASIA

Enlargement of the prostate gland is common in men over age 60 and may be detected on a digital rectal examination. The enlargement is probably related to a disturbance of hormone secretions from the sex glands that occurs as the period of reproductive activity declines. The major effect of prostatic enlargement is an inability to empty the bladder completely, leading to partial urinary tract obstruction, bilateral ureteral dilation, and hydronephrosis. On excretory urography, the enlarged prostate typically produces elevation and a smooth impression on the floor of the contrast-filled bladder (Figure 10-6). Elevation of the insertion of the ureters on the trigone of the bladder produces a characteristic J-shaped or "fish hook" appearance of the distal ureters. Residual urine in the bladder provides a growth medium for bacterial infection, which produces cystitis; the infection may ascend from the bladder to the kidney, resulting in pyelonephritis.

On MRI, benign prostatic hyperplasia causes a diffuse or nodular area of homogeneous low intensity on T1-weighted images and an inhomogeneous, mixed intermediate-high signal intensity on T2-weighted images (Figure 10-7). Focal enlargement is often accentuated by a pseudocapsule, representing compression of adjacent tissue visualized as a low-intensity rim. Diffuse enlargement shows similar intensity changes, although the pseudocapsule is not

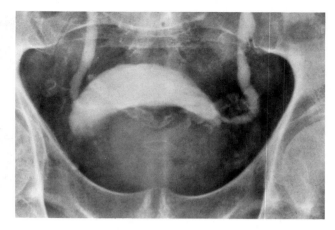

Figure 10-6 Benign prostatic hyperplasia. Large, smooth filling defect at base of bladder. Note fish-hook appearance of distal ureters and calcification in vas deferens.

present. Unfortunately, the intensity of benign prostatic hyperplasia may often be similar to that of the normal prostate or a region of prostatitis.

Surgical resection of the prostate (transurethral resection, or TUR) can relieve the obstructive symptoms.

CARCINOMA OF THE PROSTATE GLAND

Carcinoma of the prostate gland is the second most common malignancy in men. The disease is rare before the age of 50, and the incidence increases with advancing age. The tumor can be slow growing and asymptomatic for long periods or can behave aggressively with extensive metastases.

Carcinoma of the prostate is best detected by pal-

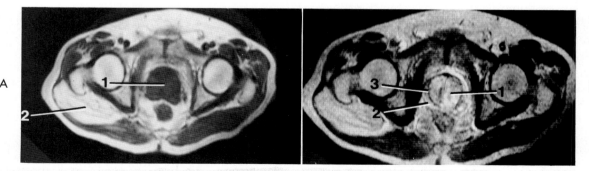

Figure 10-7 Benign prostatic hyperplasia. **A,** T1-weighted MR image shows prostatic enlargement of homogeneous low intensity. Note high signal intensity of large lipoma *(2)* in right gluteal region. **B,** On T2-weighted image, intermediate signal of enlarged transitional zone *(1)* shows increased inhomogeneity and is separated from high signal intensity peripheral zone *(2)* by low-intensity rim of pseudo-capsule. *(From McCarthy S and Fritzsche PJ: In Stark DD and Bradley WG, editors: Magnetic resonance imaging, St. Louis, The CV Mosby Co, 1988.)*

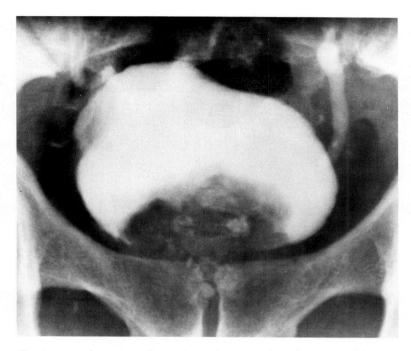

Figure 10-8 Carcinoma of prostate. Large irregular mass that elevates and impresses floor of contrast-filled bladder.

pation of a hard, nodular, and irregular mass on a routine rectal examination. Radiographically, carcinoma of the prostate often elevates and impresses the floor of the contrast-filled bladder. Unlike the smooth contour in benign prostatic hyperplasia, in carcinoma the impression on the bladder floor is usually more irregular (Figure 10-8). Bladder neck obstruction, infiltration of the trigone, or invasive obstruction of the ureters above the bladder may produce obstruction of the upper urinary tract.

Ultrasound performed by means of a probe inserted into the rectum is a new technique for detecting carcinoma of the prostate (Figure 10-9). The normal prostate has a generally homogeneous appearance with a moderate echo pattern. Early studies indicated that prostatic carcinoma appeared as hyperechoic areas. However, with the development of newer and higher frequency transducers, many carcinomas appear as areas of low echogenicity within the prostate. Up to 40% of carcinomas are isoechoic with normal prostate tissue and thus cannot be visualized on ultrasound. The most recent studies have concluded that the wide range of sonographic patterns in carcinoma indicates that ultrasound cannot reliably differentiate prostatic malignancy from benign disease.

MRI can superbly delineate the prostate, seminal vesicles, and surrounding organs to provide accurate staging of pelvic neoplasms. When the spin

echo technique is used, the central and peripheral zones of the prostate are well demonstrated and distinctly separate from the surrounding levator ani muscles. In the sagittal plane the relation of the prostate to the bladder, rectum, and seminal vesicles is clearly shown. Prostatic carcinoma is best demonstrated on long TR images, where it appears as disruption of the normally uniform high signal inten-

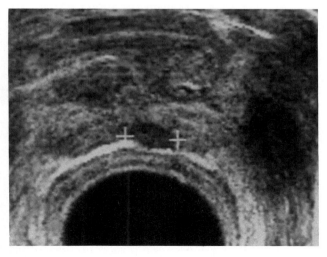

Figure 10-9 Cancer of prostate. Transrectal ultrasound demonstrates hypoechoic mass (between cursers).

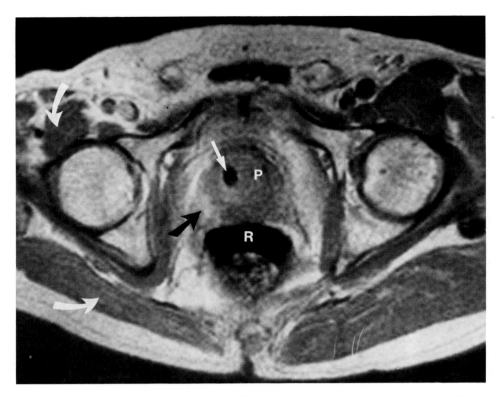

Figure 10-10 Carcinoma of prostate. Axial MR image through pelvis demonstrates abnormal area of increased signal intensity *(black arrow)* within prostate gland *(P)*. Foley catheter is in place *(straight white arrow)*, and rectum *(R)* contains air and feces. Note decreased size of pelvic musculature on right *(curved white arrows)* in this patient with above-knee amputation.

sity of the peripheral zone of the prostate (Figure 10-10). However, there is much controversy whether MRI is reliable for detection and diagnosis of prostate cancer. It has been demonstrated that a normal appearing prostate gland on MRI does not exclude the presence of a neoplasm. In addition, inhomogeneity of the gland is a common nonspecific finding that also can be seen in patients with adenoma or prostatitis.

Carcinoma of the prostate may spread by direct extension or by way of the lymphatics or the bloodstream. Spread of carcinoma of the prostate to the rectum can produce a large, smooth, concave pressure defect, a fungating ulcerated mass simulating primary rectal carcinoma, or a long, asymmetric annular stricture. Both ultrasound and CT may aid in defining extension of tumor into the bladder and seminal vesicles and in detecting metastases in enlarged lymph nodes (Figure 10-11).

The most common hematogenous metastases are to bone. They primarily involve the pelvis, thoracolumbar spine, femurs, and ribs. These lesions are most commonly osteoblastic and appear as multiple rounded foci of sclerotic density (Figure 10-12) or,

occasionally, diffuse sclerosis involving an entire bone ("ivory vertebra"). Patients with bony metastases usually have strikingly elevated levels of serum acid phosphatase. Because significant bone destruction or bone reaction must occur before a lesion can be detected on plain radiographs, the radionuclide bone scan is the best screening technique for detecting asymptomatic skeletal metastases in patients with carcinoma of the prostate. However, since the radionuclide scan is very sensitive but not specific and may show increased uptake in multiple disorders of the bone, conventional radiography of the affected site should be performed when a positive scan is obtained.

UNDESCENDED TESTIS (CRYPTORCHIDISM)

Near the end of gestation, the testis normally migrates from its intra-abdominal position through the inguinal canal into the scrotal sac. If one of the testicles cannot be palpated within the scrotum, it is important to determine whether this represents an absent testis or an ectopic position of the testis. The

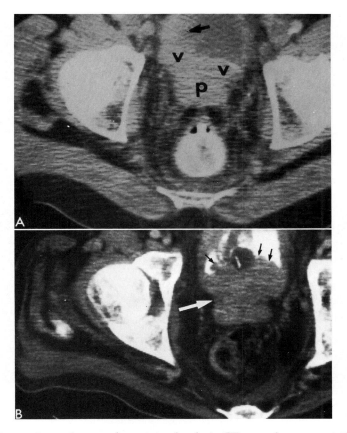

Figure 10-11 Metastatic carcinoma of prostate gland. **A,** CT scan shows prostatic carcinoma *(p)* invading wall of bladder *(arrow)* and seminal vesicles *(v)*. **B,** In another patient, CT scan shows prostatic carcinoma involving bladder *(black arrows)* and seminal vesicles. Normal sharp angle between seminal vesicles and prostate is lost *(white arrow)*. *(From Thoeni RF: In Moss AA, Gamsu G, and Genant HK, editors: Computed tomography of the body, Philadelphia, WB Saunders Co, 1983.)*

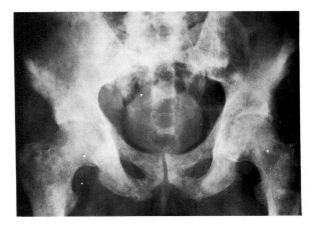

Figure 10-12 Metastatic carcinoma of prostate. Diffuse osteoblastic metastases involving bones about pelvis.

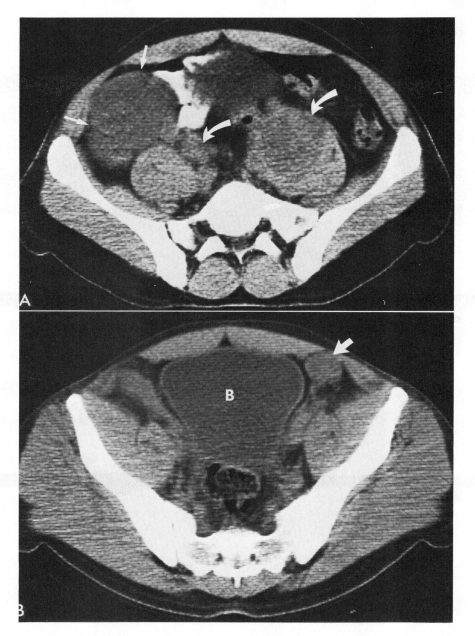

Figure 10-13 Malignant neoplasms developing in one of bilateral undescended testes. **A,** Undescended right testis is enlarged by carcinoma *(straight arrows)*. Tumor has metastasized to lymph nodes *(curved arrows),* which are enlarged. **B,** Nontumorous intra-abdominal left testis *(arrow)* appears as smaller, rounded structure adjacent to bladder *(B)*. *(From Jeffrey RB: In Moss AA, Gamsu G, and Genant HK, editors: Computed tomography of the body, Philadelphia, WB Saunders Co, 1983.)*

rate of malignancy is up to 40 times higher in the undescended (intra-abdominal) than in the descended testicle. Because of this extremely high rate of malignancy, the diagnosis of undescended testis usually leads to orchiopexy (surgical fixation of an undescended testis in the scrotum) in patients youn-

ger than 10 years of age and orchiectomy (surgical removal) in those seen after puberty.

In the absence of a palpable testicle, ultrasound is usually used as a screening technique. This modality carries no radiation risk and has a high diagnostic accuracy in demonstrating undescended

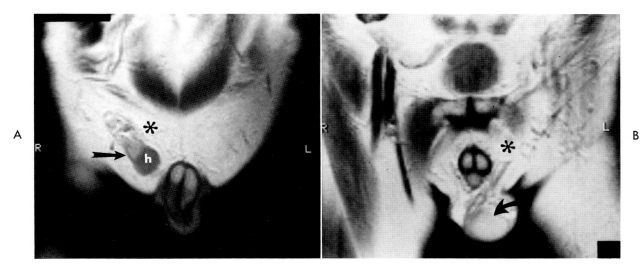

Figure 10-14 Atrophic undescended testis. **A,** Coronal MR scan shows small, intermediate signal intensity testis *(arrow)* associated with low signal intensity hydrocele *(h).* Intensity of testis is low compared with that of fat *(*).* **B,** Image slightly posterior to **A** shows normally descended contralateral testis *(curved arrow),* which has high signal intensity similar to that of fat *(*).* *(From Fritzsche PJ, et al: Radiology 164:169-173, 1987.)*

testicles that are located in the inguinal canal. However, sonography is not successful in detecting ectopic testicles in the pelvis or abdomen. If ultrasound fails to demonstrate an undescended testis, MRI or CT is indicated (Figure 10-13 and 10-14).

TESTICULAR TORSION AND EPIDIDYMITIS

Testicular torsion refers to the twisting of the gonad on its pedicle, which leads to the compromise of circulation and the sudden onset of severe scrotal

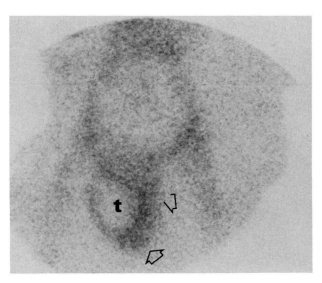

Figure 10-15 Testicular torsion. Severe diminished arterial perfusion causes testicle to appear as rounded, cold area *(t)* on radionuclide scan. Surrounding rim of increased activity represents blood supply to scrotal sac *(arrows).*

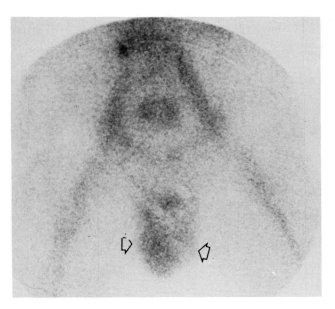

Figure 10-16 Epididymitis. Radionuclide scan shows high isotope uptake in region of testicle *(arrows)* caused by increased blood flow.

pain. Although primarily a clinical diagnosis, the scrotal pain and swelling of testicular torsion may be difficult to distinguish from that caused by inflammation of the epididymis (epididymitis). In such cases, Doppler ultrasound or radionuclide studies are of value.

Doppler ultrasound demonstrates the presence of intratesticular arterial pulsations. In testicular torsion the arterial perfusion is diminished or absent, whereas in epididymitis there is increased blood flow. Similarly, the radionuclide angiogram shows that isotope activity on the twisted side is either slightly decreased or at the normal, barely perceptible level. On the uninvolved side, the perfusion should be normal. When compared with the decreased activity on the involved side, the perfusion appears increased. Static nuclear scans demonstrate a rounded, cold area replacing the testicle in patients with torsion (Figure 10-15), but are a hot area in those with epididymitis (Figure 10-16).

TESTICULAR TUMORS

Testicular tumors are the most common neoplasms in men between the ages of 20 and 35. Almost all testicular tumors are malignant, and they tend to metastasize to the lymphatics that follow the course of the testicular arteries and veins and drain into para-aortic lymph nodes at the level of the kidneys.

There are two major types of testicular tumor. Seminomas arise from the seminiferous tubules, whereas teratomas arise from a primitive germ cell and consist of a variety of tissues. Seminomas are radiosensitive, and early diagnosis and irradiation have resulted in many cures.

Testicular tumors are best diagnosed on ultrasound examination. The normal testis has a homogeneous, medium-level echogenicity. A localized testicular tumor appears as a circumscribed mass with either increased or decreased echogenicity in an otherwise uniform testicular echo structure (Figure 10-17). Testicular tumors also can be detected on MRI (Figure 10-18).

Lymphatic metastases from testicular tumors typically occur at the level of the renal hilum (where the gonadal veins drain) and are best detected by CT (Figure 10-19). This modality also can detect spread of tumor to the lung or liver.

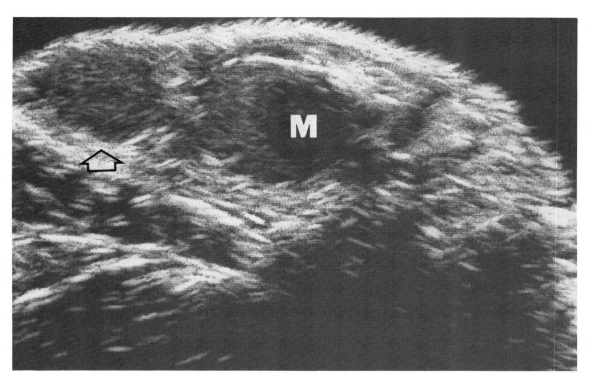

Figure 10-17   Testicular carcinoma. Transverse sonogram shows predominantly sonolucent mass (M) within enlarged left testis. Right testis (*arrow*) is normal. (*Courtesy Robert Mevorach, M.D.*)

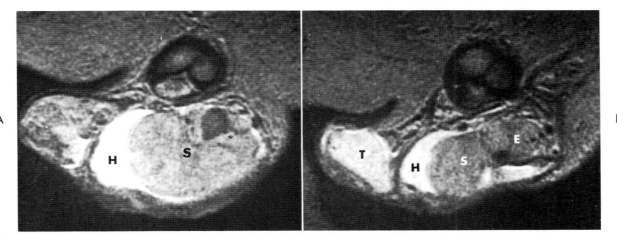

Figure 10-18 Testicular seminoma. **A,** T2-weighted MR scan shows that seminoma *(S)* in left testis has inhomogeneous signal with pronounced difference in contrast from adjacent hydrocele *(H)*. **B,** Inhomogeneous intermediate signal of intratesticular tumor *(S)* extends into epididymis *(E)*. Note that normal contralateral testis *(T)* has much higher signal intensity. *(From Baker LL et al: Radiology 163:93-98, 1987.)*

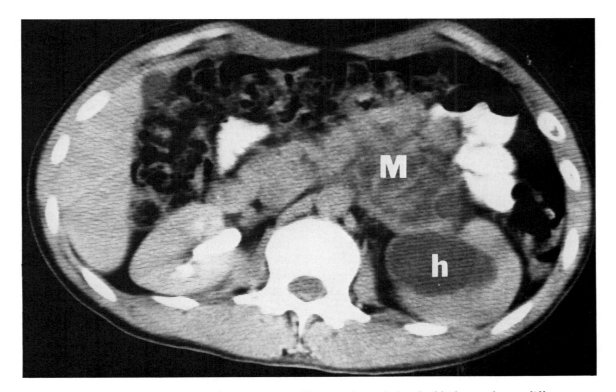

Figure 10-19 Metastatic testicular seminoma. CT scan through level of kidneys shows diffuse nodal metastases *(M)* containing characteristic low-attenuation areas. Extrinsic pressure on lower left ureter has caused severe hydronephrosis with dilation of renal pelvis *(h)*.

Female reproductive system

PHYSIOLOGY OF THE FEMALE REPRODUCTIVE SYSTEM

The ovaries are the equivalent of the testes in the male and are responsible for the production of ova and the secretion of female hormones. A woman's reproductive life begins with the onset of menstruation, the **menarche,** which generally occurs between the ages of 11 and 15. Once each month, on about the first day of menstruation, several primitive graafian follicles and their enclosed ova begin to grow and develop and the follicular cells start to secrete **estrogen.** In most cycles, only one follicle matures and migrates to the surface of the ovary, where it ruptures and expels the mature ovum into the pelvic cavity **(ovulation).**

After the release of the ovum, the remaining cells of the ruptured follicle enlarge and a golden-colored pigment (lutein) becomes deposited in their cytoplasm. This **corpus luteum** continues to grow for 7 to 8 days and secretes **progesterone** in increasing amounts. If fertilization of the ovum has not occurred, the size and secretions of the corpus luteum gradually diminish until the nonfunctional structure is reduced to a white scar (corpus albicans) that moves into the central portion of the ovary and eventually disappears. If fertilization does occur, however, the corpus luteum remains intact throughout pregnancy.

The cyclic changes in the ovaries are controlled by a variety of substances secreted by the anterior pituitary gland. Growth of the primitive graafian follicles and ova and the secretion of estrogen are controlled by follicle-stimulating hormone (FSH), whereas follicular rupture, expulsion of its ripe ovum, and the secretion of progesterone are under the control of luteinizing hormone (LH).

The fallopian tubes serve as ducts for the ovaries, even though they are not directly attached to them. The union of an ovum and a spermatozoan (fertilization) normally occurs in the fallopian tubes. About 1 day later, the resulting embryo reaches the uterus, where it begins to implant itself in the endometrium. Occasionally, implantation occurs in the fallopian tube or pelvic cavity instead of in the uterus, resulting in an **ectopic pregnancy.** Within 10 days, there is the earliest development of the placenta, which is derived in part from both the developing embryo and from maternal tissues and serves to nourish the fetus and anchor it to the

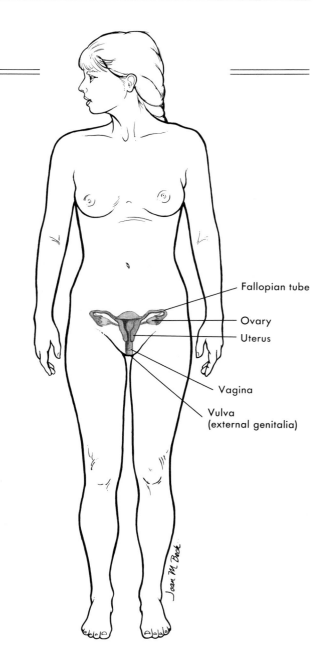

uterus. Although they are closely related, maternal and fetal blood do not mix, and the exchange of nutrients occurs across the important fetal membrane termed the **chorion.**

The menstrual cycle refers to the changes in the endometrium of the uterus that occur in women throughout the childbearing years. Each cycle lasts about 28 days and is divided into three phases: proliferative, secretory, and menstrual. Although the first day of menstruation is normally considered as the first day of the cycle, for ease of description the menstrual phase will be described last.

The **proliferative,** or **postmenstrual,** phase occurs

between the end of the menses and ovulation. Production of estrogen by ovarian follicular cells under the influence of FSH causes proliferation of the endometrium of the uterus. In a typical 28-day cycle, the proliferative phase usually includes cycle days 6 to 13 or 14. However, there is far more variability in the length of this phase than in the others.

The **secretory,** or **postovulatory,** phase occurs between ovulation and the onset of the menses. The high level of estrogen in the blood after ovulation inhibits the secretion of FSH, and the anterior lobe of the pituitary gland begins to secrete LH. This stimulates the corpus luteum to produce the hormone progesterone, which stimulates a further increase in the thickness of the endometrium and prepares the uterus for implantation of the ovum should fertilization occur. The length of the secretory phase is fairly constant and usually lasts 14 days.

If fertilization of the ovum does not occur, the high level of progesterone in the blood inhibits the secretion of LH so that the corpus luteum begins to degenerate and ceases to produce progesterone. As the superficial layers of the hypertrophied endometrium begin to break down, denuded bleeding areas are exposed. The flow of blood, mucus, and sloughed endometrium from the uterus is called the menstrual flow. This **menstrual** phase of the cycle lasts about 4 to 6 days, until the low level of progesterone causes the pituitary gland to again secrete FSH and a new menstrual cycle begins. Of course, if the ovum is fertilized, the corpus luteum does not degenerate and the endometrium remains intact throughout pregnancy.

The reproductive years terminate with the cessation of menstrual periods **(menopause),** which usually begins in the late 40s or early 50s.

PELVIC INFLAMMATORY DISEASE

Inflammation of the pelvic reproductive organs is usually the result of venereal disease (especially gonorrhea) in women of childbearing age. It can also develop from an unsterile abortion or delivery or be a complication of intrauterine devices. If pelvic inflammatory disease is not promptly and adequately treated, spread of infection to the fallopian tubes may cause fibrous adhesions that obstruct the inner portion near the uterus. If the outer ends of the tubes remain open, the spill of purulent material can lead to peritonitis and the formation of a pelvic abscess. More commonly, the outer ends close and the fallopian tubes fill with pus **(pyosalpinx).** After antibiotic therapy, the infection subsides and the tubes may remain filled with a watery fluid **(hydrosalpinx).** Obstruction of the fallopian tubes can result

in infertility or ectopic pregnancy. Spread of infection to involve the ovaries can produce tubo-ovarian abscesses, which are usually bilateral.

Ultrasound is the imaging procedure of choice for detecting pelvic inflammatory disease and pelvic abscesses. The fluid-filled urinary bladder provides an excellent acoustic window and permits confusing loops of small bowel to be displaced out of the pelvis. Pyosalpinx and tubo-ovarian abscesses typically are seen as tubular adnexal masses that are sonolucent and compatible with fluid collections (Figure 10-20). However, abscesses may also have thick and irregular, or "shaggy," walls or may contain echoes or fluid levels representing the layering of purulent debris (Figure 10-21).

The status of the fallopian tubes can be assessed radiographically by hysterosalpingography, in which the uterine cavity and fallopian tubes are opacified after the injection of contrast material into the uterus. In the normal woman with patent fallopian tubes, contrast material extravasating into the pelvic peritoneal cavity outlines the peritoneal surfaces and often loops of bowel within the pelvis (Figure 10-22). If the fallopian tubes are occluded by fibrosis from pelvic inflammatory disease or developmental

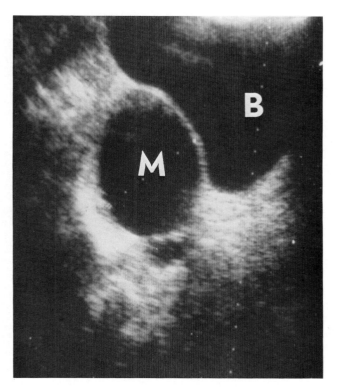

Figure 10-20 Tubo-ovarian abscess. Ultrasound demonstrates large sonolucent mass *(M)* posterior to bladder *(B).*

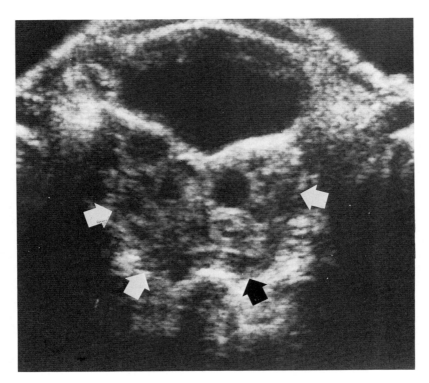

Figure 10-21 Chronic pelvic inflammatory disease. Transverse sonogram demonstrates large, complex cystic and echogenic masses *(arrows)* posterior to echo-free bladder. *(From Callen PW, editor: Ultrasonography in obstetrics and gynecology, Philadelphia, WB Saunders Co, 1983.)*

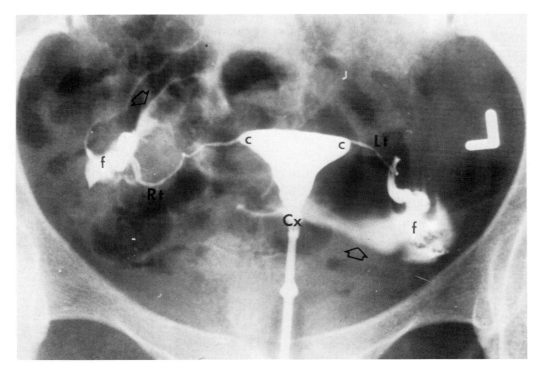

Figure 10-22 Normal hysterosalpingogram. Arrows point to bilateral spill of contrast material into peritoneal cavity. *Cx,* Internal cervical os; *c,* cornua of uterus; *RT* and *LT,* right and left fallopian tubes; *f,* fimbriated portion. *(From Yune HJ, et al: Hysterosalpingography in infertility, AJR 122:642-651, 1974.)*

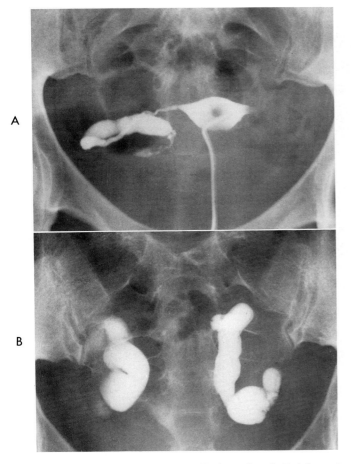

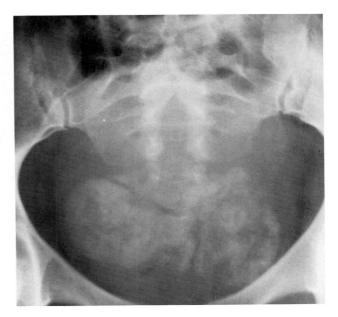

Figure 10-24 Psammomatous calcifications. Diffuse, ill-defined collections of granular amorphous calcification are visible within this cystadenocarcinoma of ovary. *(From Eisenberg RL: Diagnostic imaging in surgery, New York, McGraw-Hill Book Co, 1987.)*

Figure 10-23 Hydrosalpinx. **A,** Unilateral and, **B,** bilateral gross dilation of fallopian tubes without evidence of free spill of contrast material into peritoneal cavity.

anomalies, there is no evidence of the contrast material reaching the peritoneal cavity (Figure 10-23).

Plain abdominal or pelvic radiographs are of little value in detecting pelvic inflammatory disease and pelvic abscesses. Abnormal gas collections can be masked by fecal material in the rectum and in loops of small bowel.

CYSTS AND TUMORS

Ovarian cysts and tumors

Physiologic ovarian cysts are most common in the female infant and in women of childbearing age. They include follicular cysts (unruptured, enlarged follicles) and corpus luteum cysts, which occur after continued hemorrhage or lack of resolution of the corpus luteum. On ultrasound, cysts appear as rounded, anechoic adnexal masses.

The most common malignancies involving the ovaries are metastatic tumors, which primarily arise from carcinomas of the breast, colon, and stomach. They are frequently bilateral and often asymptomatic.

Primary cystadenocarcinoma of the ovary often contains psammomatous bodies, depositions of calcium carbonate located in the fibrous stroma of the tumor that can be detected on plain abdominal radiographs. These psammomatous calcifications appear as scattered, fine amorphous shadows that are barely denser than the normal soft tissues and can therefore be easily missed unless they are extensive (Figure 10-24). On ultrasound examination, cystadenocarcinoma typically appears as a large cystic mass with internal septa. It may be difficult to distinguish cystadenocarcinoma from cystadenoma, its benign counterpart (Figure 10-25). The more solid and irregular the areas within the mass on ultrasound, the more likely it represents a malignant tumor. In addition, the association of ascites with an ovarian mass strongly suggests underlying malignancy.

Ovarian carcinomas usually spread by implanting widely on the omental and peritoneal surfaces. This can produce the characteristic CT appearance of an "omental cake," an irregular sheet of soft-tissue densities beneath the anterior abdominal wall (Figure 10-26). CT also is of value in detecting tumor adherence to bowel, ureteral involvement, and retroperitoneal adenopathy.

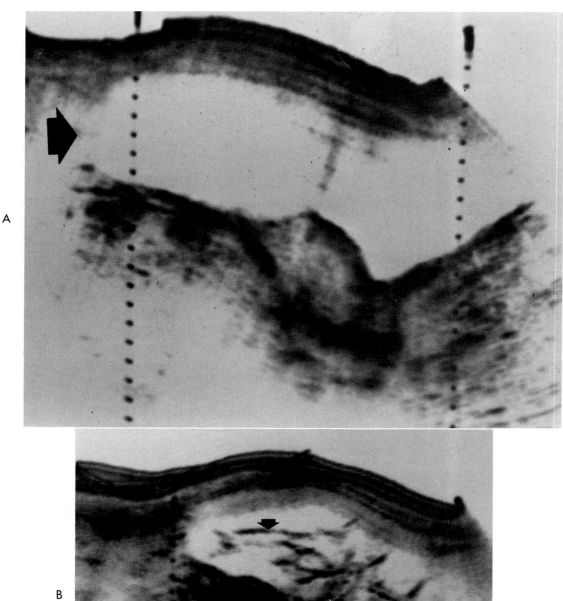

Figure 10-25   Cystadenoma. **A,** Longitudinal sonogram in asymptomatic girl demonstrates large, sonolucent, completely cystic mass *(arrow).* **B,** In another patient, longitudinal sonogram demonstrates complex, predominantly cystic mass containing several thin and well-defined septations *(arrow). (From Callen PW, editor: Ultrasonography in obstetrics and gynecology, Philadelphia, WB Saunders Co, 1983.)*

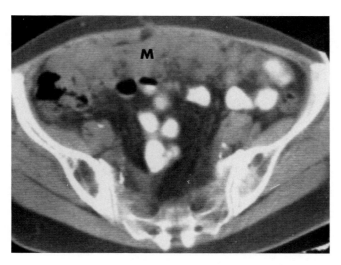

Figure 10-26 Omental cake. Metastases *(M)* resulting from cystadenocarcinoma of ovary cause irregular sheet of soft-tissue densities beneath anterior abdominal wall that posteriorly displaces adjacent contrast-filled bowel loops. *(From Lee JKT, Sagel SS, Stanley RJ, editors: Computed body tomography, New York, Raven Press, 1983.)*

Dermoid cyst (teratoma)

A dermoid cyst, the most common type of germ cell tumor, contains skin, hair, teeth, and fatty elements, all of which typically derive from ectodermal tissue. They are of no clinical significance unless they grow so large that they produce symptoms by compressing adjacent structures. About half of all ovarian dermoid cysts contain some calcification. This is usually in the form of a partially or completely formed tooth (Figure 10-27); less frequently, the wall

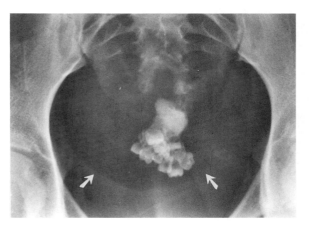

Figure 10-27 Dermoid cyst containing multiple well-formed teeth. Note relative lucency of mass *(arrows)*, which is composed largely of fatty tissue.

of the cyst is partially calcified. The characteristic calcification combined with the relative radiolucency of the lipid material within the lesion is pathognomonic of an ovarian dermoid cyst.

The most common ultrasound appearance of a dermoid cyst is a complex, primarily solid mass containing high-level echoes arising from hair or calcification within the mass (Figure 10-28). The highly echogenic nature of these masses may make it difficult to delineate the lesion completely or to distinguish it from surrounding gas-containing loops of bowel.

Uterine fibroids

Fibroids (leiomyomas) of the uterus are benign smooth-muscle tumors that are very common, often multiple, and vary greatly in size. Growth of fibroid tumors is stimulated by estrogen. They develop only during the reproductive years and tend to shrink after menopause. Abnormal bleeding between periods or excessively heavy menstrual flow is the most common symptom. Large tumors may project from the uterus to put pressure on surrounding organs and cause pelvic pain. They also can interfere with delivery or, if on a stalk (pedunculated), protrude into the vagina.

Uterine fibroids are by far the most common calcified lesions of the female genital tract. They have a characteristic mottled, mulberry, or popcorn type of calcification and appear on plain abdominal ra-

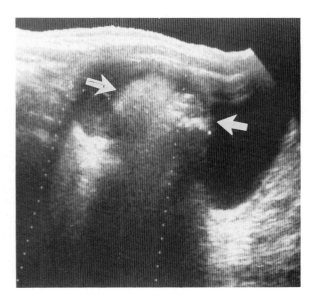

Figure 10-28 Dermoid cyst. Sagittal sonogram demonstrates only near wall of dermoid because of acoustic shadowing from hairball *(arrows)*, producing so-called tip of iceberg sign. *(From Eisenberg R: Atlas of sign in radiology, Philadelphia, JB Lippincott Co, 1984.)*

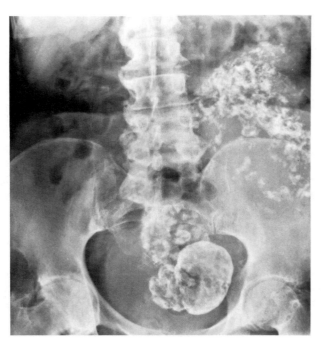

Figure 10-29 Calcified uterine fibroid. Calcified mass extends well beyond confines of pelvis.

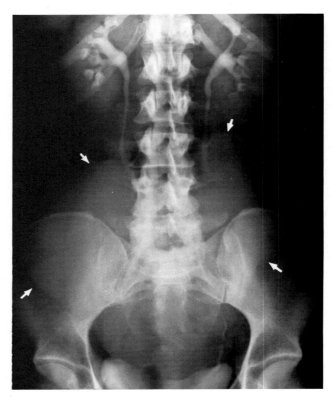

Figure 10-30 Uterine fibroid. Excretory urogram demonstrates persistent dense opacification of huge uterine leiomyoma *(arrows)*.

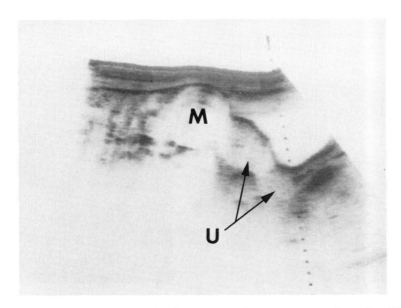

Figure 10-31 Uterine fibroid. Longitudinal sonogram demonstrates pedunculated leiomyoma as hypoechoic mass *(M)* projecting from fundus of uterus *(U)*. Decreased sound transmission through mass indicates its solid nature. *(From Callen PW, editor: Ultrasonography in obstetrics and gynecology, Philadelphia, WB Saunders Co, 1983.)*

diographs as smooth or lobulated nodules with a stippled or whorled appearance. A very large calcified fibroid occasionally occupies the entire pelvis or even extends out of the pelvis to lie in the lower abdomen (Figure 10-29).

During excretory urography, persistent uterine opacification is often seen in patients with an underlying uterine fibroid tumor (Figure 10-30). The tumor typically presses on the fundus of the bladder, causing a lobulated extrinsic impression that differs from the smooth impression usually seen with ovarian cysts. Extension of a fibroid into the adjacent tissues (parametrium) may cause medial displacement of the pelvic ureter or ureteral compression leading to hydronephrosis.

The classic ultrasound appearance of a uterine fibroid is a hypoechoic, solid contour-deforming mass in an enlarged, inhomogeneous uterus (Figure 10-31). Fatty degeneration and calcification cause focal increased echogenicity; the calcification may result in acoustic shadowing. A subserosal fibroid projecting from the uterus but attached to it by a large stalk may occasionally simulate an adnexal mass or ovarian tumor.

Endometrial carcinoma

Adenocarcinoma of the endometrium is the predominant neoplasm of the uterine body and is the most common invasive gynecologic neoplasm. It usually occurs in postmenopausal women, especially those who have never had children. Most patients are seen clinically with postmenopausal bleeding.

Excretory urography may demonstrate an enlarged uterus impressing or invading the posterior wall and fundus of the bladder. The typical ultrasound appearance of endometrial carcinoma is an enlarged uterus with irregular areas of low-level echoes and bizarre clusters of high-intensity echoes (Figure 10-32). Unless evidence of local invasion can be demonstrated, the ultrasound findings are indistinguishable from those of fibroid tumors, which often occur in patients with endometrial carcinoma. CT demonstrates focal or diffuse enlargement of the body of the uterus (Figure 10-33). This modality is especially useful in detecting clinically unsuspected omental and nodal metastases in patients with advanced disease, as well as in evaluating patients with suspected neoplastic recurrence and in checking the response to chemotherapy or radiation treatment.

MRI allows differentiation of the endometrium (inner lining) from the myometrium (muscle layer) of the uterus and has been shown to be useful in demonstrating focal or diffuse endometrial tumors (Figure 10-34). The excellent contrast resolution of this technique may allow determination of the depth of myometrial invasion.

Endometriosis

Endometriosis is the presence of normal appearing endometrium in sites other than their normal location inside the uterus. Although tissues next to the uterus (ovaries, uterine ligaments, rectovaginal septum, pelvic peritoneum) are most frequently involved in endometriosis, the gastrointestinal and urinary tracts can also be affected. Current theories

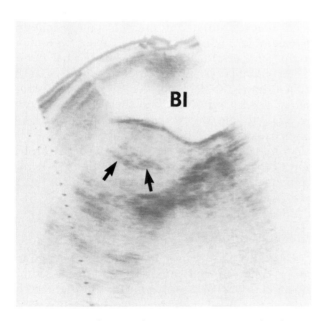

Figure 10-32 Endometrial carcinoma. Longitudinal sonogram shows uterus to be enlarged and bulbous. There are clusters of high-amplitude echoes *(arrows)* in region of central cavity echo. *Bl,* Bladder. *(From Gross BH et al: AJR 141:765-773, 1983.)*

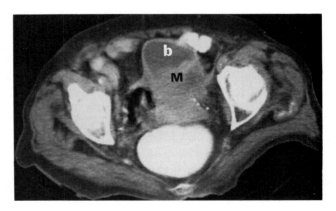

Figure 10-33 Bladder invasion by endometrial carcinoma. CT scan shows mass *(M)* obliterating fat planes between bladder *(b)* and uterus. Urine within bladder outlines thickening of posterior bladder wall. *(From Gross BH, et al: AJR 141:765-773, 1983.)*

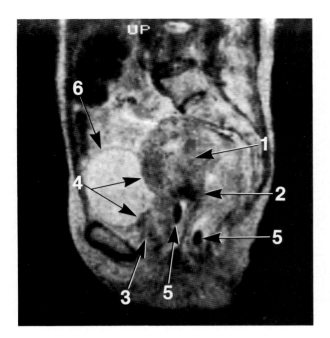

Figure 10-34 Endometrial carcinoma. Sagittal T2-weighted MR scan shows extensive tumor of mixed signal intensity *(1)* that has invaded endocervix and only permits identification of ectocervix *(2)*. Tumor has extended interiorly along serosal surface of uterus into vesicovaginal septum *(3)* and bladder wall *(4)*. Low-intensity foci in vagina represent radiotherapy implants *(5)*. Note normal urinary bladder wall superiorly *(6)*. *(From Lupetin AR: In Stark DD and Bradley WG, editors: Magnetic resonance imaging, St. Louis, The CV Mosby Co, 1988.)*

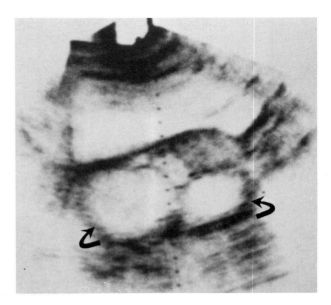

Figure 10-35 Endometrioma. Several sonolucent masses *(arrows)* simulating multiple follicular cysts arising from ovary. *(From Callen PW, editor: Ultrasonography in obstetrics and gynecology, Philadelphia, WB Saunders Co, 1983.)*

of the cause of endometriosis include (1) reflux of endometrial fragments backward through the fallopian tubes during menstruation with implantation in the pelvis; (2) transformation of multipotential cells in the abdomen and pelvis; (3) implantation of endometrial fragments during surgery or delivery; and (4) spread of endometrial tissue by way of the bloodstream or lymphatic system.

Even though the endometrial tissue lies outside the uterus, it still responds to hormonal changes and undergoes a proliferative and secretory phase along with sloughing and subsequent bleeding. Thus an endometrial implant within a closed space can continue to grow with each menstrual cycle (Figure 10-35). Clinical symptoms include abnormal bleeding, painful menstruation (dysmenorrhea), and pain during sexual intercourse (dyspareunia). Because endometriosis is usually clinically apparent only when ovarian function is active, most women who are symptomatic for endometriosis are between 20 and 45 years of age.

Endometriosis involving the urinary tract most commonly produces ureteral obstruction below the

level of the pelvis brim. The condition mimics a ureteral tumor and may appear as an intraluminal mass or stricture or as a smooth, rounded, or multilobular filling defect in the bladder. In the gastrointestinal tract, endometriosis primarily affects those segments that are situated in the pelvis (especially the rectosigmoid colon). It typically causes abdominal cramps and diarrhea during the menstrual period and may appear as single or multiple masses in the colon (Figure 10-36). Repeated shedding of endometrial tissue and blood into the peritoneal cavity can lead to the development of dense adhesive bands causing small bowel obstruction.

A rare complication of endometriosis with intrathoracic implants of endometrial tissue is recurrent catamenial pneumothorax, which is usually right-sided and occurs during menstrual flow.

Carcinoma of the cervix

Carcinoma of the cervix is the second most common form of cancer in women. Development of the tumor appears to be related to chronic irritation, infection, and poor hygiene, and there is a higher incidence in women who have begun sexual activity at an early age and have had multiple sexual partners. The development of the Pap smear examination has permitted detection of cervical carcinoma at a very early stage (carcinoma in situ) when it has not yet invaded

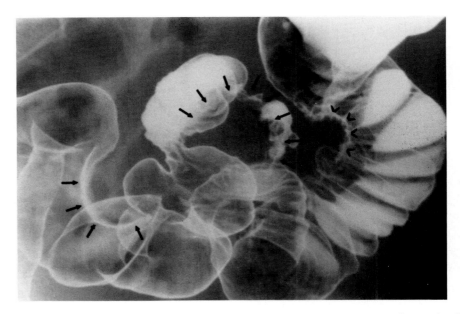

Figure 10-36 Endometriosis. Three separate endometrial implants (*arrows* and *arrowheads*) are seen in sigmoid colon. Most distal lesion has smooth interface with bowel wall, indicating no intramural invasion. The two more proximal lesions have irregular borders, indicating intramural or submucosal invasion. *(Gedgaudas RK, et al: Value of preoperative barium enema examination in the assessment of pelvic masses, Radiology 146:609-616, 1983.)*

the underlying tissues and is surgically curable. Widespread cervical cancer becomes inoperable, and radiation therapy is the usual treatment.

At the time of the initial staging, one third of patients have unilateral or bilateral hydronephrosis that can be demonstrated by excretory urography or ultrasound. Indeed, the most common cause of death in patients with carcinoma of the cervix is impairment of renal function caused by ureteral obstruction. Extension of the tumor to the bladder may cause an irregular filling defect; direct infiltration of the perirectal tissues may produce irregular narrowing of the rectosigmoid colon and widening of the retrorectal space. Distant metastases to the skeleton or lungs are uncommon, even in patients with advanced disease.

Ultrasound usually demonstrates a cervical carcinoma as a solid mass behind the bladder (Figure 10-37). CT is more accurate in detecting pelvic sidewall invasion and therefore is usually the initial staging procedure in patients in whom there is a clinical suspicion of advanced disease (Figures 10-38 and 10-39). This modality is also the procedure of choice for monitoring tumor response to treatment and for assessing suspected recurrence.

MRI can permit the cervix to be distinguished from the uterus and vagina and is thus of value in detecting and staging cervical carcinoma (Figures 10-40 and 10-41).

After radiation therapy for carcinoma of the cervix (and other types of pelvic carcinoma), it may be difficult to distinguish chronic rectal narrowing and widening of the retrorectal space caused by radiation effects from that caused by recurrence of tumor. Radiation therapy can also lead to the development of

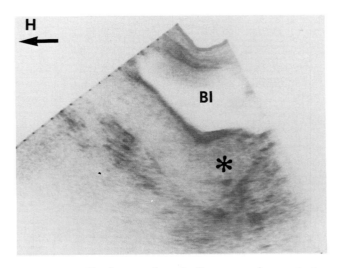

Figure 10-37 Carcinoma of cervix. Sonogram demonstrates solid, echogenic mass *(asterisk)* lying behind bladder *(Bl)* that is indistinguishable from benign cervical myoma. *(From Callen PW, editor: Ultrasonography in obstetrics and gynecology, Philadelphia, WB Saunders Co, 1983.)*

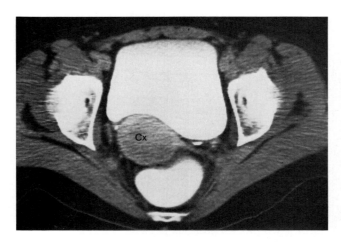

Figure 10-38 Carcinoma of cervix. CT scan demonstrates inhomogeneity of enlarged cervix *(Cx)* without evidence of bladder invasion. *(From Gross BH et al: AJR 141:765-773, 1983.)*

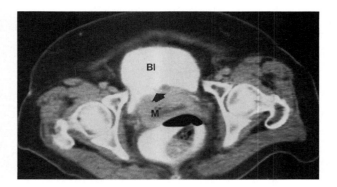

Figure 10-39 Bladder invasion by carcinoma of cervix. CT scan shows irregularity *(arrow)* of posterior margin of contrast-filled urinary bladder *(Bl)* and adjacent inhomogeneous cervical mass *(M)*. *(From Callen PW, editor: Ultrasonography in obstetrics and gynecology, Philadelphia, WB Saunders Co, 1983.)*

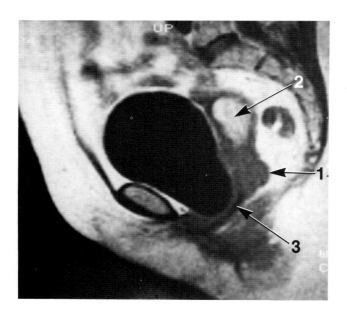

Figure 10-40 Cervical carcinoma. On this sagittal T1-weighted MR scan, posterior cervical lobulation *(1)* is only primary sign of infiltrating cervical neoplasm. Note marked widening of central uterine high-intensity zone *(2)* caused by accumulation of menstrual products in endometrial canal resulting from tumor occlusion of endocervical canal. Urine *(3)* within vagina produces low signal intensity on this imaging sequence. *(From Lupetin AR: In Stark DD and Bradley WG, editors: Magnetic resonance imaging, St. Louis, The CV Mosby Co, 1988.)*

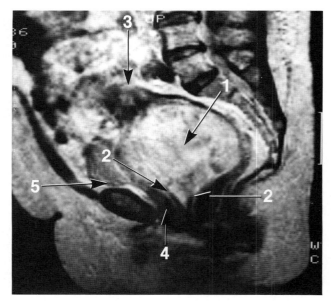

Figure 10-41 Carcinoma of cervix. Sagittal T2-weighted MR image shows bulky cervical neoplasm *(1)* with mottled high signal intensity. Lesion has invaded upper third of vaginal stroma *(2)* anteriorly and posteriorly but has spared uterus *(3)*. Urethra *(4)* and urinary bladder *(5)* are anteriorly displaced by tumor. *(From Lupetin AR: In Stark DD and Bradley WG, editors: Magnetic resonance imaging, St. Louis, The CV Mosby Co, 1988.)*

fibrous inflammatory adhesions between loops of bowel and the bladder, resulting in the development of fistulas between bowel loops (enteric-enteric) and between a bowel loop and the urinary bladder (enteric-vesical).

BREAST CANCER

Breast cancer is the most common malignancy among women. Current surgical and radiation therapy techniques provide highly effective treatment, but only if the cancers are detected when localized to the breast itself. Unfortunately, most breast tumors are discovered accidentally rather than in the course of regular survey examinations. By this time, the majority have spread either to regional lymph nodes or systemically, accounting for the current high mortality rate (about 50%) that makes breast cancer the leading cause of cancer death in women.

Periodic careful physical examination of the breast, done either by a trained health professional or by the patient herself, will discover cancers that are small and more likely to be localized. Even smaller, nonpalpable, and potentially more curable lesions can be detected by mammography, a radiographic examination that is by far the most effective breast diagnostic procedure. Indeed, routine mammography combined with physical examination is the only approach currently available that promises to significantly reduce breast cancer mortality.

The two major radiographic techniques for diagnosing breast cancer are screen-film mammography and xeromammography. Screen-film imaging uses a specially designed x-ray screen that permits the proper exposure of film by many fewer x-rays than would be otherwise necessary. This produces a conventional black-and-white image at a very low radiation dose. Xeromammography is an adaptation of the standard xerographic photocopying process; the blue-and-white x-ray images are made on paper rather than on film.

Almost all breast cancers are seen mammographically as a tumor mass or clustered calcifications, or both. Either feature, when clearly demonstrated, is so suspicious of malignancy as to require prompt biopsy whether the lesion is palpable or not. Secondary changes of breast carcinoma include skin thickening and nipple retraction. Magnification imaging and compression techniques greatly improve the diagnostic value of the image.

The typical malignant tumor mass is poorly defined, has irregular margins, and demonstrates numerous fine linear strands or spicules radiating out from the mass (Figure 10-42). This appearance is characteristic but not diagnostic of malignancy and is in stark contrast of the typical mammographic picture of a benign mass, which has well-defined, smooth margins and a round, oval, or gently lobulated contour (Figure 10-43).

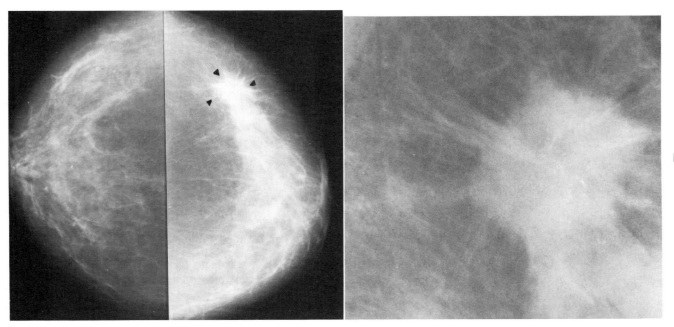

Figure 10-42 Breast cancer. **A,** Full and, **B,** magnified coned views of breast demonstrate ill-defined, irregular mass with radiating spicules *(arrowheads)*.

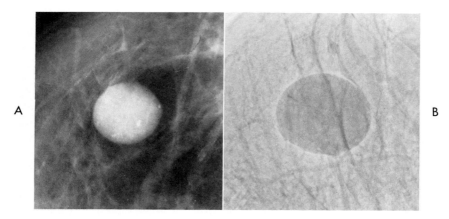

Figure 10-43   Benign breast masses. **A,** Screen-film mammogram demonstrates smooth, round fibroadenoma with clearly defined margins. **B,** Xeromammogram demonstrates smooth contour and sharply defined margins of benign cyst.

Clustered calcifications in breast cancer are typically numerous, very small, and localized to one segment of the breast. They demonstrate a wide variety of shapes, including fine linear, curvilinear, and branching forms (Figure 10-44). Although only about half of breast cancers present mammographically as clusters of calcifications, typical calcifications are seen in many of the nonpalpable intraductal cancers that often do not form mass lesions and may otherwise escape detection.

Ultrasound can differentiate a benign cyst from a solid mass and thus substantially reduces the number of biopsies done for benign cysts (Figure 10-45).

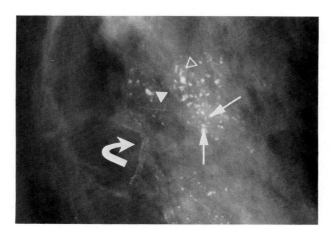

Figure 10-44   Malignant calcifications in breast cancer. Numerous tiny calcific particles with linear *(arrows)*, curvilinear *(solid arrowhead)*, and branching *(open arrowhead)* forms characteristic of malignancy. Note benign calcification in arterial wall, which is easily recognized by its large size and tubular distribution *(curved arrow).*

However, ultrasound is of limited value in detecting nonpalpable cancers, particularly those that present with calcifications alone, and thus it cannot substitute for mammography as a standard examination.

Although relatively infrequent, breast cancer also can develop in men.

Benign breast disease

Fibrocystic disease of the breast is a common benign condition occurring in about 20% of premenopausal women. It is usually bilateral with cysts of various sizes distributed throughout breasts that also contain an increased amount of fibrous tissue.

A fibroadenoma is the most common benign breast tumor. It generally appears as a smooth, well-circumscribed mass with no invasion of surrounding tissue (Figure 10-43, *A*). Ultrasound permits differentiation of a solid fibroadenoma from a fluid-filled breast cyst.

IMAGING IN PREGNANCY

Because of its noninvasive and non-ionizing character, ultrasound is the modality of choice in evaluating possible complications of pregnancy. A major role of this modality is to assess the gestational age, a measurement that is often highly inaccurate when based on the data of the last menstrual period. A knowledge of the true gestational age may be critically important for obstetric decisions, since the length of pregnancy is a major factor in interpreting the graphs that indicate the status of the fetus. Measurements of fetal age by ultrasound include the longest biparietal diameter (BPD), the crown-rump length, and the length of the fetal femur. The BPD

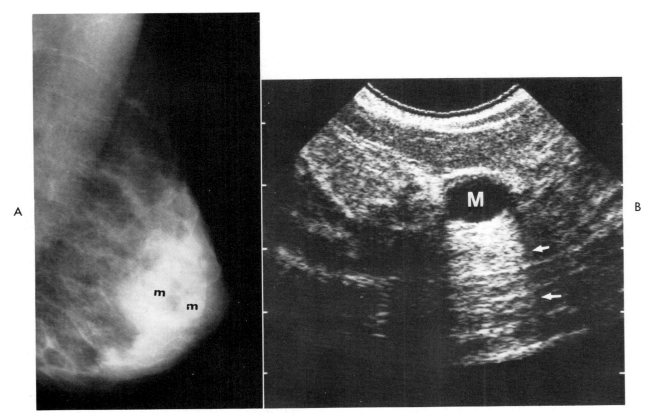

Figure 10-45 Sonography in breast disease. **A,** Mammogram shows several rounded masses *(m)* that could be solid or cystic in breast that is very dense anteriorly. **B,** Sonogram clearly shows that largest mass *(M)* is cystic, since it contains no internal echoes and shows marked posterior enhancement *(arrows).*

is measured from the outer margin of the skull on one side to the inner margin on the other side at the level of the thalami (Figure 10-46). A single measurement of the biparietal diameter has its greatest accuracy between 12 and 26 weeks; after this time, the size of the head and thus the BPD may be affected by a growth disturbance. The crown-rump length refers to the distance between the tip of the head and the bottom of the fetal trunk (Figure 10-47). This measurement is highly accurate in assessing gestational age in early pregnancy (less than 11 weeks).

An early diagnosis of multiple pregnancies can be made by ultrasound (Figure 10-48). This is essential so that therapeutic measures can be taken to reduce the high complication rate associated with twin (or more) pregnancies.

Ultrasound can be used to detect abnormalities in the volume of amniotic fluid, which is often associated with underlying fetal anomalies. **Polyhydramnios** represents the excessive accumulation of amniotic fluid that may be caused by maternal disorders such as diabetes mellitus and Rh isoimmu-

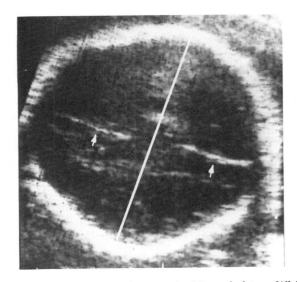

Figure 10-46 Biparietal diameter in 28-week fetus. White line indicates biparietal diameter, which is measured from outer margin of skull on one side to inner margin on other side. Arrows point to midline falx.

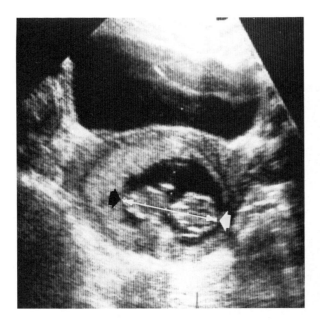

Figure 10-47 Crown-rump length. Distance between tip of head *(white arrow)* and bottom of fetal trunk *(black arrow)* measures 42 mm, equivalent to gestational age of approximately 11 weeks.

nization (Figure 10-49). Polyhydramnios is also caused by fetal abnormalities, especially those related to the central nervous system, the gastrointestinal tract, the circulatory system, and dwarfism. **Oligohydramnios** refers to a very small volume of amniotic fluid. This condition primarily results from fetal urinary tract disorders such as renal aplasia, renal dysplasia, and urethral obstruction. Oligohydramnios is also associated with intrauterine growth retardation.

Clinically significant errors of morphologic development occur in up to 5% of all children. The in utero detection of these anomalies by ultrasound may permit in utero medical or surgical therapy, provide an indication for termination of the pregnancy, or influence the mode of delivery. Although a detailed description of the rapidly expanding field of prenatal sonography is beyond the scope of this book, some of the abnormalities that can be detected, and often treated, in utero are osseous (bony) and neural anomalies of the fetal cranium and spine, gastrointestinal atresias and developmental cysts, cystic and obstructive lesions of the genitourinary tract, and congenital cardiac diseases (Figures 10-50 to 10-52).

Because ultrasound examinations can demonstrate the fetus and placenta with no apparent risk to the mother or unborn child, ultrasonography is unquestionably the imaging study of choice for eval-

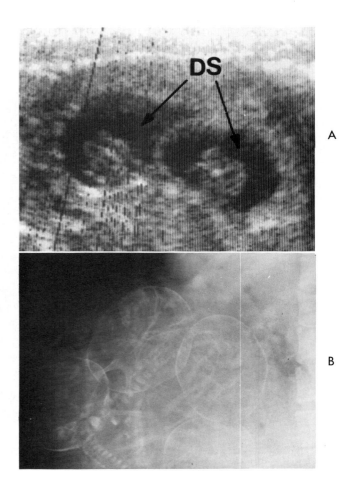

Figure 10-48 Multiple pregnancies. **A,** Ultrasound shows twin pregnancy. *DS,* Desidual sac. **B,** Lateral abdominal radiograph of woman with quadruplets clearly shows four separate fetal skulls and spines.

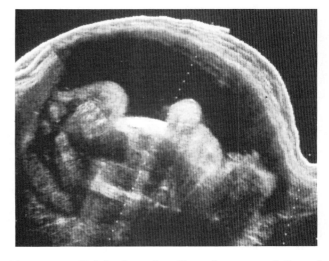

Figure 10-49 Polyhydramnios. Excessive accumulation of amniotic fluid surrounds fetus in mother with diabetes mellitus.

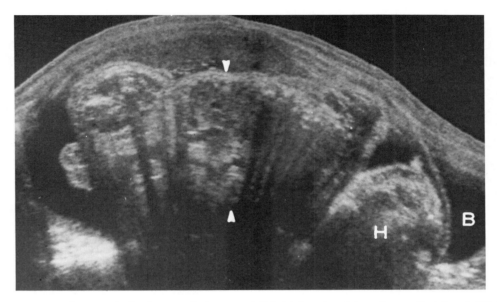

Figure 10-50 Anencephaly. Long-axis image of third-trimester fetus shows that head *(H)* is irregularly shaped, echogenic, and much smaller than body *(arrowheads)*. B, Maternal bladder. *(From Pasto ME and Kurtz AM: Semin Ultrasound CT MR 5:170-193, 1984.)*

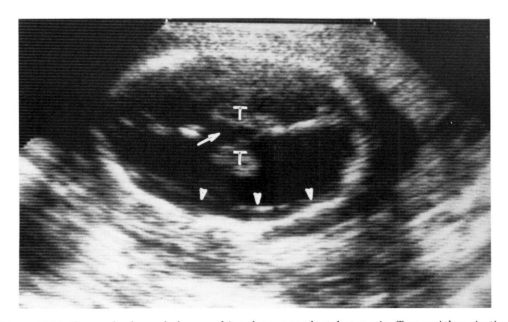

Figure 10-51 Severe hydrocephalus resulting from aqueductal stenosis. Transaxial projection demonstrates markedly dilated lateral ventricles and dilated third ventricle *(arrow)* between thalami *(T)*. Arrowheads show extremely thin residual cerebral cortex. *(From Pasto ME and Kurtz AM: Semin Ultrasound CT MR 5:170-193, 1984.)*

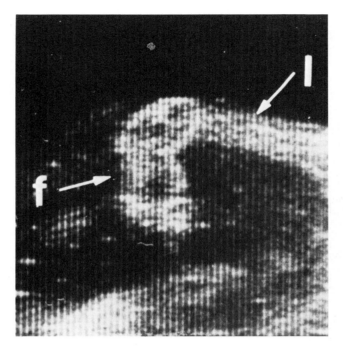

Figure 10-52 Clubfoot. Prenatal ultrasound scan shows that foot *(f)* is at right angle to leg *(From Jeanty P and Romero R: Semin Ultrasound CT Mr 5:253-268, 1984.)*

uating the gravid (pregnant) woman. In extremely rare instances, there may be justification for performing radiographic pelvimetry to demonstrate the architecture of the maternal pelvis and to compare the size of the fetal head with the size of the maternal bony pelvic outlet to determine whether the pelvic diameters are adequate for normal delivery or whether a cesarean section will be required. In almost all cases, however, the combination of careful clinical evaluation plus ultrasonography is sufficient to make these decisions without the need to resort to radiographic pelvimetry and its high radiation dose. There is absolutely no indication ever to perform fetography, the radiographic demonstration of the fetus in utero. Ultrasound can provide far better diagnostic information and is not associated with the danger of producing radiation-induced fetal malformations.

Ectopic pregnancy

Although ectopic pregnancy is a life-threatening condition, responsible for up to one fourth of maternal deaths, the diagnosis is missed by the initial examining physician in up to three fourths of the cases. More than 95% of ectopic pregnancies occur within the fallopian tubes, and more than half the patients with this complication of pregnancy have a history or pathologic evidence of pelvic inflamma-

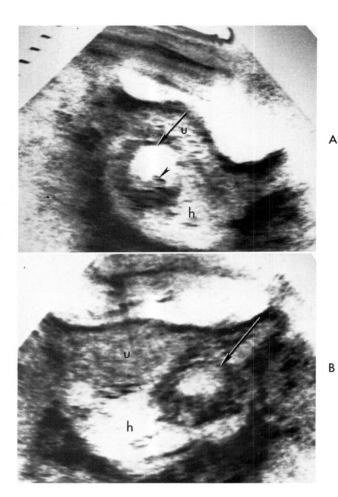

Figure 10-53 Ectopic pregnancy. **A,** Sagittal and, **B,** transverse sonograms show extrauterine gestational sac *(arrow)* on left with fetus within it *(arrowhead)*. Note complex cystic mass *(h),* which represents hematoma, in cul-de-sac. No fetal heart activity was noted. *u,* Uterus. *(From Spirt BA et al: Ectopic pregnancy: sonographic-pathologic correlations, RadioGraphics 4:821-848, 1984.)*

tory disease. Ectopic pregnancies are often associated with urine or plasma levels of human chorionic gonadotropin (HCG) that are substantially lower for the expected date of gestation than those in patients with normal intra-uterine pregnancies.

Ultrasound is the major imaging modality for diagnosing ectopic pregnancy. The classic appearance consists of an enlarged uterus that does not contain a gestational sac and is associated with an irregular adnexal mass, an "ectopic fetal head," or fluid in the cul-de-sac (Figure 10-53). The unequivocal demonstration of an intrauterine pregnancy virtually excludes an ectopic pregnancy, since the incidence of coexisting ectopic and intra-uterine pregnancies is only one in 30,000.

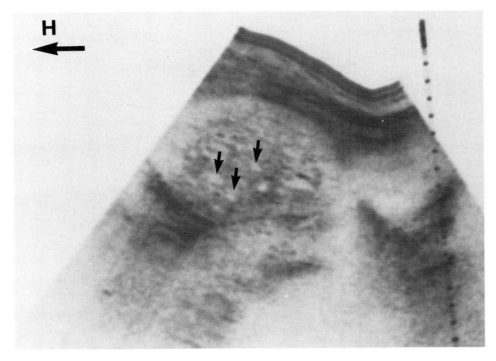

Figure 10-54 Hydatidaform mole. Longitudinal sonogram in patient in second trimester of pregnancy demonstrates large, moderately echogenic mass filling central uterine cavity. Note numerous small cystic spaces *(arrows)* that represent markedly hydropic chorionic villi. *(From Callen PW, editor: Ultrasonography in obstetrics and gynecology, Philadelphia, WB Saunders Co, 1983.)*

Trophoblastic disease

Trophoblastic disease refers to a spectrum of pregnancy-related disorders ranging from benign hydatidiform mole to the more malignant and frequently metastatic choriocarcinoma. A hydatidiform mole typically appears on ultrasound as a large, soft-tissue mass of placental (trophoblastic) tissue filling the uterine cavity and containing low-to-moderate amplitude echoes (Figure 10-54). No evidence of a developing fetus exists.

About half of choriocarcinomas follow pregnancies complicated by hydatidiform mole. The remainder occur after spontaneous abortion, ectopic pregnancy, or normal deliveries. On ultrasound, choriocarcinoma resembles benign hydatidiform mole and usually appears as a large complex mass in the expected position of the uterus. Choriocarcinoma tends to metastasize to the lungs, where it typically produces multiple large masses that rapidly regress once appropriate chemotherapy is instituted.

FEMALE INFERTILITY

The major radiographic procedure for evaluating infertile women is hysterosalpingography, in which the uterine cavity and fallopian tubes are opacified after the injection of contrast material into the uterus. In the normal woman with patent fallopian tubes, contrast material extravasating into the pelvic peritoneal cavity outlines the peritoneal surfaces and often loops of bowel within the pelvis (Figure 10-22). Developmental anomalies or fibrosis from pelvic inflammatory disease may cause occlusion of one or both of the fallopian tubes; in such cases, there is no evidence of the contrast material's reaching the peritoneal cavity (Figure 10-23). In addition to assessing tubal patency, hysterosalpingography can also demonstrate uterine abnormalities contributing to infertility, such as intrauterine fibroids, severe uterine flexion or retroversion, and other congenital and acquired malformations.

In female infertility patients receiving ovulation-induction agents, ultrasound can be used to monitor maturation of the ovarian follicles. Low-level internal echoes in mature ovarian follicles appear to be a prognostic indicator of fertility. They may represent a periovulatory state, which is an appropriate time for artificial insemination or in vitro fertilization. Ultrasound can also demonstrate the characteristic bilateral multicystic ovarian enlargement in the ovarian hyperstimulation syndrome, which may develop in women receiving menotropin (Pergonal) therapy for infertility.

QUESTIONS

1. Why has ultrasound become the major imaging modality for both the male and female reproductive systems?

2. In addition to ultrasound, what is the main radiographic study currently used for the female reproductive system?

3. The formation of sperm is known as _____.

4. What male hormone helps to regulate metabolism by promoting growth of skeletal muscles and is considered responsible for the greater degree of muscle development in males?

5. Severing of the vas deferens to create sterility is termed _____.

6. The second most common cause of malignancy in men is _____.

7. What imaging modality for demonstrating the prostate gland uses a probe inserted into the rectum?

8. Ultrasound studies of the prostate gland *cannot* always determine the malignant or benign status of prostatic disease.   TRUE   FALSE

9. Prostatic carcinoma can often spread through the bloodstream to the bone and can sometimes cause sclerosis of an entire vertebra. This pathologic condition is termed _____.

10. What screening technique is usually employed to identify the location of an undescended testicle?

11. What is the term used to describe the twisting of the male gonad on its pedicle?

12. The most common neoplasms in men between the ages of 20 and 35 are _____ tumors that tend to metastasize through the _____ system.

13. The rupture and expulsion of the mature ovum into the pelvic cavity is termed _____.

14. A pregnancy that occurs in a fallopian tube or in the pelvic cavity is termed _____.

15. What is the name of the radiographic procedure used to demonstrate the patency or status of the fallopian tubes?

16. Untreated _____ can lead to cerebral cortical lesions causing mental disorders and involvement of the skeletal system, and affects infants born to infected mothers.

17. The most common type of germ cell tumor, often containing teeth, hair, and fatty material, is called a _____.

18. Leiomyomas, more commonly referred to as _____, are benign smooth-muscle tumors of the uterus.

19. The most common malignancy among women occurs in the _____.

20. The second most common form of cancer in women is _____.

BIBLIOGRAPHY

Callen PW: Ultrasonography in obstetrics and gynecology, Philadelphia, WB Saunders Co, 1988.

Sanders RC and James AE: Ultrasonography in obstetrics and gynecology, Norwalk, Appleton-Century-Crofts, 1985.

Tabar L and Dean PB: Teaching atlas of mammography, ed 2, New York, Thieme, 1985.

CHAPTER 11

Miscellaneous Diseases

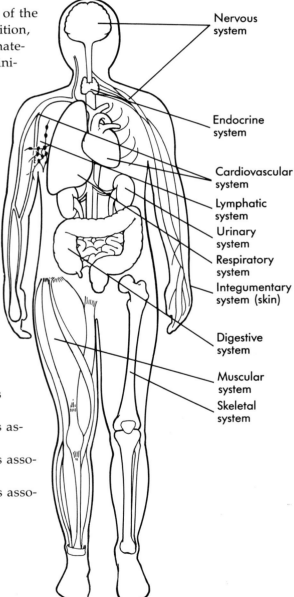

PREREQUISITE KNOWLEDGE

The student should have a basic understanding of the physiology of the various body systems. In addition, the proper learning and understanding of the material will be facilitated if the student has some clinical experience in general radiography.

GOALS

To acquaint the student with the pathophysiology and radiographic manifestations of both common and unusual disorders caused by vitamin deficiencies and some disease processes that do not fit neatly into a single body system

OBJECTIVES

1. Describe nutritional disorders and their possible relationship to disorders of other organs
2. Be able to define terminology relating to nutritional disorders
3. Be able to describe the pathologic conditions caused by various vitamin deficiencies
4. Be able to describe the pathologic conditions associated with sarcoidosis
5. Be able to describe the pathologic conditions associated with muscular dystrophy
6. Be able to describe the pathologic conditions associated with melanoma
7. Be able to describe the pathologic conditions associated with systemic lupus erythematosus

Nervous system

Endocrine system

Cardiovascular system

Lymphatic system

Urinary system

Respiratory system

Integumentary system (skin)

Digestive system

Muscular system

Skeletal system

RADIOGRAPHER NOTES

Radiography of patients with various nutritional diseases can be challenging because of the many effects these diseases have on all body systems. Some produce deformities; others can cause mental disorders. Obese patients can present unique problems in positioning or setting radiographic techniques. The radiographer must be especially empathetic when dealing with these patients, who often are embarrassed because of their size and thus difficult to deal with. Patients with melanoma that has already metastasized or those who are facing extensive surgical intervention are usually very depressed and sometimes require special handling. The manifestations of systemic lupus erythematosus cause considerable discomfort for the patient. Patients with muscular dystrophy can be easily agitated and are usually frustrated at their inability to control themselves. In general, patients suffering from the various diseases in the miscellaneous category can be very demanding and require considerable patience on the part of the radiographer.

NUTRITIONAL DISEASES

Disorders of nutrition range from malnutrition and vitamin deficiency to obesity and hypervitaminosis. In addition to inadequate intake, nutritional deficiency may be related to disorders of the liver, pancreas, and gastrointestinal tract that result in an inability of the body to digest and properly use proteins, carbohydrates, and lipids. In diabetes mellitus the absence of insulin prevents entry of glucose into the cells and thus deprives the body of its major source of energy. Abnormalities of the pancreas, liver, and gastrointestinal tract causing nutritional disease are discussed elsewhere; this section deals with diseases caused by vitamin deficiency, malnutrition, and obesity.

Vitamin deficiencies

Vitamins are an essential part of the enzymatic systems that are vital to the cellular metabolism of the body. Vitamins are formed (synthesized) only by plants, not by animals. Therefore man's supply of vitamins comes directly from eating fruits and vegetables or from animals (including fish) that have eaten plants and have stored the vitamins. Vitamins are generally divided into two categories: fat soluble and water soluble. The fat-soluble vitamins (A, D, E, and K) can be stored within body tissues. Water-soluble vitamins (B and C) cannot be stored and must be a regular part of the diet to prevent a deficiency. The major B vitamins include thiamine, riboflavin, niacin, pantothenic acid, cobalamin (vitamin B_{12}), and folic acid. Vitamin deficiency diseases are rare in the United States but are all too prevalent in underdeveloped countries.

Beriberi (thiamine)

Beriberi results from a deficiency in thiamine, a co-enzyme that is essential for carbohydrate metabolism. It primarily occurs in rice-eating countries such as China, in which the main staple is polished rice that has had the vitamin-containing skin and germ removed. Initially, peripheral vasodilation in beriberi causes increased cardiac output that produces a generalized enlargement of the cardiac silhouette and increased pulmonary vascular markings. With progression of disease, the myocardium becomes edematous and flabby and cannot function properly, leading to congestive heart failure and generalized edema (Figure 11-1). Noninflammatory degeneration of myelin sheaths caused by thiamine deficiency produces a peripheral neuropathy marked by weakness of the limbs and a "pins and needles" sensation in the extremities.

Pellagra (niacin)

Pellagra is caused by a deficiency of niacin and is characterized by reddening and scaling of the skin on exposed parts of the body, vomiting and severe diarrhea, and nervous and mental disorders (ranging from chronic depression to violent, irrational behavior).

Scurvy (vitamin C)

The deficiency of ascorbic acid (vitamin C) in scurvy leads to an inability of the supporting tissues to produce and maintain vascular endothelium and the cementing substances that hold epithelial cells together (collagen, osteoid, dentin). Scurvy was clas-

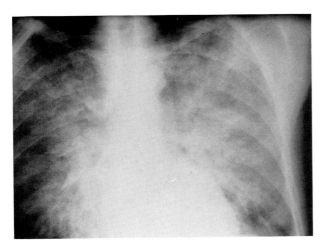

Figure 11-1 Beriberi. Diffuse pulmonary edema caused by severe high-output heart failure.

sically a disease of sailors and explorers deprived of fresh fruit and vegetables containing vitamin C.

Weakening of capillary walls in scurvy often results in bleeding into the skin, joints, and internal organs. The gums are especially affected and bleed easily. The open lesions provide an entry for bacteria, leading to necrosis of gum tissue and tooth

loosening and loss. Impaired synthesis of collagen leads to poor and delayed wound healing.

In children, disordered chondroblastic and osteoblastic activity cause radiographic bone changes that are most prevalent where growth is normally most rapid (especially about the knee and wrist). The bones are generally osteoporotic with blurring or disappearance of trabecular markings and severe cortical thinning. Widening and increased density of the zone of provisional calcification produce the characteristic "white line" of scurvy (Figure 11-2). A relatively lucent osteoporotic zone forms on the diaphyseal side of the white line. This osteoporotic zone is easily fractured, permitting the dense bone to become impacted on the shaft and jut laterally beyond it, thus giving rise to characteristic marginal spur formation (Pelken's spur). The epiphyseal ossification centers are demineralized and surrounded by dense, sharply demarcated rings of calcification (Wimberger's sign of scurvy). If epiphyseal dislocations have not occurred, the appearance of the skeletal structures usually returns to normal after appropriate therapy.

Subperiosteal hemorrhage often occurs along the shafts of the long bones. Calcification of the elevated periosteum and underlying hematoma is a radiographic sign of healing.

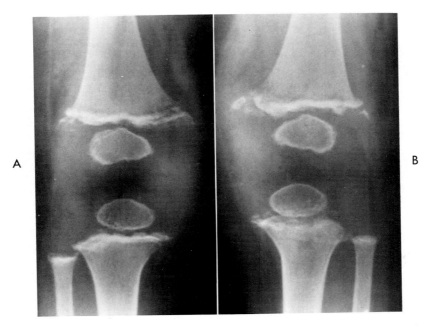

Figure 11-2 Scurvy. Frontal projections of both knees demonstrate widening and increased density of zone of provisional calcification, producing characteristic white line of scurvy. Note also submetaphyseal zone of lucency and characteristic marginal spur formation (Pelken's spur). Epiphyseal ossification centers are surrounded by dense, sharply demarcated ring of calcification (Wimberger's sign). *(From Eisenberg R: Atlas of signs in radiology, Philadelphia, JB Lippincott Co, 1984.)*

Vitamin D (rickets)

Rickets is a bone disease of young children in which a lack of vitamin D leads to decreased absorption of calcium from the gastrointestinal tract, resulting in weak, deformed bones. In adults, lack of vitamin D causes generalized softening of bones (osteomalacia). The radiographic findings of rickets and osteomalacia are found in Chapter 3.

Vitamin A

Vitamin A is essential for vision because it is a vital component of the pigment that absorbs light in the rods of the retina. A lack of vitamin A results in night blindness, an inability to see in dim light. Vitamin A also is important for maintaining the integrity of mucous membranes lining the respiratory, gastrointestinal, and urogenital tracts. A lack of vitamin A makes these membranes dry and susceptible to cracking, permitting infectious organisms to enter the underlying tissues.

Vitamin A is derived from carotene, a yellow plant pigment that is converted into vitamin A by the liver. Good sources of vitamin A include dairy products, egg yolks, and vegetables such as carrots.

Vitamin K

Vitamin K is necessary for the formation of prothrombin, an essential ingredient in the blood-clotting mechanism. It is primarily found in green leafy vegetables. A deficiency of vitamin K results in excessive bleeding.

Hypervitaminosis

Chronic excessive intake of vitamin A produces a syndrome characterized by bone and joint pain, hair loss, itching, anorexia, dryness and fissuring of the lips, hepatosplenomegaly, and yellow tinting of the skin. This condition usually affects young children, who become irritable and fail to gain weight.

Excess vitamin D causes too much calcium to be absorbed from the gastrointestinal tract. The resulting hypercalcemia leads to the deposition of calcium in the kidney, heart, lungs, and wall of the stomach (Figure 11-3).

Protein-calorie malnutrition (kwashiorkor)

Severe protein-calorie malnutrition (kwashiorkor) affects millions of young children in developing countries and produces abnormalities involving the gastrointestinal tract and nervous system. Fatty replacement of liver tissue and resulting decreased levels of albumin lead to diffuse edema and ascites and the characteristic clinical appearance of a markedly protuberant abdomen. Damage to the pancreas and intestinal mucosa prevents proper digestion and absorption of nutrients. Retarded bone growth with

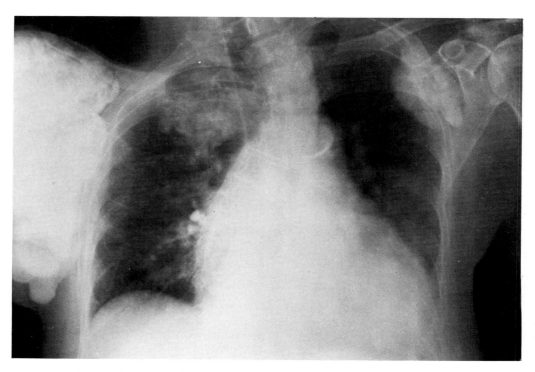

Figure 11-3 Hypervitaminosis D. Huge masses of calcification near shoulder joints bilaterally.

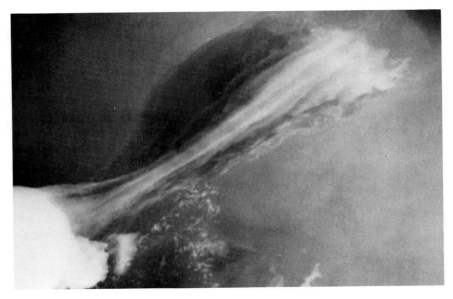

Figure 11-4 Obesity. Enlargement of retrogastric space caused by massive deposition of fatty tissue.

thinned cortices usually occurs. Atrophy of the thymus gland and lymphoid tissues diminish the child's resistance to infection from organisms that enter the body through skin lesions and the damaged mucous membranes of the gastrointestinal tract. Mental development is also impaired, and brain atrophy can be demonstrated radiographically.

Obesity

Obesity refers to an excess of adipose (fatty) tissue that develops when the caloric intake (food) consistently exceeds the amount of calories required by the body to perform its daily activities. It may be related simply to personal habits of excessive eating combined with a lack of activity or may be a result of such conditions as hypothyroidism, Cushing's disease, insulinoma, and hypothalamic disorders.

Excess adipose tissue can cause displacement of normal abdominal structures, producing such radiographic patterns as widening of the retrogastric (Figure 11-4) and retrorectal spaces. An extreme increase in the intra-abdominal volume causes diffuse elevation of the diaphragm with a relatively transverse position of the heart (simulating cardiomegaly), prominence of pulmonary markings, and atelectatic changes at the lung bases. In the most severe form of obesity (Pickwickian syndrome), the excursion of the diaphragm is limited and the lungs can barely expand with breathing. This results in profound hypoventilation, hypoxia, retention of carbon dioxide, secondary polycythemia, and pulmonary hyperten-

sion with right heart failure. An excessive deposition of fatty tissue can also appear radiographically as widening of the mediastinum and prominence of the pericardial fat pads.

Patients with morbid obesity may undergo surgical procedures in an attempt to lose large amounts of weight. Gastric restrictive operations attempt to limit gastric capacity and restrict gastric outflow, thus making the patient feel full after a small meal. This causes the patient to limit his or her oral intake and results in weight control. The major procedure is a gastroplasty, in which a small upper gastric remnant is connected to a larger lower gastric pouch by a narrow channel. Complications of gastric restrictive procedures can occur in the early and late postoperative periods and include leakage, perforation, widening of the channel, and obstruction.

SARCOIDOSIS

Sarcoidosis is a multisystem granulomatous disease of unknown cause that is most often detected in young adults. Women are affected slightly more often than men, and the disease is far more prevalent among blacks than whites.

Ninety percent of patients with sarcoidosis have radiographic evidence of thoracic involvement. Indeed, in most cases the presence of the disease is first identified on a screening chest radiograph of an asymptomatic individual.

Bilateral, symmetric hilar lymph node enlarge-

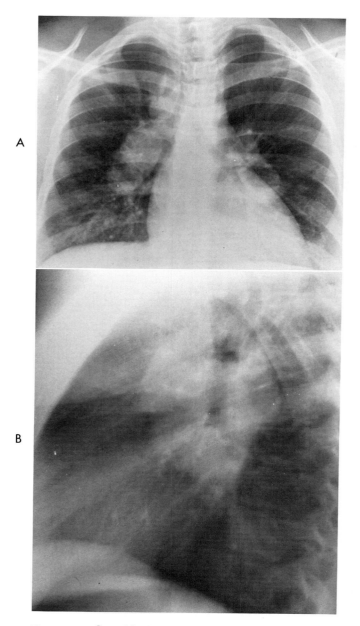

A

B

Figure 11-5 Sarcoidosis. **A,** Frontal and, **B,** lateral projections of chest demonstrate enlargement of right hilar, left hilar, and right paratracheal lymph nodes, producing classic 1-2-3 pattern of adenopathy. *(From Eisenberg R: Atlas of signs in radiology, Philadelphia, JB Lippincott Co, 1984.)*

ment, with or without diffuse parenchymal disease, is the classic radiographic abnormality in sarcoidosis. There is also usually enlargement of the right paratracheal nodes, producing the typical 1-2-3 pattern (Figure 11-5). Conventional tomography frequently reveals additional enlargement of the left paratracheal nodes, which usually cannot be seen on routine frontal radiographs because they are ob-

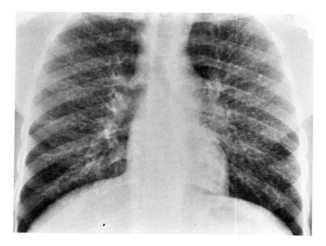

Figure 11-6 Sarcoidosis. Diffuse coarse interstitial pattern.

scured by the superimposed aorta and brachiocephalic vessels. Unilateral hilar enlargement, which is a common manifestation of primary tuberculosis or lymphoma, is rare in sarcoidosis.

Diffuse pulmonary disease develops in most patients with sarcoidosis. Although hilar and mediastinal adenopathy is often associated, there tends to be an inverse relationship between the degree of adenopathy and the extent of parenchymal disease, with the latter increasing while the adenopathy regresses. The most common appearance is a diffuse interstitial pattern that is widely distributed throughout both lungs (Figure 11-6). The alveolar pattern consists of ill-defined densities that may be discrete or may coalesce into large areas of consolidation. This pattern resembles an acute inflammatory process and may contain an air bronchogram. Infrequently, large, dense, round lesions may simulate metastatic malignancy.

Although the pulmonary lesions usually regress spontaneously or after steroid therapy, irreversible pulmonary changes develop in up to 20% of the cases. Coarse scarring is seen as irregular linear strands extending outward from the hilum toward the periphery, often associated with bulla formation (Figure 11-7). Severe fibrosis and emphysema can cause pulmonary hypertension and right heart failure.

The skeletal lesions in sarcoidosis primarily involve the small bones of the hands and feet. Granulomatous infiltration can cause destruction of the fine trabeculae, producing a mottled to lacelike, coarsely trabeculated pattern. Lytic destruction can produce sharply circumscribed, punched-out areas of lucency (Figure 11-8). About 10% of patients with sarcoidosis have elevated levels of serum calcium,

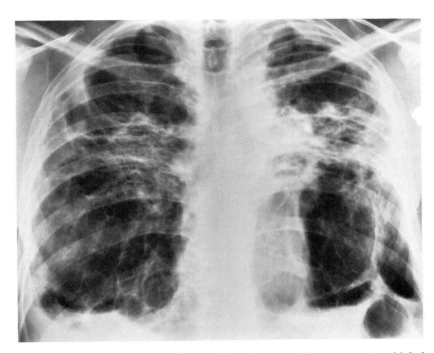

Figure 11-7 Sarcoidosis. In end-stage disease, there is severe fibrous scarring, bleb formation, and emphysema.

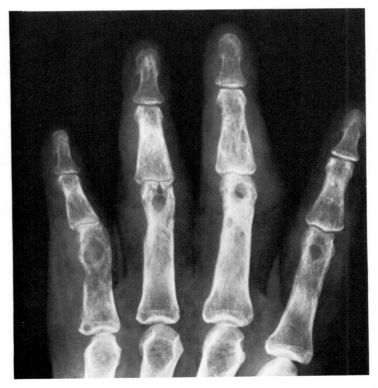

Figure 11-8 Sarcoidosis. Multiple osteolytic lesions throughout phalanges, producing typical punched-out appearance. Apparent air density in soft tissues is photographic artifact.

which may lead to nephrocalcinosis. Sarcoid involvement of the stomach can produce discrete masses or generalized luminal narrowing that predominantly involves the antrum.

SYSTEMIC LUPUS ERYTHEMATOSUS

Systemic lupus erythematosus is a connective tissue disorder that primarily involves young or middle-aged women and most likely represents an immune-complex disease. The presentation and course of the disease are highly variable. Characteristic findings include a butterfly-shaped rash over the nose and cheeks and extreme sensitivity of the skin to sunlight.

Pain in multiple muscles and joints is the most frequent clinical complaint in patients with systemic lupus erythematosus. A characteristic finding is subluxations and malalignment of joints in the absence of erosions (Figure 11-9). Cardiopulmonary abnormalities also frequently develop. Pleural effusions, usually bilateral and small but occasionally massive,

occur in about half of the patients (Figure 11-10). Enlargement of the cardiac silhouette is generally the result of pericarditis and pericardial effusion.

Although kidney involvement, often leading to renal failure, is one of the most serious manifestations of systemic lupus erythematosus, no specific urographic findings are seen. Enlargement of the liver, spleen, and lymph nodes occurs in about one fourth of patients. In the gastrointestinal system, a necrotizing inflammation of blood vessels can result in massive bleeding, multiple infarctions, and bowel perforation.

Many of the radiographic manifestations of systemic lupus erythematosus tend to disappear during spontaneous remissions or after steroid therapy.

MELANOMA

Melanoma is an extremely malignant skin cancer that metastasizes widely throughout the body. The tumor develops from a benign mole (nevus), which changes size and color and becomes itchy and sore.

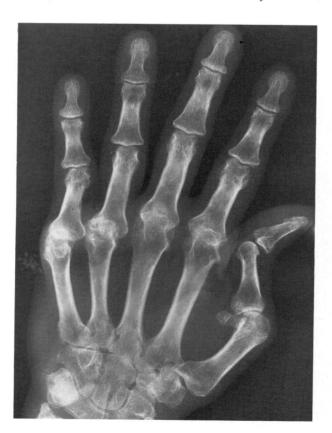
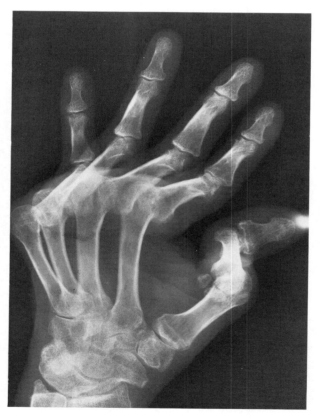

Figure 11-9 Systemic lupus erythematosus. Frontal and oblique projections of hand show subluxation of phalanges at metacarpal articulations and hyperextension deformities of proximal interphalangeal joints. Note absence of erosive changes. *(From Brown JC and Forrester DM: In Eisenberg RL and Amberg JR, editors: Critical diagnostic pathways in radiology: an algorithmic approach, Philadelphia, JB Lippincott Co, 1981.)*

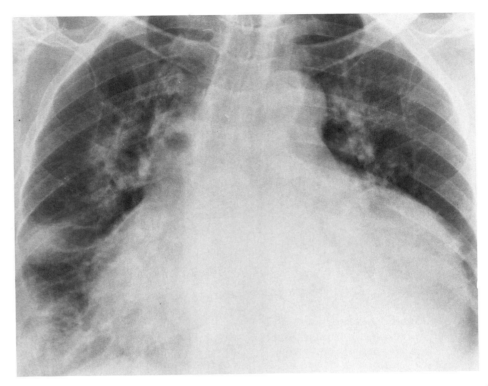

Figure 11-10 Systemic lupus erythematosus. Bilateral pleural effusions, more marked on right, with some streaks of basilar atelectasis. Massive cardiomegaly is due to combination of pericarditis and pericardial effusion.

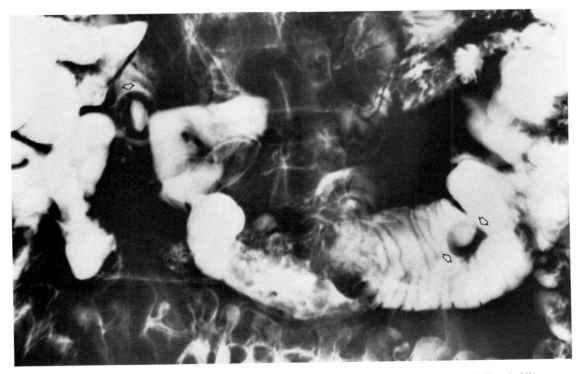

Figure 11-11 Metastatic melanoma. Large central ulcerations in two sharply defined filling defects in small bowel *(arrows)*.

Metastases from malignant melanoma frequently involve the gastrointestinal tract, usually sparing the large bowel. They are typically well-circumscribed, round or oval nodules that may develop central necrosis and ulceration to produce a dense, barium-filled central crater surrounded by a sharply marginated nodular mass (bull's-eye, or target, lesion) (Figure 11-11). Gastrointestinal metastases can be the first clinical manifestation of metastatic melanoma; at times it can be impossible to identify the primary tumor site.

Metastatic melanoma can also produce multiple nodules in the lung and destructive bone lesions with neither new bone formation nor reactive sclerosis.

MUSCULAR DYSTROPHY

Muscular dystrophy refers to a group of chronic inherited conditions in which there is replacement of muscle by fat leading to generalized weakness and eventually death caused by respiratory muscle failure or pneumonia. On radiographs of the extremities, the extensive accumulation of fat within the remaining muscle bundles produces a fine striated, or striped, appearance (Figure 11-12). Because most of the muscle tissue is replaced by fat, the fascial sheath bounding the muscles may stand out as a thin shadow or increased density as it is visualized on edge. Decreased muscular tone can lead to osteoporosis, bone atrophy with cortical thinning, scoliosis, and joint contractures.

An abnormal swallowing mechanism in muscular dystrophy can result in the failure to clear barium adequately from the pharynx; this may lead to tracheal aspiration and nasal regurgitation of contrast material (or other ingested substances).

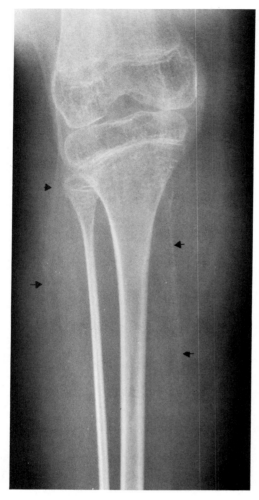

Figure 11-12 Muscular dystrophy. Thin, demineralized bones of lower leg. Increased lucency, representing fatty infiltration in muscle bundles, makes fascial sheaths appear as thin shadows of increased density *(arrows)* surrounded by fat.

QUESTIONS

1. A vitamin C deficiency that was, years ago, common among sailors because of their lack of fresh fruit and vegetables is termed _Scurvey_.

2. _Beriberi_ is a vitamin deficiency disease that occurs primarily in countries in which polished rice is the main staple.

3. A deficiency of niacin, characterized by reddening and scaling of exposed skin, vomiting, diarrhea, and nervous and mental disorders is termed _Pellegra_.

4. A bone disease of young children who have been deprived of adequate vitamin D is termed _Rickets_.

5. Vitamin _K_ is necessary in the blood-clotting mechanism.

6. A lack of vitamin _A_ can result in night blindness.

7. When caloric intake consistently exceeds the amount needed for the body to function, _Obesity_ occurs.

8. A granulomatous disease of unknown origin that usually affects women more than men and blacks more than whites and whose presence is most often identified on screening chest radiographs is _Sarcoidosis_

9. A disease of young to middle-aged women, which is most likely an immune-complex disease, can affect several systems of the body and is characterized by a butterfly-shaped rash across the nose and cheeks is _Systemic lupis ERYTHEMATOOUS_

10. A very malignant form of skin cancer, capable of metastasizing throughout the body, is _MELANOMA_

11. An inherited muscular disease characterized by severe weakness and eventual death due to respiratory muscle failure or pneumonia is _MUSCULAR DYSTROPHY_

12. The radiographer should be very alert to the possibility of _aspiration_ in patients with muscular dystrophy who lack normal swallowing ability.

BIBLIOGRAPHY

Juhl JH and Crummy AB: Essentials of radiologic imaging, Philadelphia, JB Lippincott Co, 1987.

Kirks DR, McCormick VD, and Greenspan RH: Pulmonary sarcoidosis, Am J Roentgenol 117:777-786, 1973.

Lubowitz R and Schumacher HR: Articular manifestations of systemic lupus erythematosus, Ann Intern Med 74:911-921, 1974.

achalasia Failure of the lower esophageal sphincter to relax due to absence or destruction of cells in the myenteric nerve plexus, which results in difficulty swallowing

adenopathy Enlargement of the lymphatic glands

adnexal Pertaining to the uterine appendages (ovaries, fallopian tubes, and ligaments)

amorphous Without shape or definite form

anechoic Not containing internal echoes (on ultrasound)

ankylosis Immobility and consolidation of a joint due to disease, injury, or surgical procedure

anticoagulant Substance that suppresses or delays coagulation of the blood

arteriovenous malformation Abnormal communication between an artery and vein

ascites Accumulation of fluid in the abdominal cavity

atresia Congenital absence or closure of a normal body orifice or tubular organ

Bence-Jones protein Abnormal substance typically found in the blood of patients with multiple myeloma

bougienage Passage of an instrument through a tubular structure to increase its caliber (as in the treatment of a stricture of the esophagus)

bulla Large air-containing space

callus Formation of new bone that reunites the parts about a fracture

caseation Form of necrosis in which the tissue is changed into a dry, amorphous mass resembling cheese

catamenial Pertaining to menstruation

cavitation Formation of cavities, as in pulmonary tuberculosis or neoplasm

chondroblastic Forming cartilaginous tissue

chordae tendineae Thin cords that connect each cusp of the two atrioventricular valves to papillary muscles in the heart ventricles

coalesce To merge into a single mass

colic Intermittent abdominal pain that fluctuates corresponding to smooth muscle peristalsis

collaterals Blood vessels that develop or enlarge to provide an alternative route around an obstruction

congenital Existing at birth

conjunctivitis Inflammation of the delicate membrane that lines the eyelids and covers the

exposed surface of the sclera (white part) of the eye

contracture Shortening or shrinkage of a muscle or tendon resulting in persistent flexion or distortion at a joint

cortex Outer portion of a bone or internal organ (kidney, adrenal gland, brain)

curvilinear Having a curved configuration

de novo From the beginning; anew

demarcate To set or mark the limits of

diaphysis Shaft of a long bone

diploic space Loose osseous tissue between the two tables of the skull

dysphagia Difficulty swallowing

dysplasia Disordered growth or faulty development of various tissues or body parts

dyspnea Shortness of breath

effaced Wiped out or obliterated

embolus Any foreign matter, such as a blood clot or an air bubble, carried in the blood stream

emphysema Pathologic accumulation of air in tissues or organs (especially applied to a disease of the lungs)

endemic Native to a particular country, nation, or region

endogenous Originating from within the body

engorgement Congestion of a blood vessel or tissue with blood or other fluid

epiphysis End of a long bone that at first is separated from the main part by cartilage but later fuses with it by ossification

erythropoietin Substance(s) serving as the humoral regulator of red blood cell formation

etiology Cause

exacerbation Increase in the severity of a disease or any of its symptoms

exogenous Arising from outside the body

exophthalmos Abnormal protrusion of the eyeball

extramedullary hematopoiesis Formation of red blood cells outside of the bone marrow

exudate Material such as fluid, cells, or cellular debris that has escaped from blood vessels and has been deposited in tissues or on tissue surfaces, usually as a result of inflammation

fecalith Intestinal stone formed around a center of fecal material

fibrin Essential portion of a blood clot

fibrinolysis Breaking up of a blood clot

fistula Abnormal connection, usually between two internal organs or from an internal organ to the surface of the body

focal Localized

fusiform Spindle shaped

Gram method Technique for staining microorganisms

granuloma Tumorlike mass of tissue caused by a chronic inflammatory process

Heberden's nodes Small, hard nodules at the distal interphalangeal joints of the fingers produced by calcific spurs of the articular cartilage and associated with osteoarthritis

hematogenous Spread by means of the blood stream

hemodynamic Pertaining to the movements involved in the circulation of the blood

hemoptysis Coughing up blood or blood-stained sputum

homogeneous Composed of material of similar or identical structure or quality

hydrocephalus Enlargement of the head due to an abnormal increase in fluid within the ventricular system

hyperlucency Overly black appearance on a radiograph

hyperplasia Abnormal increase in the number of cells composing a tissue or organ

hypertension High blood pressure

hypotension Low blood pressure

hypoxia Deficiency (lack) of oxygen

iatrogenic Resulting from the activity of physicians

indolent Causing little or no pain; slow to heal

infarction Death of tissue due to interruption of the normal blood supply

infundibula Thin passages connecting the calyces to the renal pelvis

inguinal Pertaining to the groin

insidious Developing in a slow or not apparent manner; more dangerous than seems evident, as in an insidious disease

intima Innermost layer of an organ or blood vessel

intraluminal Within the empty space (lumen) of a hollow viscus

intramural Within the wall of an organ

intrinsic Belonging to the real nature of a thing

ischemia Lack of blood supply in an organ or tissue

juxta-articular Adjacent to a joint

kyphosis Anterior convexity in the curvature of the thoracic spine, sacrum, and coccyx, as viewed from the side

leukocytosis Abnormal amount of white blood cells in the blood

lipoma Tumor composed of fat

lordosis Anterior concavity in the curvature of the lumbar and cervical spine, as viewed from the side

lymphangitic Spread by means of the lymphatic system

lymphoma Neoplastic disorder of lymphoid tissue

lytic Destructive

malaise Vague feeling of physical discomfort or uneasiness, as early in an illness

matrix Basic material from which a thing develops

medulla Inner substance of a bone (bone marrow) or an internal organ (kidney, adrenal gland)

mesentery Peritoneal folds attaching the small and large bowel to the back wall of the peritoneal cavity

mesothelioma Tumor developing from the surface of the pleura, pericardium, or peritoneum

metaphysis Wider part at the end of the shaft of a long bone, adjacent to the epiphyseal plate; located between the epiphysis and the diaphysis

monoclonal immunoglobulin Antibodies that are formed against a specific cell type

Morgagni hernia Protrusion of abdominal contents into the anterior and lateral aspects of the thoracic cavity

morphologic Pertaining to the form and structure of an organ

multilocular Having many cells or compartments

mycoplasma Any of a genus of tiny microorganisms, smaller than bacteria but larger than viruses, that appear to be the causative agents of many diseases

myxedema Puffy thickening of the skin with slowing down of physical and mental activity caused by failure of the thyroid gland

necrosis Death of tissue

necrotic Dead or decayed

neoplasm Any new and abnormal growth, especially when the growth is uncontrolled and progressive

nephrocalcinosis Calcium deposits within the substance of the kidney

neurogenic Originating in the nervous system

nidus Focal point, especially of a stone or inflammatory process

oligemia Decreased blood flow

osteoblastic Forming bony tissue

osteoclastic Destroying bone

osteolytic Destroying bone

palpitations Rapid or fluttering beating of the heart, of which one is aware

paradoxical Seemingly contradictory or unbelievable, but which may actually be true in fact

parenchyma Essential elements of an organ

pathognomonic Specially distinctive or characteristic of a disease or pathologic condition

pedunculated Having a stalk (pedicle)

periphery Outside or away from the central portion of a structure

peristalsis Wormlike movement by which the alimentary canal or other tubular organ propels its contents

permeative Diffusely spreading through or penetrating a substance, tissue, or organ, as by a disease process such as cancer

pinna Cartilaginous lower projecting portion of the external ear

pneumococcus Type of gram-positive bacteria

pneumoperitoneum Presence of free gas in the peritoneal cavity

postpartum After childbirth

proliferate To multiply rapidly, increase profusely

punctate Marked with dots or tiny spots

rudimentary Imperfectly developed

sclerosis Conversion of a portion of bone into an ivory-like, densely opaque mass; an abnormal hardening of body tissues or parts, especially of the walls of arteries

sequestrum Piece of dead bone that has become separated from the surrounding healthy bone

serosa Outer layer of a viscus (especially in the alimentary tract)

shock Acute peripheral circulatory failure

silhouette (cardiac) Outer border of the heart, seen against the radiolucent lungs

spirochete Spiral type of bacterium of the genus *Spirochaeta*

staging Determination of the amount of spread of a neoplasm, necessary to select appropriate therapy and to predict the future course of a disease

stasis Stagnation of some fluid in the body (as of blood in veins); reduced peristalsis of the intestines resulting in the retention of feces

subchondral Just beneath the articular margin

subluxation Incomplete or partial dislocation

telangiectasia Vascular lesion formed by dilatation of a group of small blood vessels

teratoma Neoplasm composed to various kinds of embryonic tissue

thymoma Tumor originating from the thymus gland

tortuous Full of twists, turns, or curves

trabecula Supporting or anchoring strands of connective tissue within bony structures

triradiate Radiating in three directions

trophoblastic Relating to the layer by which the fertilized ovum is attached to the uterine wall and from which the developing embryo receives its nourishment

urate Salt of uric acid

valvulae conniventes Circular folds of the small bowel

vasculitis Inflammation of a vessel

virus One of a group of minute infectious agents characterized by a lack of independent metabolism and by the ability to reproduce only within living host cells

viscous Thick, sticky

viscus Any large internal organ, especially in the abdomen

Prefixes / Suffixes / Roots

Prefix/Suffix/Root	Meaning	Example
a-, ab-	away from	abduction
a-, an-, ana-	without; not	anaplastic; asymmetric
ad-	toward	adduction
-algia	pain	arthralgia
anti-, ant-	against	antibody; antitoxin
auto-	self	autoimmune
bi-	two	bilateral; bidirectional
-blast	builder	osteoblast
cardi	heart	cardiology; cardiac; pericardium
caudal	tail	caudal
cephal	head	cephalic; hydrocephaly
chondro-	cartilage	chondroma; chondrosarcoma
-clast	destroyer	osteoclast
contra-	opposite	contralateral
cran-	skull	cranium; cranial
cyano-	dark blue	cyanotic
cyto	cell	cytoplasm; erythrocyte; leukocyte
dactyl	finger; toe	polydactyly; arachnodactyly
deci-	tenth	decimal
derm	skin	dermatology; epidermis
dys-	bad; difficult	dysplasia; dysuria
ecto-	outside of	ectoderm; ectopic
endo-, ento-	within	endoderm; endometrium
erythr-	red	erythrocyte
gastr-	stomach	gastric
-genic	causing	carcinogenic; pathogenic
gyn-, gynec-	woman	gynecology
haem-, hem-	blood	hemorrhage; hemolytic
hemi-	half	hemisphere; hemidiaphragm
hetero-	different	heterogeneous
homo-	same	homogeneous
hyper-	over; excessively	hyperthyroidism; hypertension; hyperintense
hypo-	under; too little	hypothyroidism; hypotension; hypointense

Prefix/Suffix/Root	Meaning	Example
iatro	healer, healing	iatrogenic; psychiatry
infra-	below	infratemporal
intra-	within	intramural; intradermal
ipsi-	same	ipsilateral
iso-	equal	isointense
-itis	inflammation	appendicitis, diverticulitis
juxta-	near, next to	juxta-articular
kilo-	thousand	kilogram
leuco-, leuko-	white	leukocyte; leukemia
lipo-	fat	lipoma; liposarcoma
-lysis, -lytic	dissolve	lytic; osteolytic
macro-	large	macroadenoma
magn-	great, large	magnify; magnum (foramen)
mal-	bad, ill	malunion; malalignment
mega-, megalo-	large	megadose
melan-	black	melanoma; melanin
micro-	small	microscope; microadenoma; microcirculation
milli-	thousand	milligram; milliliter
mono-	one	monostotic; monoclonal
multi-	many	multilocular; multifaceted
myelo	marrow	myelogram; osteomyelitis
myo-	muscle	myoma; myostitis
necro-	dead	necrosis
neo-	new	neovascularity; neoplasm
non-	not	nonunion; nonviable
ocul-	eye	ocular; oculomotor [nerve]
oligo-	few	oligemia
-ology	study of	radiology; pathology
onco-	tumor	oncology
ophthalm	eye	ophthalmology
-osis	condition of	diverticulosis
osteo-	bone	osteomyelitis; osteosarcoma
pan-	all	pansinusitis; pancytopenia
par-, para-	beside	para-aortic; paravertebral
path	disease	pathology; adenopathy
peri-	around	periarticular; periventricular; pericardium
plas	shape, form	neoplasm; anaplastic
pleur-	rib; side	pleural; pleurisy
pneum-	air, breath	pneumothorax; pneumonia
poly-	many	polycystic; polyostotic
post-	after, later; behind	post-traumatic; postsurgical; post-op
pre-	before	premenstrual; prepontine
pseudo-	false	pseudotumor; pseudopolyp
psych-	mind, spirit	psychiatry; psychology

Prefix/Suffix/Root	Meaning	Example
re-	again; anew	reoperate; recalcify
retro-	backward; behind	retroperitoneum
-rhea	flow, gush	diarrhea
schiz-	split	schizophrenia
sclero	hard	sclerotic; atherosclerosis
semi-	half	semicircular
sub-	under, below	suborbital; subphrenic; subhepatic
super-, supra-	above; more than	suprarenal; supraorbital
syn-, sym-	with, together	synthesis; symmetric
tachy-	fast	tachycardia
techn-	art, skill	technology; technique
tert-	third	tertiary
tetra-	four	tetralogy [of Fallot]
therm	heat	thermometer
tom	cut	tomography
trans-	across	transverse [colon]; transvenous [pacer]
tri-	three	trimalleolar; trisomy
ultra-	beyond	ultrasound
uni-	one	unilateral

Laboratory tests

↑ Acid phosphatase	Prostate cancer, metastatic to bone
↑ Alkaline phosphatase	Liver disease; Paget's disease; bone tumor
↑ Amylase	Pancreatitis
↑ Bilirubin	Liver disease
↑ Calcium	Hyperparathyroidism, bone destruction
↑ Cholesterol	Tendency toward atherosclerosis
↑ Creatinine phosphokinase (CPK)	Myocardial infarction; pulmonary infarction
↑ Creatinine	Kidney disease
↑ Glucose	Diabetes mellitus; Cushing's syndrome; glucagon-secreting pancreatic tumor
↑ Lactic dehydrogenase (LDH)	Myocardial infarction; pulmonary infarction; liver disease
↑ Total protein	Dehydration; immunoglobinopathy
↑ Serum glutamic oxaloacetic transaminase (SGOT)	Liver disease
↑ Serum glutamic pyruvic transaminase (SGPT)	Myocardial infarction; liver disease
↑ Blood urea nitrogen (BUN)	Kidney disease
↑ Uric acid	Gout; antidiuretic therapy
↓ Calcium	Hypoparathyroidism; malabsorption; osteomalacia/rickets
↓ Total protein	Chronic liver disease; malnutrition; nephrotic syndrome
↓ Cholesterol	Malnutrition; liver disease
↓ Glucose	Insulin-secreting pancreatic tumor; liver disease; hypopituitarism

Hematology results

↑ White blood cells
    Neutrophil   Bacterial infection; leukemia
    Eosinophil   Allergic/parasitic disorders
    Lymphocytes   Leukemia/lymphoma; viral infections
↑ Red blood cells   Polycythemia; COPD; cyanotic heart disease

↓ White blood cells
    Neutrophils   Acute viral infections
↓ Red blood cells   Anemia (especially hemorrhage, hemolysis)
↓ Platelets   Thrombocytopenic purpura

Gram staining

COCCI	RODS
Positive:	
Streptococci, staphylococci	*Corynebacterium diphtheriae, Clostridium tetani, Clostridium botulinum*
Negative:	
Meningococci	*Escherichia coli*
Gonococci	*Klebsiella; Pseudomonas; Shigella; Salmonella; Bordetella pertussis* (whooping cough)

Miscellaneous laboratory tests

VDRL	Syphilis
ANA (Antinuclear antibody)	Systemic lupus erythematosus (or other connective tissue or autoimmune disease)
Rheumatoid factor	Rheumatoid arthritis
HLA-B27	Rheumatoid variant (especially ankylosing spondylitis and Reiter's syndrome)
Hemoccult test	Gastrointestinal bleeding
Acid-fast bacilli stain	Tuberculosis
HIV	AIDS

Index